Handbook of Gastrointestinal Cancer

Handbook of Gastrointestinal Cancer

EDITED BY

Janusz Jankowski, MB ChB, MSc, MD, PhD, FRCP, FACG, AGAF

Sir James Black Professor of Gastrointestinal Biology and Trials
Centre for Digestive Diseases, Barts and The London School of Medicine and Dentistry
London, UK

Consultant Gastroenterologist
University Hospitals of Leicester
Leicester, UK

James Black Senior Fellow
University of Oxford
Oxford, UK

Ernest Hawk, MD, MPH

Vice President and Division Head
Division of Cancer Prevention & Population Sciences
Boone Pickens Distinguished Chair for Early Prevention of Cancer
The University of Texas MD Anderson Cancer Center
Houston, TX, USA

WILEY-BLACKWELL

A John Wiley & Sons, Ltd., Publication

Library of Congress Cataloging-in-Publication Data

Handbook of gastrointestinal cancer / edited by Janusz Jankowski, Ernest Hawk.
   p. ; cm.
   Includes bibliographical references and index.
   ISBN 978-0-470-65624-2 (pbk. : alk. paper)
   I. Jankowski, Janusz A. Z.   II. Hawk, Ernest T.
   [DNLM: 1. Gastrointestinal Neoplasms–diagnosis.   2. Gastrointestinal Neoplasms–therapy.
WI 149]
   616.99′433–dc23

                                                                            2012020844

A catalogue record for this book is available from the British Library.

Wiley also publishes its books in a variety of electronic formats. Some content that appears in print may not be available in electronic books.

Cover image: Polyp images courtesy of Mr Chris Macklin, Consultant Colorectal Surgeon; Pathology images courtesy of Andrew Wotherspoon, Consultant Histopathologist
Cover design by Andy Magee

Set in 9.25/11.5pt Minion by Aptara® Inc., New Delhi, India
Printed in Singapore by Ho Printing Singapore Pte Ltd

1   2013

Contents

List of Contributors

Shahab Ahmed, MD
Coordinator
GI Medical Oncology
The University of Texas MD Anderson Cancer Center
Houston, TX, USA

Nadir Arber, MD, MSc, MHA
Professor of Medicine and Gastroenterology
Yechiel and Helen Lieber Professor for Cancer Research
Integrated Cancer Prevention Center and Department of Gastroenterology
Tel Aviv Medical Center and Tel Aviv University
Tel Aviv, Israel

Neil Bhardwaj, MBChB, MD, FRCS
Specialist Surgical Registrar
Leicester General Hospital
University Hospitals of Leicester
Leicester, UK

Boris Blechacz, MD, PhD
Assistant Professor
Department of Gastroenterology, Hepatology and Nutrition
The University of Texas MD Anderson Cancer Center
Houston, TX, USA

Branislav Bystricky, MD
Senior Clinical Research Fellow
Gastrointestinal & Lymphoma Unit
Royal Marsden Hospital
London and Surrey, UK

Martyn Caplin, BSc Hons, DM, FRCP
Professor of Gastroenterology and GI Neuroendocrinology
Centre for Gastroenterology
Neuroendocrine Tumor Unit
Royal Free Hospital
London, UK

David Cunningham, MD, FRCP
Head
Gastrointestinal & Lymphoma Unit
Royal Marsden Hospital
London and Surrey, UK

Brian G. Czito, MD
Associate Professor
Department of Radiation Oncology
Duke University Medical Center
Durham, NC, USA

Cathy Eng, MD, FACP
Associate Professor and Associate Medical Director
Colorectal Center
Department of Gastrointestinal Medical Oncology
The University of Texas MD Anderson Cancer Center
Houston, TX, USA

Rebecca Fitzgerald, MB, BChir, MA, MD, FRCP
Group Leader and Honorary Consultant Gastroenterologist
Hutchison/MRC Research Centre
Addenbrookes Hospital
Cambridge, UK

Grant M. Fullarton, MD, FRCS (Gen)
West of Scotland Upper GI Surgical Unit
Glasgow Royal Infirmary and Southern General Hospitals
Glasgow, UK

Paul Glen, MD, FRCS (Gen)
Consultant Upper GI Surgeon
West of Scotland Upper GI Surgical Unit
Glasgow Royal Infirmary and Southern General Hospitals
Glasgow, UK

Ernest Hawk, MD, MPH
Vice President and Division Head
Division of Cancer Prevention & Population Sciences
Boone Pickens Distinguished Chair for Early Prevention of Cancer
The University of Texas MD Anderson Cancer Center
Houston, TX, USA

Eliza A. Hawkes, MBBS, FRACP
Senior Clinical Research Fellow
Gastrointestinal & Lymphoma Unit
Royal Marsden Hospital
London and Surrey, UK

Kee Wook Jung, MD
Clinical Assistant Professor
Department of Gastroenterology
Asan Medical Center
Seoul, Korea

Mohid Shakil Khan, MB, BCh, MRCP
Clinical Research Fellow
Neuroendocrine Tumor Unit
Royal Free Hospital
London, UK

Ying Li, PhD
Assistant Professor
Department of Gastroenterology-Research
The University of Texas MD Anderson Cancer Center
Houston, TX, USA

David M. Lloyd, MBBS, FRCS, MD
Honorary Senior Lecturer in Cancer Studies, University of Leicester
Consultant Hepatobiliary and Laparoscopic Surgeon
Leicester General Hospital
University Hospitals of Leicester
Leicester, UK

Jeffrey J. Meyer, MD, MS
Department of Radiation Oncology
UT-Southwestern Medical Center
Dallas, TX, USA

Lopa Mishra, MD
Chair
Department of Gastroenterology, Hepatology and Nutrition
The University of Texas MD Anderson Cancer Center
Houston, TX, USA

Menachem Moshkowitz, MD
Senior Clinical Lecturer
Integrated Cancer Prevention Center and Department of Gastroenterology
Tel Aviv Medical Center and Tel Aviv University
Tel Aviv, Israel

Christopher J. Peters, MBChB, MRCS, PhD
Specialist Registrar in Upper GI Surgery
London Deanery
London, UK

Yvonne Romero, MD
Assistant Professor of Medicine
Division of Gastroenterology and Hepatology
Department of Otolaryngology
GI Outcomes Unit
Mayo Clinic
Rochester, MN, USA

Anan H. Said, MD
Internal Medicine Resident
Department of Medicine
University of Maryland Medical Center
Baltimore, MD, USA

Kirti Shetty, MD
Director, Transplant Hepatology
Associate Professor of Medicine and Surgery
Georgetown University School of Medicine
MedStar Georgetown Transplant Institute
MedStar Georgetown University Hospital
Washington, DC, USA

Jianmin Tian, MD, MSPH
Fellow
Barrett's Esophagus Unit
Division of Gastroenterology and Hepatology
Department of Medicine
Mayo Clinic
Rochester, MN, USA

Nimish Vakil, MD, FACP, FACG, AGAF
Professor
Department of Medicine
University of Wisconsin School of Medicine and Public Health
Madison, WI, USA

Kenneth K. Wang, MD
Professor of Medicine
Department of Gastroenterology and Hepatology
Mayo Clinic
Rochester, MN, USA

Christopher G. Willett, MD
Professor and Chair
Radiation Oncology
Duke University Medical Center
Durham, NC, USA

Andrew Wotherspoon, MBChB, FRCPath
Consultant Histopathologist
Royal Marsden Hospital
London and Surrey, UK

1 Esophageal Squamous Cell Carcinoma

Jianmin Tian and Kenneth K. Wang
Mayo Clinic, Rochester, MN, USA

Key Points

- Esophageal squamous cell carcinoma (ESCC) is still more prevalent than adenocarcinoma worldwide. In western countries, high-risk individuals include smokers, patients with head and neck squamous cell carcinoma, tylosis, achalasia, lichen planus, scleroderma, Plummer–Vinson syndrome, and prior radiation of neck and chest.
- Esophagogastroduodenoscopy (EGD) with Lugol spray is currently considered as the most effective noninvasive way to identify squamous cell dysplasia and ESCC. Newer modalities such as narrow band imaging (NBI), confocal laser endomicroscopy (CLE), and autofluorescence imaging (AFI) are promising.
- Treatment for ESCC is based on the stage of the disease. Currently, ESCC that is limited in the mucosa can be managed by endoscopic mucosal resection. Patients with more advanced disease are candidates for surgery with or without neoadjuvant/adjuvant chemotherapy if it is resectable. Otherwise, for unresectable lesions, standard supportive care with or without chemotherapy is reasonable.
- The best strategies to reduce the incidence and mortality of ESCC are primary prevention and early diagnosis.

Key Web Links

http://seer.cancer.gov
US National Cancer Institute—a comprehensive database assessable to the public for various types of cancers

http://www.cancercare.on.ca
Cancer Care Ontario, Canada—updated practice guidelines for prevention and treatment of ESCC

http://www.nccn.org
US National Comprehensive Cancer Network—guidelines, education programs for heal care providers and patients

---

Handbook of Gastrointestinal Cancer, First Edition. Edited by Janusz Jankowski and Ernest Hawk.
© 2013 John Wiley & Sons, Ltd. Published 2013 by John Wiley & Sons, Ltd.

http://www.asco.org/
American Society of Clinical Oncology—practice guidelines, research
resources, education and training, public policy

http://www.asge.org/publications
The Role of Endoscopy in the Assessment and Treatment of Esophageal
Cancer

Potential Pitfalls

- Physicians should be vigilant in diagnosing ESCC particularly among the high-risk subgroups.
- Endoscopic mucosal resection (EMR) is the treatment of choice for ESCC that is T1a (limited to the mucosa) or less. Avoid excessive deep biopsies of these lesions so that EMR can be safely performed for diagnosis and potential cure.
- For more advanced ESCC lesions, coordinated care involving gastroenterologists, medical oncologists, and thoracic surgeons is essential to achieve the best clinical outcomes.

Epidemiology

On a global basis, esophageal squamous cell carcinoma (ESCC) is the leading cancer of the esophagus, and it has been ranked as eighth in incidence and sixth in mortality among tumors of all sites.[1] However, its incidence varies significantly among different geographic and ethnic subgroups (Table 1.1).[2-6] The Asian Esophageal Cancer Belt, including western and northern China, Mongolia, southern parts of the former Soviet Union, Iran, Iraq, and eastern Turkey are considered the highest risk areas. The highest rate of incidence, 700 per 100,000, was reported in Linxian, China.[3] The factors associated with esophageal cancer in these high-risk areas vary as to the population. It is interesting to note that protective factors that have been identified include increased consumption of fresh fruit and vegetables, eggs, meat, and central water supply. The risk factors for this high incidence are still to be further elucidated, but they likely include cigarette smoking, pipe smoking, excessive alcohol use, dietary habits (vitamin deficiency, etc.), differences in cooking, and environmental exposure. In Linxian, China, for example, high levels of polycyclic aromatic hydrocarbons have been found in the food that implicates cooking fuels as a potential source of this carcinogen in this high-risk area. It is important to note that risk factors such as human papilloma virus present in head and neck cancers do not seem to be a factor in squamous cell cancer in the esophagus.

The incidence of ESCC in the United States has been declining since 1973. This is in line with decrease of adult cigarette smoking rate from

Table 1.1 Incidence of esophageal squamous cancer in selected regions of the world.

Region	Locality	Incidence (per 100,000)	
		Male	Female
Asian esophageal cancer belt		>100	>100
China	Yangcheng	135.2	84.4
	Tianjin	16.6	8
India	Kashmir	42.6	27.9
	Bombay	11.4	8.9
	Bangalore	6.6	5.3
Europe			
Northern Europe		<4.0	<2.0
Eastern Europe		<4.0	<2.0
France	Calvados	26.5	–
UK	East Scotland	8.5	4.3
	England and Wales	6.5	3.2
South America			
Uruguay		40	–
Brazil	Porto Alegre	26.3	7.8
North America			
USA	Los Angeles	16.4	4.9
	Washington, DC		
	Black	16.9	4.5
	White	4.1	1.7
Africa			
Transkei		37.2	21.1

Source: Ribeiro, U.Jr., Posner, M.C., Safatle-Ribeiro, A.V. *et al.* (1996) Risk factors for squamous cell carcinoma of the oesophagus. *Br J Surg*, **83**(9), 1174–1185.

about 42% in 1960s to about 20% currently according to Centers for Disease Control and Prevention (CDC) reports. However, this decline of cigarette smoking has been stalled and caused significant public health concerns as the U.S. failed to drop below 12%, a goal set by *Healthy People 2010*. In addition, there appears to be an increase in younger smokers that may lead to a recurrence in the rate of cancer. Primary prevention of cancer is thought to be the most effective strategy in this disease in which the risk factors have been well established.

Although esophageal adenocarcinoma has surpassed ESCC since early 1990s in the United States, a high incidence is still seen among urban population and African Americans,[1] and patients with certain comorbidities such as achalasia, head and neck cancer, and tylosis (Table 1.4). The incidence among African Americans men (16.8 per 100,000) was five times higher than Caucasians (3.0 per 100,000).[4] And mortality was three times higher. In western countries, consumption of tobacco and alcohol could explain more than 90% of ESCC cases.[4] The higher ESCC rate among African Americans parallels the adult cigarette smoking rates. According to Surveillance, Epidemiology, and End Results (SEER) cancer registry data from 1992 to 1998, ESCC incidence rates for Native American and white Hispanics were not higher than general population, although select Native

American populations in specific regions of the country may have a higher incidence. Data from this group is influenced by the diversity of social and economic situations around the country.

Diagnosis

Patients with ESCC may present with dysphagia, weight loss, cough, and GI bleeding (hematemesis and/or melena). But there is no specific physical finding for ESCC, and rarely lymph nodes in the periphery could be appreciated. For cases with metastatic lesions, hepatomegaly could be present.

The following modalities are commonly used to establish the diagnosis of ESCC:

1. Esophagogastroduodenoscopy (EGD) with Lugol sprays

    Lugol solution has been used in medicine since 1985. During EGD exam, Lugol solution, approximately 10–20 mL of 1.5% Lugol iodine solution (but the concentration may vary), is applied through a catheter over the entire esophagus. Since Lugol solution contains potassium and iodine, it should be avoided in patients with hyperthyroidism, iodine allergy, and renal insufficiency. Some authors believe that patients with hypopharyngeal tumors are not candidates for Lugol's unless under endotracheal intubation due to concerns of possible laryngeal edema caused by iodine.

    The Lugol staining pattern is associated with the degree of glycogen within the squamous epithelium, and squamous cell carcinoma does not include glycogen; hence, it is not stained and a clear identification is feasible. This enables endoscopist to visualize the dysplastic areas as Lugol-voiding lesions (LVLs). Biopsies could then target these LVLs to increase the yield. The overall sensitivity is 96–100% and specificity varies from 40% to 95%. It could also be used for intraoperative determination of tumor margins to assist surgical resection.

    LVLs could also be of prognostic value. In a study of 227 patients with head and neck squamous cell carcinoma (HNSCC), those with no LVLs did not have metachronous ESCC during median follow-up of 28 months; however, 15% of those with numerous irregular LVLs lesions developed ESCC.[7] One study examined nondysplasia epithelium (NDE) from LVLs, and it found 20% of them had a *p53* hotspot mutation, and 40% among dysplasia epithelium in contrast to no *p53* mutations in 103 paired NDE samples with normal Lugol staining. It was also suggested that the chance of finding dysplasia was much higher from a patient with more LVLs than those with fewer ones.

    EGD with Lugol spray is currently considered as the most effective noninvasive way to diagnose squamous cell dysplasia and ESCC. Other newer methods such as narrow band imaging (NBI) or autofluorescence imaging (AFI) have been compared with Lugol spray to assess their accuracy. It is important to note that not all squamous cell cancers are Lugol voiding.

2. Narrow band imaging (NBI)

   NBI is a novel noninvasive endoscopic approach to visualize the microvasculature on tissue surface. Compared with white light endoscope (WLE), NBI imaging uses blue light at 415 nm and green light at 540 nm, which gives hemoglobin special absorption characteristics. Thus, it provides better visualization of superficial and subsurface vessels that helps ESCC detection. Often times, the ESCC lesion appears reddish, likely due to microvascular proliferation and/or dilation.

   In one nonrandomized study of HNSCC patients, NBI endoscope with magnification was proved to have very high sensitivity, specificity, accuracy, positive predictive value, and negative predictive value (100%, 97.5%, 97.8%, 83.3%, and 100%, respectively).[8] In another multicenter, prospective, randomized controlled trial with 320 patients, NBI was shown to have 97% sensitivity for superficial ESCC.

   As to high-grade dysplasia (HGD), one study showed the intraepithelial papillary capillary loop (IPCL) patterns were very helpful. But sensitivity and specificity were not satisfactory in contrast to a recent meta-analysis that demonstrated NBI was very sensitive (96%) and specific (94%) in detecting HGD and intramucosal adenocarcinoma for Barrett's esophagus. It is noteworthy that all studies in this meta-analysis used NBI from a GIFQ240Z scope, an instrument that maintains the capabilities of a standard video endoscope and also affords a continuous range of image magnification adjustment up to X80.

   However, NBI is not for detecting the depth of esophageal lesions based on current studies.

3. Autofluorescence imaging (AFI) videoendoscopy

   When white light from a xenon lamp travels through a special optical filter, only the blue excitation light at 390–470 nm and green reflected light at 540–560 nm penetrate through. Interestingly, the blue excitation light can cause living tissue to emit autofluorescence, which passes through another filter and then captured by the charged coupled device at the end of scope. AFI system works by combining autofluorescence (from blue light) and reflectance (from green light) to differentiate the neoplastic lesions (appears purple or magenta) from normal background (green). For the EGD scope that is equipped with AFI, the endoscopist can simply press the AFI button to switch from regular WLE to AFI. However, the flat or depressed ESCC lesions appear to be dark green, which makes it very difficult to distinguish the green color from normal squamous cell background.[9] Because of this, AFI was considered not as sensitive as NBI for these flat or depressed lesions, making it a less attractive method despite that AFI had higher ESCC detection rate (79%) compared with WLE (51%). A multicenter randomized trial showed that in detecting dysplasia and early cancer from Barrett's mucosa, the sensitivity, specificity, positive predictive value, and negative predictive value for AFI were 42%, 92%, 12%, 98.5%, respectively. Thus, at current time, AFI is best used as a complimentary method and not a screening test due to the low sensitivity.

AFI has also been used in bronchoscopy and colonoscopy for squamous cell carcinoma of lungs and dysplasia among ulcerative colitis patients in some studies with various results.

4. Confocal laser endomicroscopy (CLE)

CLE is a new technology that allows in vivo examination of histopathology at the cellular and subcellular levels by using cellular and vascular criteria. The term "confocal" refers to the alignment of both illumination and collection systems in the same focal plane. The laser light could be focused at the different layers of the tissue of interest. Then the reflected light from this layer is refocused and allowed to pass back to the lens in endoscope and to be processed and presented on the monitor. Thus, different depths of tissue can be examined in vivo, the so-called optical biopsy. Fluorescent contrasts, either intravenously or sprayed topically, can enhance the quality of CLE imaging.[10]

In a recent study, CLE provided an in vivo diagnosis in 21 patients who had known ESCC, and the sensitivity and specificity using histology as gold standard were 100% and 95%, respectively. It holds promise for determination of the depth of squamous cell esophageal cancer.[11] Another CLE study after Lugol spray and intravenous fluorescein sodium showed that the overall accuracy was 95%, and sensitivity and specificity were 100% and 87%, respectively. Intraobserver agreement was almost perfect (kappa, 0.95) and interobserver agreement was substantial (kappa, 0.79).[12]

CLE would potentially enable the endoscopist to proceed directly to endoscopic therapy, saving time and avoiding expensive and unnecessary further endoscopies. However, due to the limited tissue infiltration from the blue laser light, CLE may not be the right choice for submucosal lesions.

5. Endoscopic ultrasound (EUS)

After systematic metastatic lesions are ruled out for ESCC patients, EUS could be performed by using either conventional EUS scope or miniprobe sonography (MPS) through the regular endoscope channel. It is considered as the most accurate noninvasive method for T staging and evaluation of lymph nodes around esophagus. It could also evaluate other organs such as adrenal glands, pancreas, liver, bile ducts, and mediastinal structures. Fine needle biopsy of lymph nodes can be done if necessary. However, it is difficult to distinguish T1a and T1b lesions sometime even with MPS. When a patient has scarring from previous radiation therapy (RT), endoscopic resection, or significant ongoing inflammation, it is also very challenging to provide accurate information. Despite all these, the overall T staging accuracy of EUS is 85–90% as compared with 50–80% for CT; the accuracy of regional lymph nodes staging is 70–80% for EUS and 50–70% for CT. However, a recent review showed that T-stage from EUS had concordance of only 65% when compared with pathology specimens obtained by endoscopic mucosal resection (EMR) or surgery.

MPS is a small probe that could safely pass through a tight stricture or narrowing, and it could achieve higher resolution by using higher frequency. The use of MPS can also represent an improvement in the comfort and safety and is highly cost-effective.[13] The drawbacks for MPS are (1) unable to perform real-time ultrasound-controlled fine needle aspiration and (2) lower penetration depth due to higher frequency used, which means less satisfaction in assessing structures (lymph nodes, etc.) that are further away from GI tract.

6. Radiology: esophagraphy/CT/PET/MRI

An esophagram with barium may identify a mass lesion. However, this role has been largely supplanted by EGD exam, which could in addition provide biopsy of suspected tissues. Once HGD or mucosal ESCC are identified, chest CT with or without PET scan should be used to assess systemic involvement. This global evaluation of a patient's metastatic status (M and N staging) should be carried out before EUS.

For T staging, EUS is certainly superior to PET scan, which can only be considered when EUS or CT is inadequate. For N staging, EUS could more reliably distinguish the primary tumor from periesophageal lymph nodes based on a review in 2007. In centers with adequate experience, EUS should be the first choice unless it can not be performed due to stenosis. For M staging, PET scan has clear advantage for detection of disease beyond the celiac axis; however, it is challenging to differentiate the regional node, N1 node, and the celiac axis M1a node. As to the overall impact on the management, PET scan changed 17% of patients from curative to palliative, 4% from palliative to curative, and another 17% changed in treatment modality or delivery based on the results from a study with 68 esophageal cancer patients.

United States Preventive Services Task Force (USPSTF) recommends PET scan to improve the accuracy of M staging for patients who are potential candidates for curative therapy; however, no adequate research examined the value to predict response to neoadjuvant therapy or recurrence.

Recently, the accuracy of diffusion-weighted MR imaging for postoperative nodal recurrence of ESCC was found comparable with FDG-PET. The role of MRI certainly needs more studies to be further defined.

7. Thoracoscopy and laparoscopy

Some surgical centers use these methods for esophageal cancer staging because of the superiority over noninvasive methods. Indeed, an intergroup trial of 107 patients reported that thoracoscopy and laparoscopy could increase the detection rate of positive lymph node from 41% when using noninvasive staging tests (e.g., CT, MRI, EUS) to 56% by thoracoscopy and laparoscopy, and no major complications or deaths were reported. A more recent study in 2002 examined 111 esophageal cancer patients and compared thoracoscopy and laparoscopy versus noninvasive methods such as CT, MRI, and/or EUS, and it showed very low concordance ranging from 14% to 25% for TMN staging. This study pointed out that when compared with the final surgical pathology, a 100% specificity and positive predictive value was achieved by thoracoscopy and laparoscopy staging in diagnosis of lymph node metastasis. Although the sensitivity was about 75% (vs. 45% from noninvasive tests), the accuracy of thoracoscopy and laparoscopy could reach 90.8% and 96.4% in chest and abdomen metastases, respectively; these values were significantly higher than noninvasive staging methods (58% and 68%, respectively, for chest and abdomen).

Staging

The typical workup includes CT scan of chest (and abdomen if advanced lesions are suspected), PET (integrated PET–CT is preferred), and EUS if no metastatic lesions are found, and then surgical consult should be offered if it is resectable. The American Joint Committee on Cancer (AJCC) recently released its 7th edition of cancer staging manual (Table 1.2; Figure 1.1).

Table 1.2 TNM staging of esophageal squamous cell carcinoma (ESCC).

Part 1	
Primary tumor (T)[a]	
TX	Primary tumor cannot be assessed
T0	No evidence of primary tumor
Tis	High-grade dysplasia[b]
T1	Tumor invades lamina propria, muscularis mucosae, or submucosa
T1a	Tumor invades lamina propria or muscularis mucosae
T1b	Tumor invades submucosa
T2	Tumor invades muscularis propria
T3	Tumor invades adventitia
T4	Tumor invades adjacent structures
T4a	Resectable tumor invading pleura, pericardium, or diaphragm
T4b	Unresectable tumor invading adjacent structures, such as aorta, vertebral body, and trachea
Regional lymph nodes (N)	
NX	Regional lymph node(s) cannot be assessed
N0	No regional lymph node metastasis
N1	Metastasis in one to two regional lymph nodes
N2	Metastasis in three to six regional lymph nodes
N3	Metastasis in seven or more regional lymph nodes
Distant metastasis (M)	
M0	No distant metastasis
M1	Distant metastasis
Part 2	
Histologic grade (G)	
GX	Grade cannot be assessed—stage grouping as G1
G1	Well differentiated
G2	Moderately differentiated
G3	Poorly differentiated
G4	Undifferentiated—stage grouping as G3 squamous

Table 1.2 *Continued*

Anatomic stage/prognostic groups
Squamous cell carcinoma[c]

Stage	T	N	M	Grade	Tumor location[d]
0	Tis (HGD)	N0	M0	1, X	Any
IA	T1	N0	M0	1, X	Any
IB	T1	N0	M0	2–3	Any
	T2–3	N0	M0	1, X	Lower, X
IIA	T2–3	N0	M0	1, X	Upper, middle
	T2–3	N0	M0	2–3	Lower, X
IIB	T2–3	N0	M0	2–3	Upper, middle
	T1–2	N1	M0	Any	Any
IIIA	T1–2	N2	M0	Any	Any
	T3	N1	M0	Any	Any
	T4a	N0	M0	Any	Any
IIIB	T3	N2	M0	Any	Any
IIIC	T4a	N1-2	M0	Any	Any
	T4b	Any	M0	Any	Any
	Any	N3	M0	Any	Any
IV	Any	Any	M1	Any	Any

Source: The original source for this material is the AJCC Cancer Staging Manual, Seventh Edition (2010) published by Springer New York, Inc.
Note: cTNM is the clinical classification, pTNM is the pathologic classification.
[a]At least maximal dimension of the tumor must be recorded and multiple tumors require the T(m) suffix.
[b]High-grade dysplasia (HGD) includes all noninvasive neoplastic epithelia that was formerly called carcinoma in situ, a diagnosis that is no longer used for columnar mucosae anywhere in the gastrointestinal tract. Number must be recorded for total number of regional nodes sampled and total number of reported nodes with metastasis.
[c]Or mixed histology including a squamous component or NOS.
[d]Location of the primary cancer site is defined by the position of the upper (proximal) edge of the tumor in the esophagus.

Prognostication

The most significant prognostic factor is TMN staging, although emerging biomarkers could also explain some of the variations in survival:

1. TMN staging

   An early study in 1990s showed that early ESCC lesions that did not invade through muscularis mucosa had low lymph node metastasis rate (2–4%) or vascular invasion (8%).[14,15] And resection of such lesions yielded excellent prognosis with 5-year survival of 90–100%. It was also reported that tumor budding, that is, the isolated cancer cells or microscopic clusters of undifferentiated cancer cells (usually less than five cancer cells) outside the tumor margin, was associated with significantly lower 5-year survival rates.

   The number of lymph node metastases was found to impact the survival. In a retrospective study of 1149 ESCC patients, the overall 5-year survival rates for the patients with 0, 1, and ≥2 positive nodes were 59.8%, 33.4%, and 9.4%, respectively. And the stage-specific

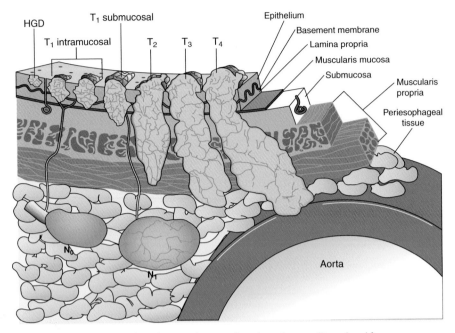

Figure 1.1 Layers of esophagus and stages of esophageal cancer. (Reproduced from Rice, W.R. (2002) Diagnosis and staging of esophageal carcinoma. In: Pearson, F.G., Cooper, J.D., Deslauriers, J. *et al.* (eds), *Esophageal Surgery*, 2nd ed, p. 687. Churchill Livingstone, New York.)

5-year survival for T2N1M0 and T3N1M0 was significantly higher in group with one positive lymph node than the group with ≥2 positive nodes (T2N1M0: 41.5% vs. 24.1%; T3N1M0: 31.2% vs. 6.8%).

Among ESCC patients with negative lymph nodes who generally have good 5-year survival, the finding of positive lymphatic invasion was linked to higher risk for hematogenous dissemination. This is from a study of 88 consecutive ESCC patients who underwent three-field lymph node dissection and no positive lymph nodes were found initially. Among those patients who eventually had lymph node invasion, the incidence of lymphatic invasion was higher than vascular invasion (79% vs. 38%), suggesting that lymphatic invasion was more commonly seen than vascular invasion. Both lymphatic and vascular invasion were independently associated with poor survival (relative risk of 4.9 and 3.5, respectively).

2. Biomarkers

CIAPIN1 is a downstream effector of the receptor tyrosine kinase–Ras signaling pathway in animal cell lines. The decreased expression of CIAPIN1 was statistically correlated with lower degree of differentiation, more depth of invasion, and lymph node metastasis among ESCC patients. Consistently, the survival rates of patients with CIAPIN1-negative tumors tended to be statistically lower than those with CIAPIN1-positive tumors.

Higher tumor-specific expression of survivin, a member of the inhibitors of apoptosis gene family, has been found to be a significant marker for poorer survival for ESCC but not esophageal adenocarcinoma. The disease-specific 5-year survival rate of patients with low survivin mRNA expression was greater than those with high survivin (43% vs. 12%).

Serum squamous cell carcinoma antigen positivity, which indicates the circulating esophageal squamous cancer cells in peripheral blood, was found more often among advanced ESCCs, but its prognostic value is limited.

Overexpression of cyclin D1, an amino acids frequently expressed in G1 phase of cell cycle, was thought to play an important role in cell growth and cancer progression. On the contrary, E-Cadherin, the most essential one of Cadherin family, which is the backbone of cell-to-cell adhesion, is also a key molecule in the initial step of cancer cell invasion. Increased cyclin D1 expression and reduced E-cadherin expression were significant prognostic factors in ESCC patients.

Prevention

1. Reduce exposure to risk factors

    Carcinogenesis of ESCC is a complex process and no single risk factor can explain the variations of incidence rates among different groups. These potential factors may also exert synergic impact on each other during this multistep carcinogenesis (Table 1.3).

    (a) Tobacco and alcohol

    It is undisputable that tobacco and alcohol, acting alone or synergistically, are the significant risks for ESCC. In one study, the significant synergistic impact of cigarette smoking and alcohol drinking on the risk of ESCC was staggering (odds ratio, 50). Population attributable risk (PAR), the difference in rate of a condition between an exposed population and an unexposed population, for the ever-smokers who consumed more than 30 alcoholic drinks per week were 56.9% and 44.9%, respectively. Tobacco and alcohol use was also associated with higher number of

Table 1.3 Risks associated with ESCC.

Environmental/dietary/behavior factors	Host factors
Tobacco	Ethnicity (African American)
Alcohol	Head and neck squamous cell carcinoma
Nitrosamines/its precursors (Barbecue)	Tylosis
Hot liquid	Achalasia
Nutritional deficiency	Lichen planus
Caustic injury (lye)	Scleroderma
Radiation	Plummer–Vinson syndrome
Agent orange (case reports)	

dysplasia lesions, and *p53* and *p21* gene mutations were also linked to ESCC during the evolving process of early stage neoplasia.

The risk varies among different types of smoking (pipe and cigar smoking have higher risk) and alcohol beverage. Interestingly, the polymorphism in acetaldehyde dehydrogenase 2 (ALDH2), which could cause flushing after alcohol use, was found to be a useful sign identifying individuals susceptible to ESCC development.

(b) Achalasia

In Greek, achalasia means "do not relax." It is a condition that causes no peristalsis in the distal segment of esophagus where the musculature is mainly smooth muscle, and inability to relax LES (lower esophageal sphincter). This is likely the result of neuron degeneration in myenteric plexuses from many reasons such as inflammation, infection, infiltration. The annual incidence is approximately 1 case per 100,000, and both genders are equally affected. The features of achalasia include dysphagia for solids and liquid, excessive belching, etc. The diagnosis can be established by symptoms, barium swallow, esophageal manometry, and EGD exam. The relationship between achalasia and esophageal carcinoma was first reported by Fagge in 1872.

Because achalasia patients often have difficulty in swallowing as baseline, clinicians should have low threshold to initiate a new workup plan for ESCC among these patients. Studies have shown that these cases were often diagnosed late and the prognosis was very dismal. However, close endoscopy surveillance does not seem cost-effective, and other modalities such as blind brush cytology still warrant research. Even so the surveillance should be carried out among those who are fit enough to undergo surgical resection if tumors are found.

One report showed 8.6% of achalasia patients could have ESCC in 15–20 years after the onset of symptoms. In another study of 1062 achalasia patients (9864 person-year follow-up), 2.3% had ESCC, a 16-fold increase of cancer risk compared with general population. It is very difficult to determine the true prevalence of ESCC among achalasia patients, and it varies from 1.7% to even 20%. Likely this variation is due to different referral base and length of follow-up. One study showed the mean interval between the diagnosis of achalasia and carcinoma was 5.7 years.

(c) Tylosis

Tylosis (focal nonepidermolytic palmoplantar keratoderma), an autosomal dominant skin disorder with thickening of the skin in the palms and soles, was associated with a high risk of squamous cell carcinoma. It was first described in 1958 in two large Liverpool families. The causative locus, the tylosis esophageal cancer (TOC) gene, has been localized to a small region on chromosome 17q25. Studies on loss of heterozygosity have indicated a role for the TOC gene in sporadic squamous cell esophageal cancer and Barrett's adenocarcinoma. About half of tylosis patients may develop ESCC by 45 years old or 95% by the age of 65.

(d) Scleroderma

Scleroderma is skin thickening and hardening associated with many different medical conditions, and it is called systemic sclerosis when other organs are also involved. Most of these patients have manifestations in GI tract and half of them may be asymptomatic. In the esophagus, it predominantly causes distal esophageal hypomotility and weak LES tone, although the upper sphincter pressure and proximal esophageal motility is normal. Clinically, it can present as heartburn and dysphagia, and it is associated with esophagitis, ulceration, strictures, Barrett's esophagus, spontaneous esophageal rupture, esophageal adenocarcinoma, or ESCC. On esophageal manometry, it has distinctive features of low contractility and weak LES.

Both ESCC and adenocarcinoma of the esophagus were found among up to 70% of scleroderma patients in an early study in 1979. However, a more recent review of seven studies showed that the link between scleroderma and cancer was not overwhelming with probably a modest increase in lung cancer. This cancer risk might be much lower among localized scleroderma (morphea) patients.

(e) Head and neck squamous cell carcinoma

It is well known that some patients with HNSCC could have either synchronous (found around the time of HNSCC diagnosis) or metachronous ESCC (diagnosed during follow-up). SEER data from 1973 to 1987 showed that the incidence of esophageal cancer was about 1.6% among 21,371 HNSCC patients, a 23 × increase of risk compared with general population. One study showed that 5% of 389 patients were found to have synchronous ESCCs within 1 year after the diagnosis of HNSCC.[16] It also revealed that metachronous ESCC was found more often among hypopharyngeal cancer patients (about 16%) than in laryngeal, oropharyngeal, or oral cancer patients. By combining seven studies with total of 25,834 HNSCC patients, the rough estimate of esophageal cancer is about 1.6%.

Although no societal guideline is available, some authors recommended panendoscopic examination (bronchoscopy, pharyngoesophagoscopy, and laryngoscopy) in patients with early-stage head and neck cancer at the time of diagnosis and then every 6 months for 5 years.

(f) Human papillomavirus (HPV)

The relationship between HPV infection and ESCC remains controversial. It was demonstrated in a high-risk population in China but not in low-risk patients in Europe.

2. Preventive measures

(a) Screening

Considerable efforts have been made in searching for optimal screening methods. The cytologic detection of ESCC or precursor

Table 1.4 Recommendations regarding endoscopy surveillance for ESCC for high-risk patients (American Society for Gastrointestinal Endoscopy).

Risk factors	EGD surveillance	
	Starting time	Intervals
Achalasia	Insufficient data for surveillance. If considered, could initiate 15 years after onset of symptoms	Undefined
Tylosis	Age 30 years old	Requires more studies; no more than every 1–3 years
Caustic ingestion	15–20 years after caustic ingestion	No more than every 1–3 years. Low threshold to evaluate swallowing problems with endoscopy

Source: This table is based on American Society for Gastrointestinal Endoscopy. (2006) *Gastrointestinal Endoscopy*, **63**, 570–580.[17]

lesions by using balloon and sponge samplers yielded very low sensitivity, although a recent study showed greater than 90% sensitivity in detecting Barrett's esophagus by cytosponge. However, the latter study also utilized trefoil factor 3, an immunostain diagnostic marker for Barrett's esophagus based on the systematic gene expression profiling, which may have enhanced the sensitivity significantly.

(b) Chemoprevention

Isotretinoin is a synthetic retinoid with chemopreventive effects that induces a differentiated state. It could potentially reduce the ESCC rate from 24% to 4% among HNSCC patients in a placebo-controlled study.

Although providing a protective effect on patients with mild esophageal squamous dysplasia after 10-month use, selenomethionine failed to inhibit esophageal squamous carcinogenesis for high-risk subjects based on a randomized, placebo-controlled study, which also demonstrated that celecoxib had no detectable protective benefit.

(c) Surveillance

The American Society for Gastrointestinal Endoscopy (ASGE) recommended surveillance on three high-risk populations: achalasia, caustic ingestion, and tylosis Table 1.4).[17]

Cancer management

In general, ESCC patients seek for medical attention when significant symptoms emerge, such as unexplained weight loss and dysphagia, at which time it is highly likely that the disease has spread to the degree that only palliative care could be provided. About 75% of patients present with stage III or IV disease. The National Comprehensive Cancer

Network (NCCN) provides a very detailed guideline in esophageal cancer management on their Web site. Based on this guideline and other publications, the current consensus can be summarized as follows:

1. Early ESCC

   Early ESCC means intramucosal lesion (T1a or less). We now have much more experience in treating them with noninvasive procedures.

   (a) EMR

   EMR is a minimally invasive endoscopic procedure to remove mucosal lesions that are less than 2 cm, or piecemeal removal of larger size lesions. Techniques can be subdivided as injection-, cap-, and ligation-assisted EMR. Specifically, EMR techniques include injection-assisted EMR, EMRC (cap with suction and then snare mucosectomy), and duette multiband mucosectomy Kit.[18] An alternative for en bloc resection of a large lesion is ESD (endoscopic submucosal dissection), but its utility in the esophagus is still under investigation as it takes much longer to perform and has higher complication rates.

   About 2–4% of mucosal ESCC (Tis or T1a) patients have lymph nodes invasion, and a few studies had shown that EMR is preferred for this population. EUS is performed first before EMR to ensure there are no lymph nodes involved. EMR could be performed for diagnostic and therapeutic purpose. In experienced hands, it has very low complications, although it can cause minor complications such as short-lived chest discomfort and pain, or minor bleeding (<2 g/dL of hemoglobin drop). Other major but fortunately rare complications include significant bleeding, perforation, and stenosis. The recurrence after EMR varies and it largely depends on the patient selection, whether or not other ablation modalities are performed. One study of 142 mucosal ESCC patients who underwent EMR showed no recurrence of diseases in 9 years of follow-up.

   The Mayo clinic researchers in the Barrett's esophagus unit conducted a study and found that antiplatelet agents can be continued after procedures to minimize cardiovascular complications among high thromboembolic risk patients. Based on the American Society of Gastroendoscopy (ASGE), patients who need to continue anticoagulation can be bridged with low-molecular-weight heparin.

   (b) Photodynamic therapy (PDT)

   Since the 1980s, PDT has been used for various medical conditions such as cancers (skin cancer, cholangiocarcinoma, and esophageal neoplasia) and wet macular degeneration. PDT uses a special agent such as sodium porfimer (approved in North America) and 5-aminolevulinic acid (5-ALA, used in Europe), either orally or intravenously to sensitize the tumor about 4 hours (oral agent) or 24 hours (intravenous agent) before photoradiation. Then laser light at 630–635 nm wavelength from a very small fiber through the endoscope channel is applied. This can activate the drug, which in turn interacts with oxygen molecule to generate a singlet oxygen state causing cell death.[19]

The response rate varies from 50% to 100% based on different studies. Severe dysplasia and superficial mucosal cancer (<2 mm in depth) can be completely ablated by PDT. However, it may not be able to eradicate the early carcinoma thicker than 2 mm in depth. A large retrospective study of 123 patients (104 ESCC, 19 adenocarcinomas) showed no difference in complete response rate and survival rate between[1] PDT alone and PDT plus multimodal treatment groups (with chemoradiation),[2] the adenocarcinoma and squamous cell carcinoma groups. PDT-related complications include stenosis (35%) and cutaneous photosensitization (13%). Other side effects may include stricture, fistula, chest pain, nausea, and vomiting; however, the perforation rate was about 1% that is lower than EMR.

However, although it is simple to perform, the role of PDT in treatment of esophageal diseases has been limited when other newer and safer methods such as EMR and radiofrequency ablation (RFA) are gaining more popularity.

(c) Other modalities

Although RFA has been used widely among Barrett's esophagus patients, the experience is still limited for ESCC. Only one case of ESCC with RFA treatment was reported in 2008. Very scarce experience with cryotherapy or argon plasma coagulation (APC) for ESCC has been reported.

2. Locally advanced ESCC

Locally advanced ESCC is defined as any T stages with local lymph nodes but no evidence of distant disease. The chemotherapy regimen should be individualized based on tumor stage and patients' performance status. Unfortunately, most of these regimens have low-to-median response rates with significant toxic profiles.

In reviewing the studies on chemoradiation and surgery, it is worth noting that (1) most clinical studies recruited not only ESCC but also esophageal adenocarcinoma, and some even stomach cancers; (2) some studies were criticized because of overall design (e.g., not randomized), small sample size, enrollment bias, uncontrolled crossover between study arms, underperformance of control arm (thus type I error), etc., so one should interpret the results with precautions; (3) these different regimens may prolong the median survival but usually no more than 12 months (most of them had benefits of 3–9 months compared with best supportive care) at the price of very serious adverse effects; (4) multimodality therapy has better response but more adverse effects; (5) surgery alone or surgery combined with other modalities, but not chemotherapy or RT alone, could be potentially curative for early-stage cancer.

(a) Chemotherapy

The most frequently investigated and clinically used regimen includes infusion of cisplatin and 5-fluorouracil (5-FU) at the first and fourth week of RT. Its response rate varies from 20% to 50%. A randomized phase II study of cisplatin and 5-FU versus cisplatin alone in advanced squamous cell esophageal cancer revealed that combined therapy failed to provide more survival benefits but had significantly more adverse effects such as grade 4 aplasia and septicemia, meningeal hemorrhage, cerebrovascular accident, and ischemia. Actually, cisplatin seems to be the most active agent (response rate of approximately 20%). But in practice, cisplatin and 5-FU are most commonly used in combination.

Other choices are ECF regimen (epirubicin, cisplatin, and 5-FU), DCF (docetaxel, cisplatin, and 5-FU), MCF (mitomycin, cisplatin, and 5-FU), irinotecan and cisplatin, and gemcitabine and cisplatin. The REAL-2 study revealed that capecitabine, an oral agent that converts into 5-FU at tumor tissue, was as effective as 5-FU, and that oxaliplatin was similar to cisplatin but with significantly less grade 3 or 4 neutropenia, alopecia, kidney toxicity, and thromboembolism, but slightly more grade 3 or 4 diarrhea and neuropathy.

(b) Radiation therapy

External plus intraluminal radiotherapy was superior to external alone in both local control and long-term survival; however, the complications such as bleeding, fistula, ulcerations, and complication-related mortality were much higher in the combined group. Up to 70–80% patients with dysphagia from the tumor could improve their symptoms.

Among postoperative ESCC patients, one retrospective study demonstrated that higher total radiation dose (>50 Gy) after surgery was associated with fewer locoregional recurrences and better diseases-free survival without more serious acute and late complications, but no improvement of overall mortality.

However, by randomizing nonsurgical patients with T1 to T4, N0/1, M0 squamous cell carcinoma, or adenocarcinoma to receive higher dose RT (64.8 Gy) or standard dose RT (50.4 Gy) while receiving the same 5-FU and cisplatin therapy, INT 0123 study showed that higher dose RT (64.8 Gy) treatment did not yield statistically significant improvement in median survival when compared with 50.4 Gy group (18.1 vs. 13.0 months), and that the locoregional failure was about the same (56% vs. 52%). More treatment-related mortality was observed in the higher dose RT group. Thus, RT with 50.4 Gy is currently considered as standard dose when combined with chemotherapy.

In a summary, the current recommendation is to use 50.4 Gy radiation together with chemotherapy.

(c) Chemoradiation therapy

Chemoradiation therapy is considered more efficacious than either chemotherapy or radiation therapy alone. For patients with significant cardiopulmonary issues who are not surgical candidates, this could be a potential cure.

A prospective trial in 1992 randomized patients to either the group with combined 5-FU and cisplatin plus 50.0 Gy of RT or to RT alone group (64.0 Gy). The results showed that combined therapy prolonged the median survival from 9 to 12.5 months, and the survival rates at 12 and 24 months were 50% and 38% in combined group versus 33% and 10% in RT alone group.

In another prospective study, 196 ESCC and adenocarcinoma patients with T1-T3, N0-N1, and M0 staging, Karnofsky score of at least 50, were randomized to chemotherapy (cisplatin and 5-FU) plus RT (50.0 Gy) versus RT (64.0 Gy) alone. It showed the 5-year survival for combined therapy was 26% compared with 0% from the RT-only group. However, due to the serious or even life-threatening adverse effects from the combined treatment, only 68% patients completed the whole chemoradiation therapy.

For potentially resectable ESCC of the mid or lower esophagus, the two- or three-stage esophagectomy with two-field dissection or chemoradiotherapy offered similar survival based on results from the prospective randomized trial—CURE study (the Chinese University Research Group for Esophageal Cancer (CURE)). The regimen they used was 5-FU 200 mg/m²/day infusion from days 1 to 42, cisplatin 60 mg/m² on days 1 and 22, and total RT of 50–60 Gy.

In a summary, chemoradiation therapy is more efficacious than either chemotherapy or radiation therapy alone. For resectable patients, surgery could provide similar benefit as chemoradiotherapy.

(d) Surgery

Cervical and cervicothoracic esophageal carcinoma located at <5 cm from the cricopharyngeus should be treated with definitive chemoradiation rather than surgery. For other appropriate candidates, surgical options include transhiatal esophagectomy or Ivor-Lewis procedure (needs thoracotomy and laparotomy) (Table 1.5).

Table 1.5 Resectability of the esophageal cancer.

Staging of esophageal cancer	Methods for resection
Tis and T1a tumors (within the mucosa)	Endoscopic mucosal resection or submucosal dissection
T1b (submucosa)	Esophagectomy
T1–T3 with regional nodal metastases (N1)	Esophagectomy
T4 with involvement in pericardium, pleural, or diaphragm	Esophagectomy
Stage IVa, distal cancer with resectable celiac nodes, but sparing the celiac artery, aorta, or other organs	Esophagectomy
Stage IVa, distal cancer with unresectable celiac nodes; involvement of celiac artery, aorta, or other organs	Unresectable
Stage IVb, unresectable tumor invading other adjacent structures, such as aorta, vertebral body, and trachea	Unresectable

The acceptable surgical options include the following[20]:

- Standard Ivor Lewis esophagogastrectomy (laparotomy and right thoracotomy) or minimally invasive Ivor Lewis (laparotomy and limited right thoracotomy).
- Standard McKeown esophagogastrectomy (laparotomy, right thoracotomy, and cervical anastomosis) or minimally invasive McKeown (limited laparotomy, right thoracotomy, and cervical anastomosis).
- Transhiatal esophagogastrectomy (laparotomy and cervical anastomosis).
- Robotic minimally invasive esophagogastrectomy.
- Left transthoracic or thoracoabdominal incision with anastomosis in the chest or neck.
- Options for reconstruction after esophagectomy include gastric pull-up, colon interposition, or jejunal interposition.

(e) Surgery with or without preoperative therapy (neoadjuvant)

A recent review (2007) of neoadjuvant therapy with chemoradiation showed better curative resection rates and lower locoregional recurrence than surgery alone, but the overall benefit for survival was not clearly demonstrated although some studies revealed such a trend. However, as eluded earlier, many of these studies were not optimally designed; study groups were mixed (gastric cancer, esophageal adenocarcinoma, and ESCC); sample size was small and under powered; and some yielded conflicting results. The multicenter, randomized trial to compare preoperative chemoradiotherapy followed by surgery with surgery alone in patients with stage I and stage II squamous cell cancer of the esophagus failed to show difference in the overall survival although it did prolong disease-free survival.

The CROSS trial is a multicenter, randomized, phase III clinical trial that compares neoadjuvant chemoradiotherapy followed by surgery with surgery alone in patients with potentially curable esophageal adenomas and ESCC with inclusion of 175 patients per arm. The results of this study are still pending.

The practice guideline from Cancer Care Ontario (http://www.cancercare.on.ca/) provided the following recommendations:

- *Bimodal regimen*: A published abstract of an individual patient data-based meta-analysis of nine randomized trials (2102 patients) comparing preoperative chemotherapy followed by surgery (CT + S) to surgery alone demonstrated a 4% (from 16% to 20%) absolute overall survival advantage for chemotherapy at 5 years. Based on seven trials (1849 patients), the disease-free survival was 10% in CT + S group versus 6% in surgery-alone group. No difference was seen in postoperative death.
- *Trimodal regimen*: A meta-analysis of 10 randomized trials comparing esophageal adenocarcinoma patients who received preoperative chemoradiotherapy followed by surgery to surgery

alone showed a 13% absolute benefit in survival at 2 years for preoperative chemoradiotherapy.

- Thus, trimodal is preferred to bimodal regimen if preoperative therapy is considered.
- Randomized trials demonstrated no survival benefit for RT given alone, either preoperatively or postoperatively, compared with surgery alone.
- Randomized trials demonstrated no survival benefit for postoperative chemotherapy compared with surgery alone.

In a summary, based on less-than-optimal studies, neoadjuvant therapy before surgery could provide small benefit in overall survival and is currently recommended.

(f) Surgery with or without postoperative therapy (adjuvant therapy)

Compared with neoadjuvant therapy, fewer studies addressed the issue of adjuvant therapy. In 2000, a study randomized 556 patients with either resectable gastric and gastroesophageal junction adenocarcinoma, to postoperative chemoradiotherapy or surgery alone. Patients in the postoperative chemoradiation arm had a median survival of 36 months and patients in the surgery alone arm had a median survival of 27 months ($p = 0.005$).

One randomized study in 2003 showed that cisplatin and 5-FU adjuvant therapy did improve the 5-year disease-free survival from 45% to 55% ($p = 0.037$) for ESCC patients with stage IIA, IIB, III, or IV with distant node involvement (M1 lymph node) after surgery.

A more recent study in 2009 prospectively randomized 151 ESCC patients (stage II–III) to surgery and adjuvant therapy versus surgery alone, and it showed significant better 5- and 10-year survival rates of 42.3% and 24.4%, respectively, for the group with adjuvant therapy versus 33.8% and 12.5%, respectively, for the surgery alone group. The local recurrence rates in the combined group and surgery alone group were 14.9% and 36.4%, respectively ($p < 0.05$).

In a summary, based on limited data, adjuvant therapy with chemoradiation may provide some survival benefit when compared with surgery alone.

(g) Target therapy

Since the current therapy has limited response for esophageal cancer patients, target therapy aiming toward certain molecules such as HER-2, VEGFR, is an area with active investigation.

The Trastuzumab for Gastric Cancer (ToGA) trial that included HER-2 positive patients with gastroesophageal and gastric adenocarcinoma demonstrated that 5-FU/cisplatin/trastuzumab was superior to 5-FU/cisplatin with median survival of 13.5 versus 11.1 months. Besides trastuzumab, other agents used in the targeted therapy include cetuximab, erlotinib, matuzumab, gefitinib (anti-HER2 antibodies), and bevacizumab (an anti-VEGFR antibody) that are also under investigations.

(h) Herbal agents

A recent Cochrane review was unable to identify a true randomized control trial among 43 articles regarding herbal use as an adjunct therapy to chemoradiation for esophageal cancer patients. The herbals in these studies were from large variety of plants and no specific brands or names were listed. This review concluded that we had no solid evidence to support or against the use of herbal agents among esophageal cancer patients.

3. Metastatic diseases and palliative care

Patients with Eastern Cooperative Oncology Group (ECOG) performance score of ≥3 could be supported by best care; if ECOG score is ≤2, chemotherapy can be considered. No regimen is considered as standard.

For space-occupying lesions, esophageal stents could be placed to restore esophageal patency, but ESCC within 2 cm of upper esophageal sphincter is a contraindication. Sometimes dilation with balloon or Savary dilators may be necessary before stent placement. Self-expanding metal stents (SEMS) have been improved continuously over the last decade in its diameter, shape, distal and proximal flanges, and types of coatings, and they are preferred over plastic one for palliative purpose. SEMS could be placed via endoscopy with or without fluoroscopy by gastroenterologists or under fluoroscopy by radiologists. The complications of stents include migration, bleeding, perforation, tumor overgrowth, pressure necrosis, etc., and the rates vary by types of stents and anatomic location of placement. The placement successful rate could be 90–97%.

Percutaneous endoscopic gastrostomy (PEG) can be considered if a patient has dysphagia. If jejunum access is needed, percutaneous endoscopic jejunostomy or PEG tube with jejunum extension can be placed.

If patients have bleeding from tumor surface, then endoscopy treatment with APC (APC) or electrocoagulation might be helpful. However, if severe bleeding is from fistulization between tumor and aorta, endoscopy intervention is insufficient and patients suffer from high mortality.

Family screening

There is no specific recommendation for family screening. However, if the family is exposed to similar environments or has similar life style as in the index case, screening seems appropriate although no formal recommendation is available.

Case Study

A 67-year-old Caucasian female has 22 years history of achalasia and underwent Heller's myotomy 12 years ago. She has had progressively worsening heartburn symptoms despite of PPI therapy. For a few years, she has intermittent vomiting especially when she lies flat. The vomitus may include undigested food from previous meal. This time she presented in your clinic with progressive dysphagia to solids, and she mainly takes liquid nutrition supplement and some mechanically soft food. She also has about 25 lb weight loss that she attributed to poor appetite. She is ambulatory and capable of all self-care but unable to carry out any work activities.

Q1. What are the possible underlying etiologies for her dysphasia?

In a different scenario, if this lady presented a few days after her Heller's myotomy, it is still possible that her symptoms are due to tissue swelling from the surgery, or possible scar formation if it is a few weeks after her operation.

However, in her current situation, she is suffering from reflux of food retained in her distal esophagus. It is possible that her achalasia had recurred. Another possible etiology for her dysphagia (the worst case scenario) is squamous cell carcinoma of esophagus, or esophageal adenocarcinoma, which could be the reason for her solid food dysphagia and significant weight loss.

Q2. What is the next step in her medical care?

One could start with esophagram, but definite diagnostic modality is EGD exam with biopsy. If cancer is found, then PET/CT scans are the next step in this investigation. If negative, then EUS can be performed for T staging.

Q3. What are the treatment options?

It certainly depends on TNM staging and her performance status. If she has metastatic diseases and space-occupying mass that caused her dysphagia, then SEMS could provide palliation. Chemotherapy or RT is also an option to reduce the tumor size.

If it is locally advanced disease, then neoadjuvant chemotherapy with ECF regimen (epirubicin, cisplatin, and 5-FU) with RT followed by esophagectomy could be offered. If it is only a mucosal lesion (which is highly unlikely given her dysphagia), series of EMR could be a potential cure and she should be under close surveillance to monitor recurrence.

Key Patient Consent Issues

Consent for EGD/EUS/EMR/Stent

Mr. (or Mrs.) X, we will perform upper endoscopy exam under sedation with ultrasonic view of your esophageal lesion and surrounding lymph nodes. If it is a shallow lesion, we may perform a procedure to resect it. It may cause some bleeding where the resection takes place, but the vast majority of patients will stop the oozing spontaneously without intervention; otherwise, cautery, coagulation, hemoclip, etc., can be utilized to stop the bleeding. Other significant, but fortunately very rare, complications are major bleeding or perforation, which may be treated with surgery or esophageal stenting.

If your lesion in esophagus is occupying the lumen, we could place a metal stent over it to relieve the trouble with swallowing. The risks include bleeding, stent migration, tumor tissue growth into the stent causing obstruction, or necrosis and even perforation.

Discussion for some chemotherapy regimens

The adverse effects could be serious for some of the agents. For example, Oxaliplatin plus capecitabine regimen could cause leukopenia (50.0%), nausea and vomiting (51.6%), diarrhea (50.0%), stomatitis (39.1%), polyneuropathy (37.5%), and hand–foot syndrome (37.5%).[21] We will closely monitor you and terminate your treatment if you are not able to tolerate it.

References

1. Jemal, A., Murray, T., Ward, E. *et al.* (2005) Cancer statistics, 2005. *Cancer J Clin*, **55**, 10–30.
2. Mahboubi, E., Kmet, J., Cook, P.J. *et al.* (1973) Oesophageal cancer studies in the Caspian Littoral of Iran: The Caspian cancer registry. *Br J Cancer*, **28**, 197–214.
3. Zheng, S., Vuitton, L., Sheyhidin, I. *et al.* (2010) Northwestern China: a place to learn more on oesophageal cancer. Part one: Behavioural and environmental risk factors. *Eur J Gastroenterol Hepatol*, **22(8)**, 917–925.
4. Brown, L.M., Hoover, R., Silverman, D. *et al.* (2001) Excess incidence of squamous cell esophageal cancer among US Black men: role of social class and other risk factors. *Am J Epidemiol*, **153**, 114–122.
5. Schottereld, D., Fraumeni, J.F. (1982) *Cancer Epidemiology and Prevention*, pp 596–604. WB Saunders, Philadelphia.
6. Cradock, V.M. (1993) *Cancer of the Esophagus*. Cambridge University Press, New York.
7. Muto, M., Hironaka, S., Nakane, M. *et al.* (2002) Association of multiple Lugol-voiding lesions with synchronous and metachronous esophageal squamous cell carcinoma in patients with head and neck cancer. *Gastrointest Endosc*, **56(4)**, 517–521.
8. Nonaka, S., Saito, Y., Oda, I. *et al.* (2010) Narrow-band imaging endoscopy with magnification is useful for detecting metachronous superficial pharyngeal cancer in patients with esophageal squamous cell carcinoma. *J Gastroenterol Hepatol*, **25(2)**, 264–269.
9. Yoshida, Y., Goda, K., Tajiri, H. *et al.* (2009) Assessment of novel endoscopic techniques for visualizing superficial esophageal squamous cell carcinoma: autofluorescence and narrow-band imaging. *Dis Esophagus*, **22(5)**, 439–446.
10. Kantsevoy, S.V., Adler, D.G., Conway, J.D. *et al.* (2009) Confocal laser endomicroscopy. *ASGE Technology Committee, Gastrointest Endosc*, **70(2)**, 197–200.
11. Iguchi, Y., Niwa, Y., Miyahara, R. *et al.* (2009) Pilot study on endomicroscopy for determination of the depth of squamous cell esophageal cancer in vivo. *J Gastroenterol Hepatol*, **24(11)**, 1733–1739.
12. Pech, O., Rabenstein, T., Manner, H. *et al.* (2008) Confocal laser endomicroscopy for in vivo diagnosis of early squamous cell carcinoma in the esophagus. *Clin Gastroenterol Hepatol*, **6(1)**, 89–94.

13. Menzel, J., Hoepffner, N., Nottberg, H. *et al.* (1999) Preoperative staging of esophageal carcinoma: miniprobe sonography versus conventional endoscopic ultrasound in a prospective histopathologically verified study. *Endoscopy*, **31**, 291–297.

14. Endo, M., Kawano, T. (1997) Detection and classification of early squamous cell esophageal cancer. *Dis Esophagus*, **10(3)**, 155–158.

15. Endo, M., Kawano, T. (1991) Analysis of 1125 cases of early esophageal carcinoma in Japan. *Dig Endosc*, **4**, 71–76.

16. Su, Y.Y., Fang, F.M., Chuang, H.C. *et al.* (2010) Detection of metachronous esophageal squamous carcinoma in patients with head and neck cancer with use of transnasal esophagoscopy. *Head Neck,* **32(6)**, 780–785.

17. American Society for Gastrointestinal Endoscopy. (2006) The role of endoscopy in the surveillance of premalignant conditions of the upper gastrointestinal tract. *Gastrointestinal Endoscopy*, **63**, 570–580.

18. Namasivayam, V., Wang, K.K., Prasad, G.A. (2010) Endoscopic mucosal resection in management of esophageal neoplasia: current status and future directions. *Clin Gastroenterol Hepatol*, **8**, 743–754.

19. Wang, K.K., Lutzke, L., Borkenhagen, L. *et al.* (2008) Photodynamic therapy for Barrett's esophagus: does light still have a role? *Endoscopy*, **40(12)**, 1021–1025.

20. National Comprehensive Cancer Network Guidelines in Oncology, v.2.2010. http://www.nccn.org/professionals/physician_gls/PDF/esophageal.pdf

21. Qin, T.J., An, G.L., Zhao, X.H. *et al.* (2009) Combined treatment of oxaliplatin and capecitabine in patients with metastatic esophageal squamous cell cancer. *World J Gastroenterol*, **15(7)**, 871–876.

2 Esophageal Adenocarcinoma

Key Web Links

http://www.refluxhelp.org/ (medical and patient support)
http://www.aga/ (research information)
http://www.youtube.com/view_play_list?p=7559F6CAAE5BA0CD

Potential Pitfalls

- The values of endoscopic surveillance for Barrett's esophagus is currently not fully elucidated and is being tested in the Barrett's Oesophagus Surveillance Study (BOSS) trial, although it can lead to detection in some patients of lower stage cancers.
- The presence of a hiatal hernia should be determined and distinguished from Barrett's esophagus during endoscopy to avoid any misdiagnosis.

Epidemiology

Nimish Vakil

University of Wisconsin School of Medicine and Public Health, Madison, WI, USA

Esophageal adenocarcinoma is one of the most important gastrointestinal cancers because its incidence has risen substantially in the United States, Western Europe (especially the United Kingdom), Australia, and other developed countries over the past four decades, and continues to rise.[1,2] Some Asian countries have also begun to report an increase in the incidence of esophageal adenocarcinoma.[3,4] In the United States, the highest incidence is seen in non-Hispanic white men, in whom the incidence is eight times higher than in non-Hispanic white women and approximately five times higher than in African American men.[5] The peak age of incidence of esophageal adenocarcinoma is in the seventh decade and beyond. In a Dutch study of 42,207 patients with Barrett's esophagus, age was a significant predictor of the development

---

Handbook of Gastrointestinal Cancer, First Edition. Edited by Janusz Jankowski and Ernest Hawk.
© 2013 John Wiley & Sons, Ltd. Published 2013 by John Wiley & Sons, Ltd.

of esophageal adenocarcinoma (hazard ratio 12; 95% CI, 8.0–18).[6] In a study from the Cleveland Clinic, the odds of those 50 years or older having a prevalent case of high-grade dysplasia or cancer was five times the odds of those younger than 50 years.[7]

Several case control studies have suggested that obesity is a risk factor for esophageal adenocarcinoma. The strongest data come from a prospective study that evaluated cancer risk in a large cohort of European subjects. 346,554 men and women participating in the European Prospective Investigation into Cancer and Nutrition were evaluated.[8] BMI, waist circumference, and waist-to-hip ratio were positively associated with the risk of esophageal adenocarcinoma: relative risk (RR), 2.60 (95% CI, 1.23–5.51); RR, 3.07 (95% CI, 1.35–6.98), and RR, 2.12 (95% CI, 0.98–4.57).

Symptomatic reflux disease is one of the best-recognized risk factors for esophageal cancer.[9] The longer the duration of reflux disease, the worse the symptoms and the more frequently they occur, the higher the risk. In one study, the odds ratios for esophageal adenocarcinoma was 43.5 (95% CI, 18.3–103.5) for patients with frequent heartburn for decades compared with patients without heartburn. Other risk factors for esophageal adenocarcinoma include cigarette smoking, which doubles the risk of esophageal adenocarcinoma.[10] A diet low in fruit and vegetables, folate deficiency, and especially low selenium have been associated with increased risk.[11,12] Alcohol intake has been associated with increased risk in some countries, but not in others. Chronic *Helicobacter pylori* infection may have a protective effect although the mechanism remains unclear.[13] One suggested mechanism is that the development of atrophy results in hypochlorhydria, reducing acid secretion and decreasing distal acid exposure.

Medications have been associated with both an increased and a decreased risk of esophageal cancer. Drugs that inhibit the lower esophageal sphincter are associated with a higher risk of esophageal cancer.[14] In contrast, proton pump inhibitors and aspirin have been associated with a decreased risk of Barrett's esophagus and cancer although these studies have several limitations.[15,16]

Family Screening and Studies

Yvonne Romero[1] and Kee Wook Jung[2]
[1]Mayo Clinic, Rochester, MN, USA
[2]Asan Medical Center, Seoul, Korea

Screening for Barrett's esophagus and esophagus cancer

Your patient was just diagnosed with Barrett's esophagus or esophageal adenocarcinoma. Should you recommend that their family members be screened for Barrett's esophagus or early cancer? Will your recommendation be based on whether the family member reports heartburn or acid regurgitation? Before attempting to provide data to inform your clinical recommendations, it is necessary to understand some basic genetic concepts, and the limitations of family studies performed to date, especially as differences in study design may have contributed to mixed results. Understanding these concepts will help you explain the rationale behind your recommendations for each unique patient and their family.

Many of the known risk factors for Barrett's esophagus and the adenocarcinoma cell type of esophagus cancer have a heritable (also known as germline) genetic component including male sex and white ethnicity. In this regard the world's first genome wide paper has shown that several SNPs lead to Barrett's esophagus.[17] Obesity, which is a strong risk factor for esophageal adenocarcinoma, is thought to be 33% attributable to germline genetics, with environment (e.g., the foods available) and behavior (e.g., the portion size the person chooses to eat) playing major roles in the development of obesity. Central obesity, in which the person demonstrates an elevated waist-to-hip circumference ratio, is mildly associated with Barrett's esophagus. On the basis of twin studies, it has been estimated that 31% of gastroesophageal reflux disease (GERD) symptoms, namely, heartburn and acid regurgitation, also have a heritable component.[18]

Conversely, somatic genomic changes are due to the accumulation of genetic mutations over time. Somatic mutations are not inherited. A major risk factor for esophageal adenocarcinoma is advancing age. The average age at which esophageal adenocarcinoma is diagnosed in the United States is 68 years.[19] When a person's risk of a specific cancer increases as they age, this implies that a time-related accumulation of somatic mutations is playing a role. Usually, cancers that are inherited due to germline genetic factors are diagnosed at a younger age when compared with people who develop sporadic, nonfamilial cancer.

Most people with Barrett's esophagus are unaware that they have an abnormal lining of their swallowing tube that increases their risk for the adenocarcinoma type of esophagus cancer. Although heartburn and acid regurgitation are the hallmark symptoms of GERD, not all people with Barrett's esophagus or esophageal adenocarcinoma (diseases thought to be due to reflux) perceive GERD symptoms. GERD symptoms cannot be used in the general population to direct screening as 20% of US adults report weekly symptoms, and esophageal adenocarcinoma is rare (fewer than 10,000 cases per year among 300 million people in the United States). As a result, millions of patients with reflux would need to be screened to find a relatively small number of patients with Barrett's. Conversely, 40% of people with esophageal adenocarcinoma in a background of Barrett's esophagus deny ever experiencing GERD symptoms and are astounded to learn they have been diagnosed with a reflux-induced malignancy.[20] As a result, patients would not be detected by screening programs based on symptoms.

Aging clearly increases the risk of esophageal adenocarcinoma, suggesting that nonheritable (somatic) factors are important in the development of this highly lethal malignancy. However, the precise relationship between age and Barrett's esophagus is not clear, hampered largely by the need for endoscopy to diagnose Barrett's esophagus. Thus, how much of Barrett's esophagus is heritable (germline) versus sporadic (somatic) is not known. Barrett's esophagus is rarely diagnosed in infants and children.[21] Although Barrett's esophagus is commonly diagnosed in the sixth and seventh decades of life, it is possible that the person had Barrett's esophagus for decades prior to its diagnosis as endoscopy is infrequently recommended for young adults and children, especially those who lack GERD symptoms.

The attributable risk of family history of Barrett's esophagus and/or esophageal adenocarcinoma on the predisposition to the development of Barrett's esophagus and esophageal adenocarcinoma is an area of active investigation. As people in a family tend to eat similar foods and share similar behaviors, family studies have to be interpreted with caution, keeping environmental and behavioral factors in mind.

GERD symptoms

Three independent studies have shown that GERD symptoms tend to aggregate in families.[22-24] One study compared how frequently people with a first-degree relative with esophageal adenocarcinoma or long-segment (greater than 3 cm in length) biopsy-proven Barrett's esophagus (having intestinal metaplasia with goblet cells on their biopsies from the tubular esophagus) reported GERD symptoms compared with people who did not have a first-degree relative with esophageal adenocarcinoma or Barrett's esophagus. The key strength of the study design was that they compared the first-degree relatives of patients with esophagus cancer or Barrett's esophagus with the first-degree relatives of the SPOUSE of the person with the positive family history. By doing so, the researchers were attempting to adjust for environmental factors as it is quite likely that members of the entire extended family eat similar types of foods. Thus, there is very good evidence that GERD symptoms aggregate in families, but how much is due to shared environment and behavior versus germline genetics is not yet clear.

Hiatal hernia, reflux esophagitis, Barrett's esophagus and esophageal adenocarcinoma

Case reports have described families in which multiple members have been diagnosed with GERD symptoms, hiatal hernia, reflux esophagitis, Barrett's esophagus, or esophageal adenocarcinoma.[25,26] Whether this is due to shared inherited germline mutations, or shared environmental and behavioral factors (contributing to somatic mutations) is under investigation. It also remains possible that the appearance of familial clustering of disease is merely due to chance. Reflux esophagitis is a chemical burn of the inner lining of the esophagus caused by the backward motion of stomach contents (e.g., acid, bile, and food) into the esophagus. It has been postulated that years of inflammation from reflux esophagitis may contribute to the formation of Barrett's esophagus, especially in genetically predisposed individuals. The presence of a hiatal hernia, where the stomach has migrated from the abdomen into the chest, increases a person's propensity to reflux. Studies investigating the prevalence of GERD and its complications in families in which at least one person has Barrett's esophagus and/or esophageal adenocarcinoma have generated mixed results.

One investigative group conducted a study in which they offered a research upper endoscopy to first-degree relatives of patients with long-segment biopsy-proven Barrett's esophagus and/or adenocarcinoma of the tubular esophagus (not the gastroesophageal junction or proximal stomach), who had never before been endoscoped.[27] People with and without GERD symptoms were invited to undergo endoscopy. For comparison, the research group also asked patients scheduled for a clinically indicated endoscopy to complete a questionnaire about their family history and their personal GERD symptoms. The original manuscript describing the details of this study was under review at the time of this publication. The unpublished results of this prospective study of 315 first-degree relatives and 360 controls found that advancing age ($p = 0.001$), male sex ($p = 0.005$), and GERD symptoms of prolonged duration ($p = 0.001$) are independent predictors of Barrett's esophagus. Strikingly, even after adjusting for age, sex, and GERD symptoms, first-degree relatives were over twice as likely to have Barrett's esophagus compared with controls without such a family history. Reflux esophagitis was frequently found in both relatives and controls who reported weekly GERD symptoms of prolonged duration, who were not using proton pump inhibitors or histamine receptor antagonist medications. Somewhat surprisingly, among people who denied experiencing GERD symptoms, first-degree relatives were three times more likely to have reflux esophagitis compared with controls. This study suggests that a person who has a first-degree relative with long-segment Barrett's esophagus has an increased chance of having Barrett's esophagus and reflux esophagitis themselves compared with people who do not have this family history. People with a family history who reported GERD symptoms had the highest chance of having Barrett's esophagus and reflux esophagitis. Importantly, lack of GERD symptoms did not confer absence of reflux esophagitis or Barrett's esophagus. People with a family history who denied GERD symptoms still had a moderately high chance of having reflux esophagitis, with a few also having Barrett's esophagus.

The group of first-degree relatives who participated in this research study have been prospectively followed. Three of these people with a family history of long-segment biopsy-proven Barrett's esophagus, with or without esophageal adenocarcinoma, who have Barrett's esophagus themselves, have progressed to esophageal adenocarcinoma in their 50s. This is nearly two decades younger than the average age of diagnosis of sporadic esophageal adenocarcinoma, raising the possibility of germline genetic factors.

In contrast, a separate family study found that the age of diagnosis of esophageal adenocarcinoma was not different in people with a family history of Barrett's esophagus or cancer compared with people without a known family history.[28] These two major studies differed in their criteria for family history. The first study required a family history of long-segment biopsy-proven Barrett's esophagus, while the second study was more liberal and included people with shorter segment disease. The second study included people with gastroesophageal and tubular esophageal adenocarcinoma, while the first study excluded families with gastroesophageal junction tumors for the theoretical possibility that tumors found at that location might behave more like stomach cancers than reflux-induced esophagus cancer. Importantly, both studies confirmed the importance of obesity as a risk factor for esophageal adenocarcinoma. Currently, at least two large genome-wide collaboratives are in the final stages of reporting their findings in ~5000 cases each (EAGLE using a UK and North European cohort and BEACON using a more dispersed worldwide cohort).

From a collaboration of EAGLE and BEACON – 8,000 patients with Barrett's and 18,000 controls, we have identified 2 genetic regions predisposing to hereditary predisposition. These genetic regions termed single nucleotide polymorphisms (SNPs) are located on 6p and 16q. This important discovery will lay the foundation for genetic stratification of risk.[17]

When counseling your patient and their family, it is best to keep the following in mind: The results of the first study have not yet undergone peer review, and their results have not been confirmed by a separate independent group. With these caveats in mind, applying the results of both studies, if three or more members in a family have objective evidence of long-segment Barrett's esophagus and/or adenocarcinoma of the esophagus, one may consider offering screening endoscopy to other first-degree relatives, especially if the relative reports heartburn or acid regurgitation, and the affected family member with Barrett's esophagus or cancer was diagnosed before age 50 (young onset disease). Until the results of these studies are confirmed, there is not enough data to support recommending screening endoscopy to relatives who deny GERD symptoms. It is important to remember that the report of difficulty in swallowing (dysphagia) is considered an alarm symptom. People reporting new onset dysphagia, especially if accompanied by a second alarm symptom, unintentional weight loss, should undergo diagnostic endoscopy. Endoscopy prompted to investigate an alarm symptom is not a screening procedure.

Esophageal squamous cell carcinoma

Although extremely rare, there are families in whom multiple members have the squamous cell type of esophagus cancer (as opposed to the adenocarcinoma type of cancer discussed in the Barrett's esophagus section).[29] The esophagus is lined by stratified squamous epithelium, which is very similar to the cells of your skin. Tylosis is a germline heritable disease that predisposes to esophageal squamous cell carcinoma. People with tylosis have very thick skin (hyperkeratosis) on the palms of their hands and soles of their feet. People with Type-A tylosis are usually diagnosed by age 15, and commonly progress to esophageal squamous cell carcinoma before age 50 (thus, demonstrating early onset disease). The average age at diagnosis for patients with sporadic esophageal squamous cell carcinoma is 68 years.[19] Tylosis is a rare autosomal dominant disease with studies showing linkage on chromosome 17. As people with tylosis A have a 60–90% lifetime risk of esophageal squamous cell carcinoma, screening and surveillance are recommended by the American Society of Gastrointestinal Endoscopy.[30] For example, if someone in a tylosis family developed cancer at age 33, all other family members with palmoplantar hyperkeratosis are urged to begin endoscopic evaluation by age 23, at least one decade before the affected family member was diagnosed. Recent data indicate RHBDF2 mutations are associated with tylosis and opens up the way for screening.[31] Because environmental factors play a major role in the development of esophageal squamous cell carcinoma, people in tylosis families should be strongly cautioned against the use of tobacco, alcohol, nitrosamine-rich foods (e.g., barbeque, grilled/charred meat, and hot dogs), and scalding hot temperature beverages.

In China, Iran, and Afghanistan, families have been described in which more than one member develops a nontylosis esophageal squamous cell carcinoma. It is currently thought that these clusters are likely due to environmental factors particularly, nutritional deficiencies, the cultural practice of drinking beverages at scalding hot temperatures, preparing and consuming nitrosamine-rich foods, and heavy use of tobacco products. Investigation as to potential germline mutations contributing to esophageal squamous cell carcinoma in Asia are in progress.

In summary, further elucidation as to the germline mutations and chromosome abnormalities contributing to familial Barrett's esophagus, esophageal adenocarcinoma, and esophageal squamous cell carcinoma will impact screening, surveillance, and treatment recommendations.

Prognostication

Christopher J. Peters[1] and Rebecca C. Fitzgerald[2]
[1]London Deanery, London, UK
[2]Hutchison/MRC Research Centre, Cambridge, UK

The overall 5-year survival for all patients diagnosed with esophageal adenocarcinoma is less than 8%,[32] but this rises to 17–23% in patients who are operative candidates.[33] Chances of survival vary greatly depending on the stage of disease and a number of other patient factors, mainly related to medical fitness. While 5-year survival has approximately doubled in the last 30 years, this is largely ascribed to decreased perioperative mortality.[32] Predicting prognosis is important as surgery for esophageal adenocarcinoma still has associated mortality and significant morbidity. Furthermore, it is important to identify patients who might benefit from additional oncological treatments.

Staging

Esophageal adenocarcinoma is staged using the internationally recognized TNM (tumor, node, metastasis) system, which continues to evolve over time as our understanding of the disease develops. Preoperatively, T-stage and N-stage are typically assessed with endoscopic ultrasound,[34] whereas CT and PET can best clarify M-stage and can provide extra information about T-stage and N-stage.[35] Patients with a significant intra-abdominal component to the tumor may also undergo a staging laparoscopy.[36] Postoperatively, the definitive TNM stage is derived from histopathological analysis of the specimen. Historically, the sixth edition of TNM[37] required the esophageal staging system to be used for all Siewert Type-I tumors and Type-II tumors where the bulk of cancer lied in the esophagus, and the gastric system for the remaining Type-II and all Type-III tumors. In contrast, the recently published seventh edition of TNM has created a harmonized system for all junctional cancers[38,39]. The T-stage divides cancers according to the depth of invasion [T0, no evidence of primary; Tis, high-grade dysplasia; T1, invades into lamina propria or submucosa; T2, invades into muscularis propria; T3, invades into adventitia; T4, invades into adjacent structures (T4a, operable; T4b, inoperable)]; N-stage is based on the number of involved regional lymph nodes (N, 0 involved lymph nodes; N1, 1–2 involved lymph nodes; N2, 3–6 involved lymph nodes; and N3, 7 or more); and M-stage is based on distant metastasis (M0, no distant metastasis; M1, distant metastasis). The TNM staging is combined into four stages of disease (I, II, III, and IV) with significant differences in outcome.

Pathological features

It is entirely predictable that, in general, more advanced tumors tend to have a worse prognosis. There is a good deal of evidence to suggest T-stage is prognostic in esophageal adenocarcinoma,[40,41] probably because increasing depth of invasion is associated with increasing likelihood of tumor spread.[42] In terms of N-stage, patients with no nodal disease do considerably better than those with lymph node metastases (5-year survival 70% vs. 21%).[43] There is also a considerable body of evidence suggesting that the number of positive lymph nodes has prognostic value.[43,44] The current staging system takes this into account using the cutoffs derived from the gastric cancer system[38]. Historically, the TNM sixth edition considered tumors M1a if the celiac lymph node was involved, but there was little evidence for this being significant in esophageal adenocarcinoma.[45] The latest TNM system has removed this classification and reserves M1 for spread to distant lymph nodes and other organs, both of which are established as poor prognostic signs.[38,39]

Tumors are graded microscopically into well, moderately or poorly differentiated categories. It has been demonstrated that poor differentiation is a predictor of N-stage,[42] but when combined with other pathological features, it does not appear to be important on its own[46]. There is good evidence that involvement of the proximal and distal margins after surgery is a poor prognostic sign,[47] but the evidence regarding the circumferential margin is less clear.[48,49] This may be due to differing histopathological analyses and differing rates of R0 (clear margin) resections between centers. Similarly, both vascular and perineural invasion are possibly poor prognostic signs but with unclear independent significance.[50,51]

Patient factors

There is some evidence that advanced age has a negative impact on prognosis, but when combined with other features, including comorbidities and use of chemotherapy, it has not been shown to independently predictive of outcome.[52] There is evidence that cancers detected de novo in an unscreened population tend to be more advanced and have a worse prognosis.[53] Preoperative malnutrition and dysphagia are also negative prognostic factors,[54] again most likely because they are surrogates for advanced disease.

Future

Increasing importance is being placed on the molecular changes that occur during cancer development and the influence these may have on prognosis. This is both looking at individual genes[55,56] and patterns of molecular changes.[57,58] At present, there are no molecular staging systems for esophageal adenocarcinoma in routine clinical use though prospective clinical trials are underway for some.[57] It is highly likely that, akin to advances in other cancers such as breast, in the future molecular changes will be established as a useful tool for prognostication in esophageal adenocarcinoma. A more refined approach to prognosis should inform the choice of patient treatment and ultimately improve outcomes for patients.

Key Issues in Patient Informed Consent

Grant M. Fullarton and Paul Glen
Glasgow Royal Infirmary and Southern General Hospitals, Glasgow, UK

Informed consent implies patients are fully updated with relevant information about their condition allowing them to make an informed decision about their treatment.

There have been significant advances in the management of both the precursor of esophageal adenocarcinoma Barrett's high-grade dysplasia and early (mucosal) adenocarcinoma (T1m) and established esophageal adenocarcinoma, which are relevant to this discussion.

Barrett's esophagus with high-grade dysplasia and early esophageal adenocarcinoma (T1m)

- Currently, the gold standard treatment for patients is esophagectomy; however, this is associated with significant overall morbidity and mortality even in centers of excellence (range 0–8% with mean of 3%). There has been significant progress in less invasive endoscopic ablative techniques as an alternative option in these cases. There is randomized controlled evidence of decreased cancer progression shown initially with photodynamic laser therapy and more recently with radiofrequency ablation.[59,60] Although photodynamic therapy (PDT) carries risks of complications such as short-lived photosensitization (100%) and postprocedure stricture formation (30%), radiofrequency ablation with much more controlled mucosal ablation appears safer with fewer side effects and demonstrates high rates of ablation of both dysplastic and nondysplastic Barrett's up to 3 years post-therapy.[61]
- Early (mucosal) adenocarcinoma may also be effectively treated by endoscopic mucosal resection followed by ablation of residual Barrett's to decrease the risk of subsequent malignant transformation in any remaining Barrett's tissue.[62,63] Observational studies suggest the long-term survival is similar in endoscopic and surgically treated groups.[64]

Key Points

- All patients undergoing therapy should be discussed in a multidisciplinary team meeting.
- All patients should be treated in specialist centers with full access to all treatment modalities.

Esophageal adenocarcinoma

Potentially curative treatment
Before discussing treatment, all patients should be appropriately staged and discussed at a multi-disciplinary team meeting (MDT) where staging investigations and fitness should be reviewed. The recommendation of MDT will then be communicated to the patients, and the consent process will begin.

Surgical resection
A significant morbidity and mortality is associated with resections of esophageal cancer, and patients should be aware of this to aid their decision making. In-hospital mortality is around 3–5% even in high-volume centers; specific scoring systems have been developed to

allow a more individual assessment of risk. Postoperative complications are also reported to occur in 40–50% of patients with major morbidity in around 24% of patients.[65]

There is currently no randomized controlled trial (RCT) evidence that there is a survival advantage in either minimally invasive or conventional open surgery. Perioperative benefits have been reported with minimally invasive surgery.

The current standard of care is neoadjuvant chemotherapy with epirubicin, cisplatin, and fluorouracil; associated adverse effects are well documented from the prospective study establishing this treatment.[66] This confers a 13% improvement in 5-year survival (5-year survival with treatment 36%).

Key Points

- Patients undergoing resection of an esophageal cancer should have neoadjuvant chemotherapy.
- Esophageal resection is associated with a mortality of around 3–5%.
- Anastomotic leak rate around 11%.
- Pneumonia occurs in around 8%.
- Prolonged intubation occurs in 10%.

Radical chemoradiotherapy

Many patients diagnosed with esophageal cancer have a level of fitness that precludes surgery, and others may not wish an operation with the associated morbidity and mortality. With localized disease there is an option of radical chemoradiotherapy. This often involves administration of chemotherapy as an induction phase in an attempt to sensitize the tumor to radiotherapy, then radiotherapy to the tumor and surrounding margins over a period of 4–6 weeks alongside chemotherapy. One- and two-year survival following radical chemoradiotherapy is 47% and 21%.[67]

It is difficult to compare directly the outcomes from resection and radical chemoradiotherapy as the reported cohorts are different, with more advanced stage and increased comorbidity in the nonsurgical group. No randomized controlled studies have been performed comparing radical chemoradiotherapy against resection in patients deemed suitable for surgical resection.

Key Points

- 1-Year survival around 21%.
- Side effects from chemotherapy include nausea, bone marrow suppression, and mucositis.
- Radiotherapy can cause sore throat and difficulty swallowing, nausea, reduced appetite and tiredness.

Palliative therapy

Unfortunately, the majority of patients presenting will be deemed suitable only for palliation, which means provide care to treat symptoms rather than underlying cancer, and after this has been established by MDT consensus this should be carefully and appropriately discussed. There is no current RCT evidence demonstrating clear benefit of one method over another. Palliative options include oncological—chemotherapy, radiotherapy, and endoscopic—laser, PDT, and other ablative techniques and radiological stenting. The optimal palliation should be decided by the MDT with agreement by the patient.

References

1. Brown, L.M., Devesa, S.S., Chow, W.H. (2008) Incidence of adenocarcinoma of the esophagus among white Americans by sex, stage, and age. *J Natl Cancer Inst*, **100**, 1184–1187.
2. Bollschweiler, E., Wolfgarten, E., Gutschow, C., Holscher, A.H. (2001) Demographic variations in the rising incidence of esophageal adenocarcinoma in white males. *Cancer*, **92**, 549–555.
3. Fernandes, M.L., Seow, A., Chan, Y.H., Ho, K.Y. (2006) Opposing trends in incidence of esophageal squamous cell carcinoma and adenocarcinoma in a multi-ethnic Asian country. *Am J Gastroenterol*, **101**, 1430–1436.
4. Shibata, A., Matsuda, T., Ajiki, W., Sobue, T. (2008) Trend in incidence of adenocarcinoma of the esophagus in Japan, 1993–2001. *Jpn J Clin Oncol*, **38**, 464–468.
5. Cook, M.B., Chow, W.H., Devesa, S.S. (2009) Oesophageal cancer incidence in the United States by race, sex, and histologic type, 1977–2005. *Br J Cancer*, **101(5)**, 855–859.
6. de Jonge, P.J., van Blankenstein, M., Looman, C.W., Casparie, M.K., Meijer, G.A., Kuipers, E.J. (2010) Risk of malignant progression in patients with Barrett's oesophagus: a Dutch nationwide cohort study. *Gut*, **59(8)**, 1030–1036.
7. Guardino, J.M., Khandwala, F., Lopez, R. *et al.* (2006) Barrett's esophagus at a tertiary care center: association of age on incidence and prevalence of dysplasia and adenocarcinoma. *Am J Gastroenterol*, **101(10)**, 2187–2193.
8. Steffen, A., Schulze, M.B., Pischon, T. *et al.* (2009) Anthropometry and esophageal cancer risk in the European prospective investigation into cancer and nutrition. *Cancer Epidemiol Biomarkers Prev*, **18(7)**, 2079–2089.
9. Lagergren, J., Bergström, R., Lindgren, A., Nyrén, O. (1999) Symptomatic gastroesophageal reflux as a risk factor for esophageal adenocarcinoma. *N Engl J Med*, **340(11)**, 825–831.
10. Tramacere, I., La Vecchia, C., Negri, E. (2011) Tobacco smoking and esophageal and gastric adenocarcinoma: A meta-analysis. *Epidemiology*, **22(3)**, 344–349.
11. Chen, J., Zhang, N., Ling, Y. *et al.* (2011) Alcohol consumption as a risk factor for esophageal adenocarcinoma in North China Tohoku. *J Exp Med* **224(1)**, 21–27.
12. Pandeya, N., Williams, G., Green, A.C., Webb, P.M., Whiteman, D.C.; Australian Cancer Study. (2009) Alcohol consumption and the risks of adenocarcinoma and squamous cell carcinoma of the esophagus. *Gastroenterology*, **136(4)**, 1215–1224.
13. Ye, W., Held, M., Held, M. *et al.* (2004) *Helicobacter pylori* infection and gastric atrophy: Risk of adenocarcinoma and squamous-cell carcinoma of

the esophagus and adenocarcinoma of the gastric cardia. *J Natl Cancer Inst*, **96(5)**, 388–396.

14. Lagergren, J., Bergström, R., Adami, H.O., Nyrén O. (2000) Association between medications that relax the lower esophageal sphincter and the risk for esophageal adenocarcinoma. *Ann Intern Med*, **133(3)**, 165–175.

15. Hillman, L.C., Chiragakis, L., Shadbolt, B., Kaye, G.L., Clarke, A.C. *et al.* (2008) Effect of proton pump inhibitors on markers of risk for high-grade dysplasia and oesophageal cancer in Barrett's oesophagus. *Aliment Pharmacol Ther*, **27(4)**, 321–326.

16. Nguyen, D.M., Richardson, P., El-Serag, H.B. (2010) Medications (NSAIDs, statins, proton pump inhibitors) and the risk of esophageal adenocarcinoma in patients with Barrett's esophagus. *Gastroenterology*, **138(7)**, 2260–2266.

17. Su, Z., Gay, L.J., Strange, A., *et al.* (2012) Common variants at the MHC locus and at chromosome 16q24.1 predispose to Barrett's esophagus. *Nat Genet*, **9**, doi:10.1038/ng.2048.

18. Cameron re 31% GERD twins Cameron, A.J., Lagergren, J., Henricksen, C., Nyren, O., Locke, G.R., III, Pedersen, N.L. (2002) Gastroesophageal reflux disease in monozygotic and dyzogitic twins. *Gastroenterology*, **122**, 55–59.

19. National Cancer Institute, Surveillance Epidemiology and End Results (S.E.E.R.) http://seer.cancer.gov/statfacts/html/esoph.html

20. Lagergren, J., Bergstrom, R., Lindgren, A., Nyren O. (1999) Symptomatic gastroesophageal reflux as a risk factor for esophageal adenocarcinoma. *N Engl J Med* **340**, 825–831.

21. Nguyen, D.M., El-Serag, H.B., Shub, M. *et al.* (2011) Barrett's esophagus in children and adolescents without neurodevelopmental or tracheoesophageal abnormalities: a prospective study. *Gastroint Endosc*, **73(5)**, 875–880.

22. Romero, Y., Cameron, A.J., Locke, G.R., III, *et al.* (1997) Familial aggregation of gastroesophageal reflux in patients with Barrett's esophagus and esophageal adenocarcinoma. *Gastroenterology*, **113**, 1449–1456.

23. Chak, A., Lee, T., Kinnard, M.F. *et al.* (2002) Familial aggregation of Barrett's oesophagus, oesophageal adenocarcinoma, and oesophagogastric junctional adenocarcinoma in Caucasian adults. *Gut*, **51**, 323–328.

24. Trudgill, N.J., Kapur, K.C., Riley, S.A. (1999) Familial clustering of reflux symptoms. *Am J Gastroenterol*, **94**, 1172–1178.

25. Fahmy, N., King, J.F. (1993) Barrett's esophagus: an acquired condition with genetic predisposition. *Am J Gastroenterol* **88**, 1262–1265.

26. Everhart, C.W., Jr., Holzapple, P.G., Humphries, T.J. (1978) Occurrence of Barrett's esophagus in three members of the same family: first report of familial incidence. *Gastroenterology*, **74**, A1032.

27. Romero, Y., Slusser, J.P., de Andrade, M. *et al.*; the Barrett's Esophagus Genomic Study Group. (2006) Evidence from linkage analysis for susceptibility genes in familial Barrett's esophagus and esophageal adenocarcinoma. *Gastroenterology*, **130(4, Suppl 2)**, A-106.

28. Chak, A., Falk, G., Grady, W.M. *et al.* (2009) Assessment of familiality, obesity, and other risk factors for early age of cancer diagnosis in adenocarcinomas of the esophagus and gastroesophageal junction. *Am J Gastroenterol*, **104**, 1913–1921.

29. Brage Varela, A., Blanco Rodriguez, M.M., Estevez Boullosa, P., Garcia, S.J. (2011) Tylosis A with squamous cell carcinoma of the oesophagus in a Spanish family. *Eur J Gastroenterol Hepatol*, **23(3)**, 286–288.

30. American Society of Gastrointestinal Endoscopy. (1998) The role of endoscopy in the surveillance of premalignant conditions of the upper gastrointestinal tract. *Gastroint Endosc*, **48**, 663–668.

31. Blaydon, D.C., Etheridge, S.L., Risk, J.M. *et al.* (2012) RHBDF2 mutations are associated with tylosis, a familial esophageal cancer syndrome. *Am J Hum Genet*, **1090(2)**, 340–346.

32. Cancer Stats. Cancer Research UK. (2009) Available from http://info.cancerresearchuk.org/cancerstats/.

33. Allum, W.H., Stenning, S.P., Bancewicz, J., Clark, P.I., Langley, R.E. (2009) Long-term results of a randomized trial of surgery with or without preoperative chemotherapy in esophageal cancer. *J Clin Oncol*, **27(30)**, 5062–5067.

34. Choi, J., Kim, S.G., Kim, J.S., Jung, H.C., Song, I.S. (2009) Comparison of endoscopic ultrasonography (EUS), positron emission tomography (PET), and computed tomography (CT) in the preoperative locoregional staging of resectable esophageal cancer. *Surg Endosc*, **24(6)**, 1380–1386.

35. Pramesh, C.S., Mistry, R.C. (2005) Role of PET scan in management of oesophageal cancer. *Eur J Surg Oncol*, **31(4)**, 449.

36. de Graaf, G.W., Ayantunde, A.A., Parsons, S.L., Duffy, J.P., Welch, N.T. (2007) The role of staging laparoscopy in oesophagogastric cancers. *Eur J Surg Oncol*, **33(8)**, 988–992.

37. Sobin, L.H., Wittekind, C. (eds) (2002) *TNM Classification of Malignant Tumours* (6th edition). Wiley-Liss, New York.

38. Rice, T.W., Blackstone, E.H., Rusch, V.W. (2010) 7th edition of the AJCC Cancer Staging Manual: esophagus and esophagogastric junction. *Ann Surg Oncol*, **17(7)**, 1721–1724.

39. Rice, T.W., Rusch, V.W., Ishwaran, H., Blackstone, E.H. (2010) Cancer of the esophagus and esophagogastric junction: data-driven staging for the seventh edition of the American Joint Committee on Cancer/International Union against Cancer Staging Manuals. *Cancer*, **116(16)**, 3763–3773.

40. Wijnhoven, B.P., Tran, K.T., Esterman, A., Watson, D.I., Tilanus, H.W. (2007) An evaluation of prognostic factors and tumor staging of resected carcinoma of the esophagus. *Ann Surg*, **245(5)**, 717–725.

41. Holscher, A.H., Bollschweiler, E., Bumm, R., Bartels, H., Hofler, H., Siewert, J.R. (1995) Prognostic factors of resected adenocarcinoma of the esophagus. *Surgery*, **118(5)**, 845–855.

42. Rice, T.W., Zuccaro, G., Jr., Adelstein, D.J. Rybicki, L.A., Blackstone, E.H., Goldblum, J.R. (1998) Esophageal carcinoma: depth of tumor invasion is predictive of regional lymph node status. *Ann Thorac Surg*, **65(3)**, 787–792.

43. Peters, C.J., Hardwick, R.H., Vowler, S.L., Fitzgerald, R.C. (2009) Generation and validation of a revised classification for oesophageal and junctional adenocarcinoma. *Br J Surg*, **96(7)**, 724–733.

44. Rizk, N., Venkatraman, E., Park, B., Flores, R., Bains, M.S., Rusch, V. (2006) The prognostic importance of the number of involved lymph nodes in esophageal cancer: implications for revisions of the American Joint Committee on Cancer Staging System. *J Thorac Cardiovasc Surg*, **132(6)**, 1374–1381.

45. Schomas, D.A., Quevedo, J.F., Donahue, J.M., Nichols, F.C., III, Romero, Y., Miller, R.C. (2009) The prognostic importance of pathologically involved celiac node metastases in node-positive patients with carcinoma of the distal esophagus or gastroesophageal junction: a surgical series from the Mayo Clinic. *Dis Esophagus*, **23(3)**, 232–239.

46. Wayman, J., Bennett, M.K., Raimes, S.A., Griffin, S.M. (2002) The pattern of recurrence of adenocarcinoma of the oesophago-gastric junction. *Br J Cancer*, **86(8)**, 1223–1219.
47. Mulligan, E.D., Dunne, B., Griffin, M., Keeling, N., Reynolds, J.V. (2004) Margin involvement and outcome in oesophageal carcinoma: a 10-year experience in a specialist unit. *Eur J Surg Oncol*, **30(3)**, 313–317.
48. Sujendran, V.A., Baron, R., Warren, B.F., Maynard, N. (2008) Effect of neoadjuvant chemotherapy on circumferential margin positivity and its impact on prognosis in patients with resectable oesophageal cancer. *Br J Surg*, **95(2)**, 191–194.
49. Khan, O.A., Fitzgerald, J.J., Soomro, I., Beggs, F.D., Morgan, W.E., Duffy, J.P. (2003) Prognostic significance of circumferential resection margin involvement following oesophagectomy for cancer. *Br J Cancer*, **88(10)**, 1549–1552.
50. Robey-Cafferty, S.S., el-Naggar, A.K., Sahin, A.A., Bruner, J.M., Ro, J.Y., Cleary, K.R. (1991) Prognostic factors in esophageal squamous carcinoma. A study of histologic features, blood group expression, and DNA ploidy. *Am J Clin Pathol*, **95(6)**, 844–849.
51. Paraf, F., Flejou, J.F., Pignon, J.P., Fekete, F., Potet F. (1995) Surgical pathology of adenocarcinoma arising in Barrett's esophagus. Analysis of 67 cases. *Am J Surg Pathol*, **19(2)**, 183–191.
52. Vallbohmer, D., Holscher, A.H., Brabender, J. *et al.* (2008) Clinicopathologic and prognostic factors of young and elderly patients with esophageal adenocarcinoma: is there really a difference? *Dis Esophagus*, **21(7)**, 596–600.
53. Mariette, C., Finzi, L., Fabre, S., Balon, J.M., Van Seuningen, I., Triboulet, J.P. (2003) Factors predictive of complete resection of operable esophageal cancer: a prospective study. *Ann Thorac Surg*, **75(6)**, 1720–1726.
54. Micheli, A., Mariotto, A., Giorgi Rossi, A., Gatta, G., Muti, P. (1998) The prognostic role of gender in survival of adult cancer patients. *Eur J Cancer*, **34(14)**, 2271–2278.
55. Miller, C.T., Moy, J.R., Lin, L. *et al.* (2003) Gene amplification in esophageal adenocarcinomas and Barrett's with high-grade dysplasia. *Clin Cancer Res*, **9(13)**, 4819–4825.
56. Wang, K.L., Wu, T.T., Choi, I.S. *et al.* (2007) Expression of epidermal growth factor receptor in esophageal and esophagogastric junction adenocarcinomas: association with poor outcome. *Cancer*, **109(4)**, 658–667.
57. Peters, C.J., Rees, J.R., Hardwick, R.H. *et al.* (2010) A four gene signature predicts survival in resected adenocarcinoma of the esophagus, junction and gastric cardia. *Gastroenterology*, **139(6)**, 1995–2004.
58. Lagarde, S.M., Ver Loren van Themaat, P.E., Moerland, P.D. *et al.* (2008) Analysis of gene expression identifies differentially expressed genes and pathways associated with lymphatic dissemination in patients with adenocarcinoma of the esophagus. *Ann Surg Oncol*, **15(12)**, 3459–3470.
59. Overholt, B.F., Lightdale, C.J., Wang, K.K., *et al.* (2005) Photodynamic therapy with porfimer sodium for ablation of high-grade dysplasia in Barrett's esophagus: international, partially blinded, randomised phase III trial. *Gastrointest Endosc*, **62(4)**, 488–498.
60. Shaheen, N.J., Sharma, P., Overholt, B.F. *et al.* (2009) Radiofrequency ablation in Barrett's esophagus with dysplasia. *N Engl J Med*, **360**, 2277–2288.

61. Shaheen, N.J., Overholt, B.F., Sampliner, R.E. *et al.* (2011) Durability of radiofrequency ablation in Barrett's esophagus with dysplasia. *Gastroenterology*, **141**, 460–468.

62. Pech, O., Behrens, A., May, A. *et al.* (2008) Long-term results and risk factor analysis for recurrence after curative endoscopic therapy in 349 patients with high-grade intraepithelial neoplasia and mucosal adenocarcinoma in Barrett's oesophagus. *Gut*, **57**, 1200–1206.

63. Pouw, R.E., Wirths, K., Eisendrath, P. *et al.* (2010) Efficacy of radiofrequency ablation combined with endoscopic resection for Barrett's esophagus with early neoplasia. *Clin Gastroenterol Hepatol*, **8**, 23–29.

64. Prasad, G.A., Wu, T.T., Wigle, D.A. *et al.* (2009) Endoscopic and surgical treatment of mucosal (T1a) esophageal adenocarcinoma in Barrett's esophagus. *Gastroenterology*, **137**, 815–823.

65. Wright, C.D., Kucharczuk, J.C., O'Brien, S.M., Grab, J.D., Allen, M.S. (2009) Predictors of major morbidity and mortality after esophagectomy for esophageal cancer: a society of thoracic surgeons general thoracic surgery database risk adjustment model. *J Thoracic Cardiovascular Surg*, **137**, 587–596.

66. Cunningham, D., Allum, W.H., Stenning, S.P., Thompson, J.N. *et al.* (2006) Perioperative chemotherapy versus surgery alone for resectable gastroesophageal cancer. *N Engl J Med*, **355**, 11–22.

67. Combined chemotherapy and radiotherapy (without surgery) compared with radiotherapy alone in localized carcinoma of the esophagus (2006). *Cochrane Database Syst Rev*, **1**, CD002092.

3 Gastric Cancer

Branislav Bystricky and David Cunningham
Royal Marsden Hospital, London and Surrey, UK

Key Points

- Gastric cancer is the fourth most common malignancy in the world and is diagnosed at an advanced stage in more than 50% cases in the West.
- Upper GI endoscopy with biopsy remains the gold standard in diagnosis.
- Five-year overall survival is halved for every stage progression, with 5-year survival of 50–60% in stage I and 6–8% in stage IV.
- The main risk factors for gastric cancer are *Helicobacter pylori* infection, cigarette smoking, chronic atrophic gastritis, gastric ulcers, prior partial gastrectomy, and gastroesophageal reflux disease.
- Standard treatment approaches for resectable gastric and gastroesophageal junction tumors are perioperative chemotherapy, adjuvant S1 in East Asia, and postoperative chemoradiotherapy in North America.
- Palliative combination chemotherapy improves survival and quality of life and is indicated for patients with metastatic disease, with the addition of trastuzumab in patients with HER-2 overexpressing tumors.

Key Web Links

http://www.cancerresearchuk.org
UK cancer information, funding and research

http://www.bsg.org.uk/
British Society of Gastroenterology—education, training, research resources, and patient information

http://www.macmillan.org.uk
UK patient support and information site

http://www.esmo.org
European Society of Medical Oncology—updated clinical practice guidelines, educational manuscripts, and fellowship opportunities

Handbook of Gastrointestinal Cancer, First Edition. Edited by Janusz Jankowski and Ernest Hawk.
© 2013 John Wiley & Sons, Ltd. Published 2013 by John Wiley & Sons, Ltd.

http://www.nccn.org
US National Comprehensive Cancer Network—clinical practice guidelines in oncology

http://www.asco.org/
American Society of Clinical Oncology—education, public policy, and research resources

http://www.cancer.net/
Patient support and information site supported by the ASCO Cancer Foundation

Potential Pitfalls

- Treatment of gastric cancer requires multidisciplinary input from pathology, gastroenterology, radiology, surgery, oncology, as well as allied health professionals.
- Adjuvant treatment should be given after gastrectomy to patients who did not receive any neoadjuvant treatment.
- Patients with metastatic disease in good performance status should be referred for palliative chemotherapy.
- Specialists in palliative medicine should be involved with patients failing chemotherapy.

Epidemiology

Gastric adenocarcinoma is the most frequent histological type of gastric malignancy (90%); other types include non-Hodgkin's lymphomas (Chapter 10), leiomyosarcomas, gastrointestinal (GI) stromal tumors, and neuroendocrine tumors (Chapter 9). Gastric cancer remains the second leading cause of cancer death worldwide: the estimated incidence is 1 million new cases a year, making it the fourth most common malignancy in the world, after lung, breast, and colorectal cancers.[1] Incidence rates are twice as high in men as in women, with the highest rates occurring in Eastern Asia and Eastern Europe and the lowest rate in Northern and Western Africa (Figure 3.1). In the European Union, there were approximately 86,000 new cases of gastric cancer diagnosed in 2006. Regional differences have been attributed to environmental factors, such as high dietary intake of salt, smoked, and cured meats; in addition, there are significant differences in incidence across socioeconomic groups. Gastric cancer incidence increases with age and rises rapidly from the age of 60 years onward. Although the age-standardized incidence of gastric cancer in the United Kingdom has been steadily decreasing since 1975, the incidence of tumors of gastroesophageal junction (GEJ) is rising.

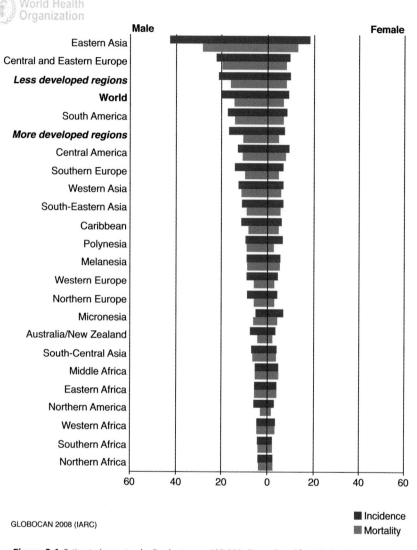

International Agency for Research on Cancer

World Health
Organization

GLOBOCAN 2008 (IARC)

■ Incidence
■ Mortality

Figure 3.1 Estimated age-standardized rates per 100,000. (Reproduced from Ferlay, J., Shin, H.R., Bray, F., Forman, D., Mathers, C. and Parkin, D.M.: GLOBOCAN 2008, *Cancer Incidence and Mortality Worldwide: IARC CancerBase No. 10 [Internet].* Lyon, France, International Agency for Research on Cancer, 2010, http://globocan.iarc.fr)[1]

Diagnosis

Patients with early gastric cancers can be relatively asymptomatic and are often picked up incidentally with iron-deficiency anemia. Locally advanced disease can present with anorexia, early satiety, abdominal discomfort, or pain. Tumors involving the gastric cardia can cause dysphagia, whereas distal tumors involving the pylorus can manifest with nausea and vomiting caused by gastric-outlet obstruction. The most common sites of distant metastases are the liver, lungs, and bone; symptoms that may suggest distant spread include weight loss, shortness of breath, and bone pain. All advanced cancers, especially involving the upper GI tract, can cause weight loss. Melena and hematemesis are usually signs of bleeding locally advanced cancer.

Physical examination in the early stages is often unrevealing. In more advanced stages of disease, patients may have an upper abdominal mass, palpable peritoneal deposits, or hepatomegaly secondary to liver metastases. A classical sign of metastatic gastric cancer is the Virchow's node, a palpable left supraclavicular lymph node that develops when thoracic duct is blocked by metastases from abdominal cancers. Signet-ring, mucin-producing diffuse gastric cancer often metastasizes to the ovaries, a finding called Krukenberg tumor. A palpable metastatic nodule in the umbilicus known as Sister Mary Joseph nodule is thought to arise by lymphatic spread along the hepatoduodenal and falciform ligaments. Blood tests reveal iron-deficiency anemia in more than 50% of patients and patients with liver metastases may have abnormal liver function tests. Tumor markers including carcinoembryonic antigen (CEA) and carbohydrate antigen 19-9 (Ca19-9) have been found to have a low sensitivity and specificity for the detection of gastric cancer but can be used for monitoring of response to treatment.[2]

Guidelines for urgent referral for upper GI endoscopy have been published in an attempt to improve early diagnosis and are summarized in Table 3.1.[3] However, patients with a high clinical suspicion including those 55 years and older with unexplained, persistent recent onset of dyspepsia who do not fulfill guideline criteria should still be urgently referred for upper GI endoscopy. Direct visualization of tumor with endoscopy and biopsy remains the gold standard for diagnosis of gastric cancer. In addition to upper GI endoscopy with biopsies, double-barium GI series can be helpful in defining gastric distensibility and obliteration of the gastric folds, especially in linitis plastica tumors.

The UICC 2009 TNM classification (7th edition) clinically and pathologically stages primary gastric cancers into four T stages (based

Table 3.1 National Institute for Health and Clinical Excellence (NICE) guidelines for referral for urgent upper GI endoscopy.[3]

Patients of any age with dyspepsia presenting with
Chronic gastrointestinal bleeding
Progressive unintentional weight loss
Progressive difficulty swallowing
Persistent vomiting
Iron-deficiency anemia
Epigastric mass
Suspicious barium meal

Table 3.2 UICC TNM classification of gastric cancer (7th edition).[4]

T1a	Lamina propria, muscularis mucosae				
T1b	Submucosa				
T2	Muscularis propria	**N1**	1–2 nodes		
T3	Subserosa	**N2**	3–6 nodes		
T4a	Perforates serosa	**N3a**	7–15 nodes	**M0**	No distant metastasis
T4b	Adjacent structures	**N3b**	16 or more	**M1**	Distant metastasis

on depth of invasion), three N stages (with minimum of 16 lymph nodes recovered to accurately assign pN stage), and M stage (the presence of metastatic disease), which is usually based on the clinical or radiological findings. The regional lymph node of the stomach includes perigastric (along lesser and greater curvature), the nodes along the left gastric, common hepatic, splenic and coeliac arteries, and hepatoduodenal nodes. Involvement of all other lymph nodes is classified as distant metastasis (M1 stage) (Table 3.2).[4]

Computerized tomography (CT) of the chest and abdomen is used for staging gastric cancers and although it can be difficult to accurately assess the thickness of gastric cancer (T stage) on the CT due to variability in gastric filling, CT scans provide important information regarding the lymph node (N stage) and distant organ (M stage) involvement. CT scanning can determine lymph nodes greater than 5 mm; however, its sensitivity for tumor involvement is only 40–50% (Figures 3.2 and 3.3). Endoscopic ultrasound (EUS) is being used more

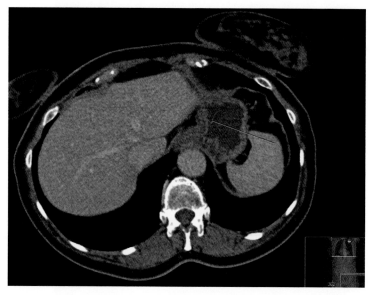

Figure 3.2 Primary tumor is not easily visualized on this CT scan and is confined to the wall of the stomach (Case 1).

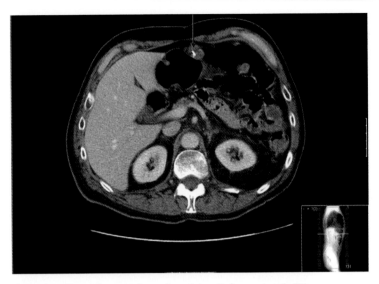

Figure 3.3 CT scan demonstrating peritoneal deposits from metastatic GEJ adenocarcinoma (Case 2).

frequently to complement upper GI endoscopy and CT scans in the staging of gastric cancer (Figure 3.4). EUS can accurately assess the invasion of any of the five stomach layers and define distal and proximal extent of the tumor. This is especially useful in assessing early tumors

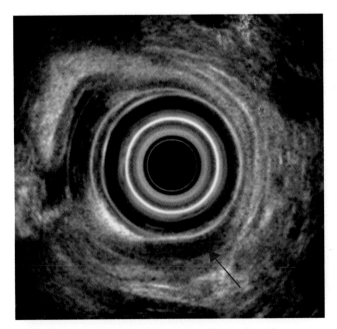

Figure 3.4 EUS of gastric wall, demonstrating a T2 lesion (Case 1).

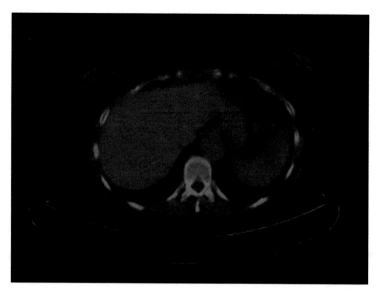

Figure 3.5 Low-grade [18]FDG uptake on CT/PET scan localized on the lesser curvature (Case 1).

and tumors arising at the GEJ. Studies demonstrate 92% accuracy of EUS in T staging compared with 42% for CT.[5] Nevertheless, the use of EUS for N staging is suboptimal due to low penetration of transducer and lymph node visualization. Although 18-fluorodeoxyglucose positron emission tomography ([18]FDG-PET) scans have revolutionized imaging in oncology in the last decade, only 41–83% of gastric cancers are [18]FDG avid. Mucinous and signet-ring cells tumors have less prominent [18]FDG uptake; tumors at the GEJ tend to be more avid and [18]FDG-PET positive.[6] [18]FDG-PET scans remain a valuable tool complementing CT in detection of distant metastases (Figures 3.5 and 3.6).[7] There is evidence to suggest that [18]FDG-PET is a useful predictor of early response to neoadjuvant

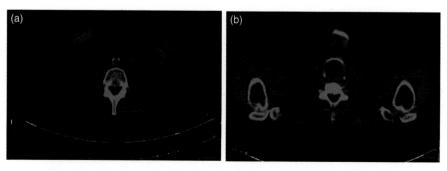

Figure 3.6 CT/PET scan demonstrating avid [18]FDG uptake in the rectus abdominis (a) and trapezius (b) muscle (Case 2).

chemotherapy and a strong prognostic indicator; in a trial of 35 patients with [18]FDG avid tumors, the 2-year survival rate in metabolic responders after 2 weeks of neoadjuvant chemotherapy was 90% compared with 25% in the patients who did not achieve a metabolic response.[8] A staging laparoscopy should be performed in all patients being considered for radical resection as staging CT scans can underestimate the extent of disease in up to 37% of patients.[9] Laparoscopy allows direct visualization of peritoneal cavity and peritoneal cytology can be performed. The detection of malignant cells in peritoneal washings identifies patients at very high risk of recurrence and is associated with poor prognosis.[10] Other histological factors that predict for worse prognosis include poorly differentiated tumors, lymphovascular invasion, and tumors with an infiltrative, diffuse growth pattern.

Prevention

The incidence of gastric cancer in the offspring of immigrants from countries with high incidence falls to that of the new home country, suggesting that development of gastric cancer depends on environmental exposure, with external and dietary carcinogens being the most likely factors. The main identified risk factors for gastric cancer are *Helicobacter pylori* (*H. pylori*) infection, various dietary and occupational exposures, medical conditions, and family history (Table 3.3). Observational cohort studies and meta-analysis suggest that aspirin use might reduce risk of adenocarcinoma of stomach, particularly distal, intestinal type[11-13]; however, further research on the potential of chemoprevention with aspirin or other nonsteroidal anti-inflammatory drugs is needed in high-risk populations.

Table 3.3 Risk factors for development of gastric cancer.

Infection	*Helicobacter pylori*
Environmental	Dietary factors
	Cigarette smoking
Medical	Chronic atrophic gastritis
	Gastric ulcers
	Prior partial gastrectomy
	GERD
	Pernicious anemia
	Gastric atrophy
Hereditary	HDGC
	Li–Fraumeni syndrome
	HNPCC
	Cowden's syndrome
	Peutz–Jeghers syndrome

GERD, gastroesophageal reflux disease; HDGC, hereditary diffuse gastric cancer; HNPCC, hereditary nonpolyposis colorectal cancer.

H. pylori is defined as gastric carcinogen by WHO and is the most important known risk factor for noncardiac gastric cancer[14]; infection with *H. pylori* doubles the risk of gastric cancer. Early *H. pylori* eradication in patients with peptic ulcer disease lowers the incidence of gastric cancer to that of the general population.[15] Interestingly, there is a suggestion that *H. pylori* may have a protective effect in the development of GEJ adenocarcinomas.

A typically Mediterranean diet consisting of high dietary intake of olive oil, unrefined cereals, fruit and vegetables—with moderate consumption of cheese, yogurts, fish, and wine—and low intake of meat not only provides protection against heart disease and diabetes but also reduces incidence of stomach cancer by 33%.[16] An active program of gastric cancer prevention is justified only in countries with high incidence, such as in East Asia. Nationwide screening of gastric cancer has been conducted since 1983 in Japan and has resulted in earlier diagnosis and declining mortality rates.[17] Outside Japan, mass screening has not proven to be cost-effective.

Hereditary diffuse gastric cancer (HDGC) is a genetic syndrome characterized by a high risk of stomach and breast cancers. Gastric cancers occurring in this syndrome are typically diffuse, infiltrating the entire stomach (linitis plastica) and tend to have a signet-ring appearance. Hereditary gastric cancer is inherited in an autosomal dominant pattern and a germline mutation of the E-cadherin gene (*CDH1*), a tumor suppressor gene, has been identified in 30–50% of these families. Affected individuals have a lifetime risk up to 80% of developing gastric cancer. The average age for diagnosis of gastric cancer in these individuals is 38 years and affected individuals with a *CDH1* mutation should be counseled regarding a prophylactic gastrectomy. Table 3.4 lists the criteria for referral for *CDH1* testing.[18]

Gastric cancer predisposition has also been described in the Li–Fraumeni syndrome (due to an underlying *p53* mutation), hereditary nonpolyposis colorectal cancer (HNPCC, caused by mutations in DNA mismatch repair genes), Cowden's syndrome (also known as multiple hamartoma syndrome, caused by *PTEN* mutation), and Peutz–Jeghers syndrome (hereditary intestinal polyposis, caused by *STK11/LKB* mutation).

Table 3.4 Updated consensus guidelines on HDGC, International Gastric Cancer Linkage Consortium, Cambridge 2008.[18]

1. Two or more cases of gastric cancer in a family, with at least one diffuse gastric cancer diagnosed before the age of 50 years
2. Three or more cases of diffuse gastric cancer in first- or second-degree relatives diagnosed at any age
3. An individual diagnosed with diffuse gastric cancer before 40 years of age
4. An individual diagnosed with both diffuse gastric cancer and lobular breast cancer
5. Family history of diffuse gastric cancer and lobular breast cancer (one diagnosis before 50 years of age)
6. Detection of signet-ring cells in situ next to diffuse-type gastric cancer

Cancer management

Resectable gastric cancer

The prognosis of patients with gastric cancer remains poor even following radical gastrectomy with a D2 lymph node dissection, with a 5-year survival rate of 31% for stage II and 11% for stage III.[19]

Surgery

Surgery is critical in the curative treatment of gastric cancer. Endoscopic mucosal resection (EMR) is a minimally invasive procedure offered only to patients with very early gastric cancer (T1a) of intestinal type without ulceration and up to 2 cm in size.[20] Annual endoscopic surveillance following treatment is necessary in these patients to detect local recurrence and metachronous gastric cancer.[21,22] The incidence of lymph node involvement increases to 20% in tumors involving submucosa (T1b) and these patients require gastrectomy with lymph node dissection.[23] The extent of lymph node dissection performed during gastrectomy for gastric cancer has been a matter of controversy. Lymph node dissection is classified according to lymph nodal groups removed during surgery: a D1 dissection involves removal of perigastric lymph nodes directly attached to greater and lesser curvature, D2 involves removal of lymph nodes around the branches of the coeliac axis, and D3 involves removal of additional distant abdominal lymph nodes (at the posterior aspect of the head of the pancreas and at the root of the mesentery).[24] The current UICC TNM staging (7th edition) is based upon dissection of 16 or more lymph nodes to assign the pN stage. Two large trials in the West have evaluated the role of extent of surgery by randomizing gastric cancer patients to either a D1 or D2 lymph node dissection. The Medical Research Council (MRC) trial of 400 patients with resectable gastric adenocarcinoma demonstrated equivalent 5-year survival rates in both groups, with increase in postoperative morbidity and mortality reported in the D2 resection arm.[19] Pancreatico-splenectomy combined with D2 dissection was demonstrated as an adverse factor affecting survival of patients in the D2 arm in this trial. A more recent Dutch trial of D1 versus D2 dissection demonstrated lower locoregional recurrence and gastric cancer-related death in the patients who underwent a D2 lymphadenectomy with an increase in postoperative mortality and morbidity.[25,26] Pancreatico-splenectomy was frequently performed as a part of the D2 lymphadenectomy in this trial and the overall survival (OS) in the D2 group of patients without pancreatectomy or splenectomy has almost doubled (from 5 years in pancreatico-splenectomy D2 group to 9 years in D2 group without organ resection). Further support for the role of radical lymph node resection was demonstrated in a large German gastric cancer study of more than 1600 patients, which reported radical lymph node resection (defined as removal of more than 26 lymph nodes) to be the strongest independent predictor of survival.[27] Japanese studies have consistently showed low perioperative mortality with D2 dissection; however, greater morbidity has been reported following more extensive para-aortic nodal dissection without improvement in survival.[28]

For medically fit patients treated in specialized centers with access to adequate postoperative care, D2 dissection without resection of the pancreas and spleen (unless directly invaded by the tumor) is now the standard in patients with resectable tumors.

Approximately 40% of patients will die as a result of disease recurrence, half of them suffering both local and distant recurrences.[25,29] Several approaches incorporating chemotherapy and radiotherapy have been investigated in an attempt to reduce local and distant recurrences and improve the outcome of patients with gastric cancer.

Perioperative chemotherapy

The role of perioperative chemotherapy was investigated by the MRC Adjuvant Gastric Infusional Chemotherapy (MAGIC) trial in which 503 patients with adenocarcinoma of stomach, GEJ, or lower third of the esophagus were randomized to receive three cycles of preoperative chemotherapy with epirubicin, cisplatin, and 5-FU (ECF) followed by three cycles postoperatively or to surgery alone.[30] There was a significant improvement in the 5-year OS from 23% in the surgery-only group to 36.3% in perioperative chemotherapy group (Table 3.5). In addition, patients in the perioperative chemotherapy group had higher rates of curative surgery, tumor down staging, and had less advanced nodal disease. The incidence of postoperative complications was similar between the two arms. The benefit of perioperative chemotherapy was also demonstrated in the French ACCORD07/FFCD 9703 trial, which randomized 224 patients with resectable adenocarcinoma of stomach, GEJ, and lower esophagus to either two to three cycles of neoadjuvant chemotherapy with cisplatin and 5-FU and further three to four cycles of adjuvant chemotherapy in responding patients or patients with positive lymph nodes versus surgery only. The improvement in 5-year survival was similar to the MAGIC trial with a 14% absolute improvement in OS in the perioperative chemotherapy arm. Similarly, a higher proportion of

Table 3.5 Summary of practice changing trials in operable gastric cancer.

Author & study	Treatment arm	Median OS (months)	5-year OS (%)	p value (for OS)
Cunningham et al. MAGIC[30]	Surgery	20	23.0	
	Perioperative ECF	24	36.3	0.009
Ychou et al. ACCORD07/ FFCD 9703[31]	Surgery	nr	24	
	Perioperative CF	nr	38	0.02
Macdonald et al. INT-0116[33,34]	Observation	27	41 (3-year)	
	Adjuvant chemoradiotherapy	35	50 (3-year)	0.005
Sakuramoto, Sasako et al. ACTS-GC[46,47]	Observation	nr	61	
	Adjuvant S1	nr	72	HR 0.67 95% CI: 0.54-0.83

C, cisplatin; E, epirubicin; F, 5-FU; nr, not reported.

patients receiving neoadjuvant chemotherapy underwent R0 resection and there was slightly less advanced nodal involvement than in the patients in the surgery-alone arm.[31] The REAL-2 trial[32] of palliative chemotherapy in patients with advanced disease demonstrated noninferiority of the oral fluoropyrimidine prodrug capecitabine when substituted for infused 5-FU in the ECF regimen, and based on extrapolation from this trial, epirubicin, cisplatin, and capecitabine (ECX) is now a commonly used perioperative chemotherapy regimen.

Adjuvant chemoradiotherapy

Adjuvant chemoradiotherapy was investigated by US Southwest Oncology Group (Intergroup-0116) trial, which randomized 556 patients with resected adenocarcinoma of stomach or GEJ to adjuvant chemoradiotherapy or observation only. Patients in chemoradiotherapy arm received three cycles of 5-day bolus 5-FU and leucovorin, one cycle was given before and two cycles after concomitant chemoradiotherapy with 5-FU and leucovorin during the first 4 and last 3 days of the radiation schedule.[33] The median survival was 36 months in the chemoradiotherapy arm compared with 27 months in the observation. After 10 years follow-up, the survival benefit was maintained.[34] Only 10% of the patients in this study underwent recommended D2 dissection and 54% had less than D1 dissection. Three toxicity-related deaths occurred and a high incidence of grade 3–4 hematological and GI toxicity was reported in the treatment arm.

The North American CALGB 80101 study randomized 546 patients to adjuvant ECF chemotherapy and 5-FU chemoradiotherapy versus 5-FU bolus chemotherapy and 5-FU chemoradiotherapy. A safety analysis revealed a 3% mortality and 40% grade 4 adverse events in the 5-FU bolus arm compared with 0% mortality and 26% grade 4 adverse events in the ECF arm; however, no improvement in median OS was demonstrated by the addition of adjuvant ECF chemotherapy to 5-FU chemoradiotherapy.[35] Although postoperative chemoradiotherapy is considered one of the accepted approaches in the United States, it has not gained wide acceptance in Europe due to the concerns regarding the abdominal radiation and quality of surgery used in the Intergroup-0116 trial. The Korean ARTIST study randomized 458 curatively resected gastric cancer patients with D2 lymphadenectomy to six cycles of adjuvant cisplatin/capecitabine chemotherapy or chemoradiotherapy with capecitabine administered between four cycles of cisplatin/capecitabine chemotherapy. The addition of chemoradiotherapy did not prolong disease-free survival (74.2% compared with 78.2% with the addition of chemoradiotherapy).[36]

Adjuvant chemotherapy

Adjuvant chemotherapy in gastric cancer has been investigated in more than 31 trials using various agents, either alone or in combination. Most of these trials demonstrated either no or small benefit only.[37] Several meta-analyses of adjuvant chemotherapy trials have been performed and demonstrate a reduction in risk of death of 17–28%,[38-44] the higher rates were seen in Japanese trials investigating oral fluoropyrimidines.[42] A large meta-analysis of individual patient data of 3838 patients from 17 trials reported a benefit from adjuvant chemotherapy compared with surgery alone, with 18% reduction in the risk of death (hazard ratio, 0.82; 95% confidence intervals, 0.75–0.90; $p < 0.001$) and estimated median OS of 4.9 years compared with 7.8 years following surgery only and adjuvant chemotherapy, respectively.[37] The absolute survival benefit with adjuvant chemotherapy was 5.8% at 5 years.

Eight cycles of adjuvant capecitabine and oxaliplatin chemotherapy was investigated in CLASSIC trial from East Asia and demonstrated improvement in disease-free survival (hazard ratio, 0.56; 95% confidence intervals, 0.44—0.72; $p < 0.001$) in 1035 patients analyzed in intent-to-treat population.[45] In a large Japanese trial of adjuvant chemotherapy with an oral drug, 1059 patients were randomized after gastrectomy with a D2 resection to treatment with S1 (a combination of tegafur and enzyme inhibitors gimeracil and oteracil) for 1 year versus observation after curative R0 resection. The majority of patients (89%) had lymph node-positive disease; however, more than 50% had only T2 tumor. A significant improvement in OS was demonstrated—from 70% to 80% at 3 years and 61% to 72% at 5 years[46,47] in the treatment arm. Treatment was well tolerated with low rates of grades 3–4 adverse events reported. Adjuvant S1 is now the standard of care in Japan; however, the results from trials in the Japanese population are often not reproduced in Western populations; treatment with S-1 and cisplatin in advanced gastroesophageal cancers did not demonstrate superior OS to 5-FU/cisplatin combination in non-Asian populations.[48] A retrospective study compared survival between the Caucasian and Asian population with gastric cancer living in the United States using Los Angeles County Cancer Surveillance registry. Asian patients with localized gastric adenocarcinoma had significantly better survival than Caucasians, independent of the tumor location or number of lymph nodes retrieved.[49] These findings suggest that there may be differences in tumor biology between these two populations and results from Asian trials might not be directly comparable with Caucasian population.

In summary, treatment of resectable gastric cancer should be multimodal with the use of systemic chemotherapy in addition to surgical resection with D2 lymphadenectomy. Administration of preoperative chemotherapy is better tolerated than postoperative treatment and perioperative chemotherapy using epirubicin, cisplatin, and capecitabine has become one of the standard approaches in the West and Australia[50] while adjuvant S1 is commonly used in Asia and postoperative chemoradiotherapy in the United States.

Locally advanced and metastatic gastric cancer

Despite greater awareness, earlier investigation, and advances in treatment, approximately 50% of patients still present with inoperable disease and 40% will recur after radical treatment.

Surgery

Patients with symptomatic gastric outlet obstruction due to tumor can gain rapid symptomatic benefit from palliative gastroenterostomy or metal expandable stent placement through the obstruction.[51] Endoscopic stenting is the preferred treatment method over a surgical bypass, with lower cost, faster recovery of oral intake, and shorter postprocedure hospital stay.[52,53] Palliative gastrectomy can extend survival and can be considered in highly selected patients with only one metastatic site; however, higher morbidity and mortality needs to be taken into consideration for these patients with limited life span.[54–56]

Radiotherapy

Palliative radiotherapy can provide symptomatic relief from tumor obstruction, painful bony metastases, and bleeding. In two studies, palliative radiotherapy improved dysphagia due to inoperable gastric carcinoma in more than 75% of patients.[57,58] Pain was controlled in 86% and half of these patients did not require further intervention. A retrospective review of 30 patients receiving 30 Gy in 10 fractions for bleeding tumor has reported symptomatic relief in 68–91% and decreased transfusion requirements.[59,60] Median time to rebleeding after palliative radiotherapy using 30 Gy was reported to be 3.3 months.[61]

First-line chemotherapy

Several randomized trials and meta-analyses have confirmed the benefit of palliative chemotherapy in gastric cancer patients with prolongation of OS and improvement in quality of life.[62] Almost 400 patients were randomized on the European Organization for Research and Treatment of Cancer (EORTC) study to three different combination regimens (doxorubicin, 5-FU, and modified methotrexate (FAMTX); etoposide, leucovorin, and 5-FU (ELF); or 5-FU with cisplatin). Response rates were disappointedly low at 9–20% with median survival ranging from 6.7 to 7.2 months without significant difference between the arms.[63]

In 1990s, ECF regimen was developed and demonstrated encouraging activity with objective tumor responses documented in 71%, complete response was reported in 12% and a median OS of 8.2 months.[64] Due to the high incidence of line complications during 5-FU infusion, its inconvenience, and frequent contraindications of cisplatin administration due to nephrotoxicity or ototoxicity, the REAL-2 phase III trial evaluated noninferiority of the oral fluoropyrimidine capecitabine to infusional 5-FU and oxaliplatin to cisplatin. This four arm study recruited 1002 patients with locally advanced or metastatic esophagogastric cancer to one of the triplet chemotherapy regimens: standard ECF, with capecitabine (ECX), with oxaliplatin (EOF), or with both oxaliplatin and the capecitabine (EOX).[32] Noninferiority was demonstrated for both of these agents with the median OS given in Table 3.6. As compared with cisplatin, oxaliplatin was associated with less neutropenia and alopecia, but more diarrhea and peripheral neuropathy. The rate of thromboembolic events and elevation of serum creatinine was lower in oxaliplatin groups than in the

Table 3.6 Summary of trials in advanced gastric cancer.

Author & study	Regimen	RR (%)	PFS (months)	OS (months)	p value (for OS)
Cunningham et al. REAL-2[32]	ECF	41	6.2	9.9	
	EOF	42	6.5	9.3	
	ECX	46	6.7	9.9	
	EOX	48	7.0	11.2	0.02
Kang et al. ML17032[65]	CF	32	5.0	9.3	
	CX	46	5.6	10.5	0.008
Al-Batran et al.[67]	FLP	25	3.9	8.8	
	FLO	35	5.8	10.7	ns
Van Cutsem et al. V325[69]	CF	25	3.7 (TTP)	8.6	
	DCF	37	5.6 (TTP)	9.2	0.02
Dank et al.[71]	CF	26	4.2 (TTP)	8.7	
	IF	32	5.0 (TTP)	9.0	0.53
Koizumi et al. SPIRITS[72]	S1	31	4.0	11.0	
	S1 + C	54	6.0	13.0	0.04
Boku et al. JCOG9912[73]	S1	28	4.2	11.4	
	5-FU	9	2.9	10.8	
	IC	38	4.8	12.3	0.055
Narahara et al.[74]	S1	27	3.6 (TTF)	10.5	
	I + S1 (IRI-S)	42	4.5 (TTF)	12.8	0.233
Ajani et al. FLAGS[48]	CF	32	5.5	7.9	
	S1 + C	29	4.8	8.6	0.2
Ohtsu et al. AVAGAST[75]	CF/CX	37	5.3	10.1	
	CF/CX + bevacizumab	46	6.7	12.1	0.1
Bang et al. ToGA[76]	CF/CX	35	5.5	11.1	
	CF/CX + trastuzumab	47	6.7	13.8	0.004

C, cisplatin; D, docetaxel; E, epirubicin; F, 5-FU; I, irinotecan; IRI-S, irinotecan and S1; L, leucovorin; ns, not significant; O, oxaliplatin; TTF, time to treatment failure; TTP, time to tumor progression; X, capecitabine.

cisplatin groups. As expected, a modest increase of hand–foot syndrome was observed in the ECX group. However, there were no significant differences in quality of life. Noninferiority of cisplatin/capecitabine (CX) combination to cisplatin/5-FU (CF) was confirmed in a phase III trial, which reported a median OS of 10.5 months compared with 9.3 months in capecitabine- and 5-FU-containing arms, respectively.[65] A meta-analysis of these trials reported a modest survival benefit of capecitabine compared with infused 5-FU.[66] The substitution of oxaliplatin has been explored in another phase III randomized trial of 2-weekly oxaliplatin, leucovorin and 24-hour 5-FU infusion (FLO) versus same 5-FU/leucovorin schedule with cisplatin (FLP).[67] No significant difference in median OS was noted (10.7 compared with 8.8 months for FLO and FLP, respectively), but FLO regimen was associated with less serious adverse events related to treatment. The benefit of the addition of anthracycline has been confirmed in a meta-analysis of three randomized trials demonstrating a 2-month survival benefit with anthracycline in combination with cisplatin/5-FU chemotherapy.[62,68]

A large phase III study investigated the activity of docetaxel in combination with cisplatin/5-FU (DCF) compared with cisplatin/5-FU (CF).[69] The addition of docetaxel resulted in prolongation of OS from 8.6 months to 9.2 months; however, more grade 3–4 neutropenia (82% compared with 57%) and febrile neutropenia (29% vs. 12% in CF arm) were reported with 3-weekly DCF regimen. A randomized phase II study demonstrated maintained activity with reduced toxicity when a weekly docetaxel was added to CF or to capecitabine.[70]

Other combination regimens explored include irinotecan with leucovorin and infusional 5-FU. A phase III trial randomized 333 patients to receive either weekly irinotecan regimen given with leucovorin and a 22-hour infusion of 5-FU (IF) or monthly cisplatin with 5-day continuous infusion of 5-FU (CF). Treatment with IF chemotherapy did not yield significant superiority over CF treatment in time to progression or OS (9.0 months vs. 8.7 months, respectively).[71] Patients treated in the IF arm experienced less neutropenia, thrombocytopenia, stomatitis but had similar rates of diarrhea. IF regimen has shown similar activity to CF and represents a viable option for selected patients.

The oral fluoropyrimidine S-1 has been extensively investigated in Japan as a monotherapy or in combination. Combination with cisplatin significantly improved median OS over monotherapy (13 compared with 11 months).[72] Three arm study investigating single agent S-1 compared with infusional 5-FU or with combination of irinotecan/cisplatin demonstrated noninferiority of S-1 compared with 5-FU (median OS 11.4 months compared with 10.8 months, respectively) and no superiority of irinotecan/cisplatin (median OS 12.3 months).[73] S-1 has also been compared with irinotecan and phase III study demonstrated higher response rates in the combination arm over S1 alone; however, this did not translate into a longer 1-year survival.[74] The encouraging results of S-1 in combination with cisplatin prompted investigation of this combination to 5-FU and cisplatin in the Western population. Interestingly, S1 in combination with cisplatin did not significantly prolong survival compared with cisplatin/5-FU (8.6 months vs. 7.9 months, respectively), although lower rates of neutropenia, stomatitis, hypokalemia, and treatment-related deaths were reported.[48] The results from Japanese trials with S1 have not been replicated in a Western population and S1 is not used outside of East Asia.

Targeted agents

Despite numerous trials of doublet and triplet combination regimens, the median OS for patients with advanced gastric cancer is less than a year. Attempts to intensify treatment in order to improve outcomes have included the combination of cytotoxic chemotherapy with targeted agents. The addition of bevacizumab, an anti-VEGF-A (vascular endothelial growth factor A) monoclonal antibody to fluoropyrimidine/cisplatin combination did not significantly improve OS in the AVAGAST study (10.1 months for control arm compared with 12.1 for bevacizumab arm).[75]

Treatment with the monoclonal antibody trastuzumab, which targets the HER-2 receptor, was investigated in a large randomized phase III study (ToGA) in patients with advanced gastric and GEJ tumors.[76] HER-2 is a transmembrane tyrosine kinase receptor involved in signal transduction, cell proliferation, migration, and survival. It is overexpressed in approximately 20% of gastric and GEJ tumors. The addition of trastuzumab to cisplatin/fluoropyrimidine resulted in a 2.7-month improvement in median survival. The treatment was well tolerated with no increase in grades 3 and 4 toxicities or cardiac adverse events. The addition of trastuzumab to chemotherapy in gastric and GEJ tumors has now become the standard of care in patients overexpressing HER-2 receptor. The REAL-3 trial is currently evaluating the effectiveness of EOX in combination with panitumumab, a humanized monoclonal antibody against the epidermal growth factor receptor (EGFR). There is urgent need for integration of translational research and identification of biomarkers to predict which patients will benefit from targeted agents, chemotherapy, and radiotherapy in order to personalize treatment rather than the current unselected approach.

Second-line chemotherapy

There is currently no standard second-line treatment. Several phase II trials have investigated second-line chemotherapy using irinotecan and taxanes demonstrating response rates of 20% with median OS from initiating second-line treatment of 4–6 months in this highly selected population.[77,78] There are currently several clinical trials evaluating second-line treatment with cytotoxic chemotherapy and targeted agents and patients with good performance status should be considered for entry into these trials.

Family screening

In patients with HDGC with *CDH1* mutation, a prophylactic gastrectomy (without radical lymph node dissection) is strongly advised and patients should be appropriately counseled.[18] Annual surveillance with gastroscopy and minimum of 30 biopsies is recommended for patients unwilling to undergo radical surgery or for those who meet clinical criteria for HDGC without detected *CDH1* mutation. In addition, annual mammography and breast MRI is recommended for women from 35 years old given the higher incidence of lobular breast cancer with HDGC (60% in their lifetime). There is increasing evidence of signet-ring cell colon cancers in these families and colonoscopic screening (every 3–5 years) starting at age 40 or 10 years less than the age of the youngest affected member is now recommended.

Key patient consent issues

Families meeting criteria for HDGC should be counseled regarding the benefits of *CDH1* testing and its limitations. Given the autosomal dominant pattern of inheritance, patient with *CDH1* have 50% chance of passing the mutation to their offspring. The recommended age for consideration of genetic testing of relatives is from 16 to 18 years of age, as HDGC is rare below this age.

Individuals with *CDH1* mutation at risk of HDGC are advised to undergo prophylactic gastrectomy once their growth and development has stopped, approximately at age 20. Decision regarding prophylactic surgery and exact timing should be discussed with patient in detail after discussion at multidisciplinary meeting. It is important that these patients consult with a genetic counselor and dietician before making their final decision.[18] Following gastrectomy, patients need to change their eating habits and often require ongoing dietician support. Patients postgastrectomy require monitoring of hematological parameters and life-long vitamin B_{12} substitution. Fat, folate, calcium, iron, and vitamins A, D, E, K malabsorption, lactose intolerance, and dumping syndrome are potential complications of gastrectomy. Patients with diagnosed gastric cancer should meet with a dietician prior to therapeutic gastrectomy.

Acknowledgments

Branislav Bystricky and David Cunningham acknowledge National Health Service funding to the National Institute for Health Research (NIHR) Biomedical Research Centre. The authors would like to thank Professor Gordon Stamp for providing histopathology photomicrographs.

Case Studies

Case 1

A 77-year-old lady presented to her GP with intermittent abdominal pain every 2 weeks lasting for 3 days and occasional vomiting. Upper GI endoscopy revealed small lesion in the body of stomach with histology confirming moderately to poorly differentiated invasive adenocarcinoma. HER-2 immunohistochemistry and brightfield double in situ hybridization was focally positive (Figure 3.7). Patient underwent a CT scan (Figure 3.2) and a PET scan (Figure 3.5), demonstrating low-grade [18]FDG uptake centered on the lesser curvature of the gastric body. There was no other metabolically active regional adenopathy or distant metastases. The EUS showed a lesion measuring 15 mm across on the

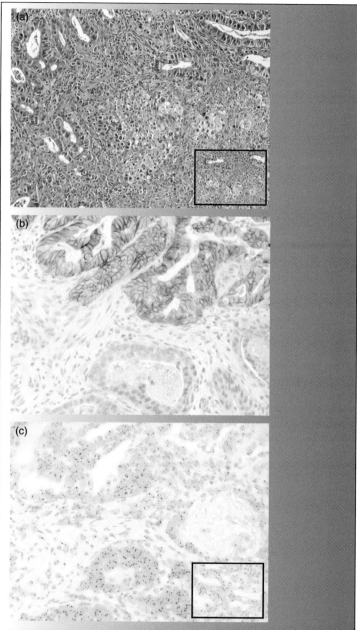

Figure 3.7 Histopathology H&E, demonstrating poorly differentiated adenocarcinoma with areas of necrosis and heterogeneity (a), higher power (a-inset). (b) HER-2 staining by immunohistochemistry (score 3+), demonstrating intratumoral heterogeneity in staining characteristic of gastric adenocarcinomas. (c) HER-2 labeling by brightfield double in situ hybridization, an automated technique using two probes targeting *HER-2* gene (*black*) and chromosome 17 centromere (*red*). Size differences and color contrast allow for visual separation and analysis of morphological features using brightfield microscope. (c-inset) Higher power, gain 2-3 *HER-2* copies/cell (Case 1).

lesser curvature of the stomach extending into the muscularis propria with two small 2–3 mm adjacent lymph nodes (Figure 3.4). Staging laparoscopy was negative for distant metastases. After completion of the staging investigations, her TNM staging was T2N0Mx, stage IB. Performance status was 0, past medical history included hypertension and a pacemaker insertion for bradycardia. Cardiac function was adequate on echocardiogram (ejection fraction, 66%) as well as her kidney function (creatinine clearance by EDTA of 95 mL/min). She was enrolled in ST03 trial investigating addition of bevacizumab to standard perioperative chemotherapy ECX. After three cycles of ECX chemotherapy, restaging CT scan did not reveal any tumor. She underwent radical gastrectomy and lymphadenectomy with final pathology demonstrating pathological complete response to chemotherapy. She continues with further three cycles of chemotherapy as per trial protocol.

Case 2

A 67-year-old gentleman presented with vomiting, retrosternal pain, and weight loss of approximately 6 kg in 3 months. For this period, he has been struggling with regurgitation of undigested food. At presentation, he was managing only soft foods. Diagnostic investigations demonstrated bulky adenocarcinoma of the GEJ type III with locally enlarged lymph nodes. Biopsy confirmed moderately differentiated adenocarcinoma. After the completion of staging investigations, TNM stage was T3N1Mx, IIIA. Patient declined participation in neoadjuvant trial and received two cycles of cisplatin and 5-FU chemotherapy. Restaging investigations demonstrated some response to chemotherapy, but without significant impact on his dysphagia. Dysphagia had deteriorated prior to planned surgery and radiologically guided gastrostomy tube was inserted. A CT scan had demonstrated rapid local and nodal progression of disease. The surgery was abandoned in view of progressive disease and he underwent definitive chemoradiotherapy (54 Gy in 30 fractions) with capecitabine as a radiosensitizer. Excellent response was seen on restaging endoscopy, and biopsies from the site of previous tumor demonstrated chronic active inflammation without malignancy. Restaging CT and PET scans demonstrated [18]FDG avidity in small cervical lymph nodes as well as multiple sites of radiotracer uptake in the left trapezius and the right rectus abdominis muscle (Figure 3.6), corresponding to clinical findings of palpable soft-tissue deposits. Biopsy from the abdominal wall lesion revealed poorly differentiated mucinous adenocarcinoma, consistent with the gastroesophageal origin. HER-2 staining was negative (Figure 3.8). Palliative radiotherapy with 20 Gy had a good effect on the left shoulder pain. Palliative chemotherapy with EOX was commenced. After three cycles, which had to be dose reduced for grade 3 diarrhea, CT scan has demonstrated progression of abdominal lymphadenopathy and development of new peritoneal deposits (Figure 3.3). Patient's performance status remained good and he was keen to pursue further treatment. He commenced a phase I study with ABT-263 (Bcl-2 family inhibitor) in combination with docetaxel chemotherapy.

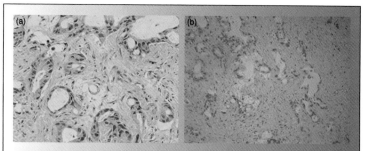

Figure 3.8 Histopathology H&E, demonstrating poorly differentiated adenocarcinoma with pleomorphic cells and desmoplasia (a). (b) HER-2 staining by IHC (negative) (Case 2).

References

1. Ferlay, J., Shin, H.R., Bray, F. *et al.* (2010) *GLOBOCAN 2008, Cancer Incidence and Mortality Worldwide: IARC Cancer Base No. 10 [Internet].* International Agency for Research on Cancer, Lyon, France. http://globocan.iarc.fr

2. Horie, Y., Miura, K., Matsui, K. *et al.* (1996) Marked elevation of plasma carcinoembryonic antigen and stomach carcinoma. *Cancer*, **77**, 1991–1997.

3. NICE. (2004) *Dyspepsia: Management of Dyspepsia in Adults in Primary Care.* National Institute for Clinical Excellence, London.

4. Sobin, L.H., Gospodarowicz, M.K., Wittekind, C.H. (2009) *TNM Classification of Malignant Tumours* (7th edition), 256pp. Wiley-Blackwell, Oxford.

5. Botet, J.F., Lightdale, C.J., Zauber, A.G. *et al.* (1991) Preoperative staging of gastric cancer: comparison of endoscopic US and dynamic CT. *Radiology*, **181**, 426–432.

6. Stahl, A., Ott, K., Weber W.A. *et al.* (2003) FDG PET imaging of locally advanced gastric carcinomas: correlation with endoscopic and histopathological findings. *Eur J Nucl Med Mol Imaging*, **30**, 288–295.

7. Podoloff, D.A., Ball, D.W., Ben-Josef, E. *et al.* (2009) NCCN task force: clinical utility of PET in a variety of tumor types. *J Natl Compr Canc Netw*, **7(Suppl 2)**, S1–S26.

8. Ott, K., Fink, U., Becker, K. *et al.* (2003) Prediction of response to preoperative chemotherapy in gastric carcinoma by metabolic imaging: results of a prospective trial. *J Clin Oncol*, **21**, 4604–4610.

9. Muntean, V., Mihailov, A., Iancu, C. *et al.* (2009) Staging laparoscopy in gastric cancer. Accuracy and impact on therapy. *J Gastrointestin Liver Dis*, **18**, 189–195.

10. Bentrem, D., Wilton, A., Mazumdar, M. *et al.* (2005) The value of peritoneal cytology as a preoperative predictor in patients with gastric carcinoma undergoing a curative resection. *Ann Surg Oncol*, **12**, 347–353.

11. Epplein, M., Nomura, A.M., Wilkens, L.R. *et al.* (2009) Nonsteroidal antiinflammatory drugs and risk of gastric adenocarcinoma: the multiethnic cohort study. *Am J Epidemiol*, **170**, 507–514.

12. Abnet, C.C., Freedman, N.D., Kamangar, F. *et al.* (2009) Non-steroidal anti-inflammatory drugs and risk of gastric and oesophageal adenocarcinomas: results from a cohort study and a meta-analysis. *Br J Cancer*, **100**, 551–557.

13. Wang, W.H., Huang, J.Q., Zheng, G.F. *et al.* (2003) Non-steroidal anti-inflammatory drug use and the risk of gastric cancer: a systematic review and meta-analysis. *J Natl Cancer Inst*, **95**, 1784–1791.

14. IARC Working Group on the Evaluation of Carcinogenic Risks to Humans. (1994) Schistosomes, liver flukes and *Helicobacter pylori*. *IARC Monogr Eval Carcinog Risks Hum*, **61**, 1–241.

15. Wu, C.Y., Kuo, K.N., Wu, M.S. *et al.* (2009) *Early Helicobacter pylori* eradication decreases risk of gastric cancer in patients with peptic ulcer disease. *Gastroenterology*, **137**, 1641–1648, e1–e2.

16. Buckland, G., Agudo, A., Lujan, L. *et al.* (2010) Adherence to a Mediterranean diet and risk of gastric adenocarcinoma within the European Prospective Investigation into Cancer and Nutrition (EPIC) cohort study. *Am J Clin Nutr*, **91**, 381–390.

17. Hamashima, C., Shibuya, D., Yamazaki, H. *et al.* (2008) The Japanese guidelines for gastric cancer screening. *Jpn J Clin Oncol*, **38**, 259–267.

18. Fitzgerald, R.C., Hardwick, R., Huntsman, D. *et al.* (2010) Hereditary diffuse gastric cancer: updated consensus guidelines for clinical management and directions for future research. *J Med Genet*, **47**, 436–444.

19. Cuschieri, A., Weeden, S., Fielding, J. *et al.* (1999) Patient survival after D1 and D2 resections for gastric cancer: long-term results of the MRC randomized surgical trial. Surgical Co-operative Group. *Br J Cancer*, **79**, 1522–1530.

20. Nakajima, T. (2002) Gastric cancer treatment guidelines in Japan. *Gastric Cancer*, **5**, 1–5.

21. Nakajima, T., Oda, I., Gotoda, T. *et al.* (2006) Metachronous gastric cancers after endoscopic resection: how effective is annual endoscopic surveillance? *Gastric Cancer*, **9**, 93–98.

22. Kobayashi, M., Narisawa, R., Sato, Y. *et al.* (2010) Self-limiting risk of metachronous gastric cancers after endoscopic resection. *Dig Endosc*, **22**, 169–173.

23. Adachi, Y., Shiraishi, N., Kitano S. (2002) Modern treatment of early gastric cancer: review of the Japanese experience. *Dig Surg*, **19**, 333–339.

24. Hermanek, P. (1999) The second English edition of the Japanese classification of gastric carcinoma. A Western commentary. *Gastric Cancer*, **2**, 79–82.

25. Songun, I., Putter, H., Kranenbarg, E.M. *et al.* (2010) Surgical treatment of gastric cancer: 15-year follow-up results of the randomised nationwide Dutch D1D2 trial. *Lancet Oncol*, **11**, 439–449.

26. Bonenkamp, J.J., Songun, I., Hermans, J. *et al.* (1995) Randomised comparison of morbidity after D1 and D2 dissection for gastric cancer in 996 Dutch patients. *Lancet*, **345**, 745–748.

27. Siewert, J.R., Bottcher, K., Roder, J.D. *et al.* (1993) Prognostic relevance of systematic lymph node dissection in gastric carcinoma. German Gastric Carcinoma Study Group. *Br J Surg*, **80**, 1015–1018.

28. Sasako, M., Sano, T., Yamamoto, S. *et al.* (2008) D2 lymphadenectomy alone or with para-aortic nodal dissection for gastric cancer. *N Engl J Med*, **359**, 453–462.

29. Bonenkamp, J.J., Hermans, J., Sasako, M. *et al.* (1999) Extended lymph-node dissection for gastric cancer. *N Engl J Med*, **340**, 908–914.

30. Cunningham, D., Allum, W.H., Stenning, S.P. *et al.* (2006) Perioperative chemotherapy versus surgery alone for resectable gastroesophageal cancer. *N Engl J Med*, **355**, 11–20.

31. Ychou, M., Boige, V., Pignon, J.P. *et al.* (2011) Perioperative chemotherapy compared with surgery alone for resectable gastroesophageal adenocarcinoma: an FNCLCC and FFCD multicenter phase III trial. *J Clin Oncol*, **29**, 1715–1721.

32. Cunningham, D., Starling, N., Rao, S. *et al.* (2008) Capecitabine and oxaliplatin for advanced esophagogastric cancer. *N Engl J Med*, **358**, 36–46.

33. Macdonald, J.S., Smalley, S.R., Benedetti, J. *et al.* (2001) Chemoradiotherapy after surgery compared with surgery alone for adenocarcinoma of the stomach or gastroesophageal junction. *N Engl J Med*, **345**, 725–730.

34. Smalley, S.R., Benedetti, J., Macdonald, J.S. *et al.* (2012) Updated analysis of SWOG-directedi intergroup study 0116:a phase III trial of adjuvant radiochemotherapy versus observation after curative gastric cancer resection. *J Clin Oncol*, **30**, 2327–2333.

35. Fuchs, C.S., Tepper, J.E., Niedzwiecki, D. *et al.* (2011) Postoperative adjuvant chemoradiation for gastric or gastroesophageal junction (GEJ) adenocarcinoma using epirubicin, cisplatin, and infusional (CI) 5-FU (ECF) before and after CI 5-FU and radiotherapy (CRT) compared with bolus 5-FU/LV before and after CRT: intergroup trial CALGB 80101. *J Clin Oncol*, **29(Suppl)**, abstract 4003.

36. Lee, J., Lim do, H., Kim, S. *et al.* (2012) Phase III trial comparing capecitabine plus cisplatin versus capecitabine plus cisplatin with concurrent capecitabine radiotherapy in completely resected gastric cancer with D2 lymph node dissection: the ARTIST trial. *J Clin Oncol*, **30**, 268–273.

37. Paoletti, X., Oba, K., Burzykowski, T. *et al.* (2010) Benefit of adjuvant chemotherapy for resectable gastric cancer: a meta-analysis. *JAMA*, **303**, 1729–1737.

38. Mari, E., Floriani, I., Tinazzi, A. *et al.* (2000) Efficacy of adjuvant chemotherapy after curative resection for gastric cancer: a meta-analysis of published randomised trials. A study of the GISCAD (Gruppo Italiano per lo Studio dei Carcinomi dell'Apparato Digerente). *Ann Oncol*, **11**, 837–843.

39. Gianni, L., Panzini, I., Tassinari, D. *et al.* (2001) Meta-analyses of randomized trials of adjuvant chemotherapy in gastric cancer. *Ann Oncol*, **12**, 1178–1180.

40. Earle, C.C., Maroun, J.A. (1999) Adjuvant chemotherapy after curative resection for gastric cancer in non-Asian patients: revisiting a meta-analysis of randomised trials. *Eur J Cancer*, **35**, 1059–1064.

41. Janunger, K.G., Hafstrom, L., Nygren, P. *et al.* (2001) A systematic overview of chemotherapy effects in gastric cancer. *Acta Oncol*, **40**, 309–326.

42. Oba, K., Morita, S., Tsuburaya, A. *et al.* (2006) Efficacy of adjuvant chemotherapy using oral fluorinated pyrimidines for curatively resected gastric cancer: a meta-analysis of centrally randomized controlled clinical trials in Japan. *J Chemother*, **18**, 311–317.

43. Liu, T.S., Wang, Y., Chen, S.Y. *et al.* (2008) An updated meta-analysis of adjuvant chemotherapy after curative resection for gastric cancer. *Eur J Surg Oncol*, **34**, 1208–1216.

44. Zhao, S.L., Fang, J.Y. (2008) The role of postoperative adjuvant chemotherapy following curative resection for gastric cancer: a meta-analysis. *Cancer Invest*, **26**, 317–325.

45. Bang, Y., Kim, Y.W., Yang, H. *et al.* (2012) Adjuvant capecitabine and oxaliplatin for gastric cancer after D2 gastrectomy (CLASSIC): a phase 3 open-label, randomised controlled trial. *Lancet*, **379**, 315–321.

46. Sakuramoto, S., Sasako, M., Yamaguchi, T. *et al.* (2007) Adjuvant chemotherapy for gastric cancer with S-1, an oral fluoropyrimidine. *N Engl J Med*, **357**, 1810–1820.

47. Sasako, M., Sakuramoto, S., Katai, H. *et al.* (2011) Five-year outcomes of a randomized phase III trial comparing adjuvant chemotherapy with S-1 versus surgery alone in stage II or III gastric cancer. *J Clin Oncol*, **29**, 4387–4393.

48. Ajani, J.A., Rodriguez, W., Bodoky, G. *et al.* (2010) Multicenter phase III comparison of cisplatin/S-1 with cisplatin/infusional fluorouracil in advanced gastric or gastroesophageal adenocarcinoma study: the FLAGS trial. *J Clin Oncol*, **28**, 1547–1553.

49. Kim, J., Sun, C.L., Mailey, B. *et al.* (2010) Race and ethnicity correlate with survival in patients with gastric adenocarcinoma. *Ann Oncol*, **21**, 152–160.

50. Okines, A., Verheij, M., Allum, W. *et al.* (2010) Gastric cancer: ESMO Clinical Practice Guidelines for diagnosis, treatment and follow-up. *Ann Oncol*, **21**, v50–v54.

51. Gaidos, J.K., Draganov, P.V. (2009) Treatment of malignant gastric outlet obstruction with endoscopically placed self-expandable metal stents. *World J Gastroenterol*, **15**, 4365–4371.

52. Siddiqui, A., Spechler, S.J., Huerta, S. (2007) Surgical bypass versus endoscopic stenting for malignant gastroduodenal obstruction: a decision analysis. *Dig Dis Sci*, **52**, 276–281.

53. Ly, J., O'Grady, G., Mittal, A. *et al.* (2010) A systematic review of methods to palliate malignant gastric outlet obstruction. *Surg Endosc*, **24**, 290–297.

54. Hartgrink, H.H., Putter, H., Klein Kranenbarg, E. *et al.* (2002) Value of palliative resection in gastric cancer. *Br J Surg*, **89**, 1438–1443.

55. Schwarz, R.E., Zagala-Nevarez, K. (2002) Gastrectomy circumstances that influence early postoperative outcome. *Hepatogastroenterology*, **49**, 1742–1746.

56. Scheidbach, H., Lippert, H., Meyer, F. (2010) Gastric carcinoma: when is palliative gastrectomy justified? *Oncol Rev*, **4**, 127–132.

57. Mantell, B.S. (1982) Radiotherapy for dysphagia due to gastric carcinoma. *Br J Surg*, **69**, 69–70.

58. Kim, M.M., Rana, V., Janjan, N.A. *et al.* (2008) Clinical benefit of palliative radiation therapy in advanced gastric cancer. *Acta Oncol*, **47**, 421–427.

59. Lee, J.A., Lim do, H., Park, W. *et al.* (2009) Radiation therapy for gastric cancer bleeding. *Tumori*, **95**, 726–730.

60. Hashimoto, K., Mayahara, H., Takashima, A. *et al.* (2009) Palliative radiation therapy for hemorrhage of unresectable gastric cancer: a single institute experience. *J Cancer Res Clin Oncol*, **135**, 1117–1123.

61. Asakura, H., Hashimoto, T., Harada, H. *et al.* (2010) Palliative radiotherapy for bleeding from advanced gastric cancer: is a schedule of 30 Gy in 10 fractions adequate? *J Cancer Res Clin Oncol*, **137(1)**, 125–130.

62. Wagner, A.D., Grothe, W., Haerting, J. *et al.* (2006) Chemotherapy in advanced gastric cancer: a systematic review and meta-analysis based on aggregate data. *J Clin Oncol*, **24**, 2903–2909.

63. Vanhoefer, U., Rougier, P., Wilke, H. *et al.* (2000) Final results of a randomized phase III trial of sequential high-dose methotrexate, fluorouracil, and doxorubicin versus etoposide, leucovorin, and fluorouracil versus infusional fluorouracil and cisplatin in advanced gastric cancer: a trial of the European Organization for Research and Treatment of Cancer

Gastrointestinal Tract Cancer Cooperative Group. *J Clin Oncol*, **18**, 2648–2657.

64. Findlay, M., Cunningham, D., Norman, A. *et al.* (1994) A phase II study in advanced gastroesophageal cancer using epirubicin and cisplatin in combination with continuous infusion 5-fluorouracil (ECF). *Ann Oncol*, **5**, 609–616.

65. Kang, Y.K., Kang, W.K., Shin, D.B. *et al.* (2009) Capecitabine/cisplatin versus 5-fluorouracil/cisplatin as first-line therapy in patients with advanced gastric cancer: a randomised phase III noninferiority trial. *Ann Oncol*, **20**, 666–673.

66. Okines, A.F., Norman, A.R., McCloud, P. *et al.* (2009) Meta-analysis of the REAL-2 and ML17032 trials: evaluating capecitabine-based combination chemotherapy and infused 5-fluorouracil-based combination chemotherapy for the treatment of advanced oesophago-gastric cancer. *Ann Oncol*, **20**, 1529–1534.

67. Al-Batran, S.E., Hartmann, J.T., Probst, S. *et al.* (2008) Phase III trial in metastatic gastroesophageal adenocarcinoma with fluorouracil, leucovorin plus either oxaliplatin or cisplatin: a study of the Arbeitsgemeinschaft Internistische Onkologie. *J Clin Oncol*, **26**, 1435–1442.

68. Ross, P., Nicolson, M., Cunningham, D. *et al.* (2002) Prospective randomized trial comparing mitomycin, cisplatin, and protracted venous-infusion fluorouracil (PVI 5-FU) with epirubicin, cisplatin, and PVI 5-FU in advanced esophagogastric cancer. *J Clin Oncol*, **20**, 1996–2004.

69. Van Cutsem, E., Moiseyenko, V.M., Tjulandin, S. *et al.* (2006) Phase III study of docetaxel and cisplatin plus fluorouracil compared with cisplatin and fluorouracil as first-line therapy for advanced gastric cancer: a report of the V325 Study Group. *J Clin Oncol*, **24**, 4991–4997.

70. Tebbutt, N.C., Cummins, M.M., Sourjina, T. *et al.* (2010) Randomised, non-comparative phase II study of weekly docetaxel with cisplatin and 5-fluorouracil or with capecitabine in oesophagogastric cancer: the AGITG ATTAX trial. *Br J Cancer*, **102**, 475–481.

71. Dank, M., Zaluski, J., Barone, C. *et al.* (2008) Randomized phase III study comparing irinotecan combined with 5-fluorouracil and folinic acid to cisplatin combined with 5-fluorouracil in chemotherapy naive patients with advanced adenocarcinoma of the stomach or esophagogastric junction. *Ann Oncol*, **19**, 1450–1457.

72. Koizumi, W., Narahara, H., Hara, T. *et al.* (2008) S-1 plus cisplatin versus S-1 alone for first-line treatment of advanced gastric cancer (SPIRITS trial): a phase III trial. *Lancet Oncol*, **9**, 215–221.

73. Boku, N., Yamamoto, S., Fukuda, H. *et al.* (2009) Fluorouracil versus combination of irinotecan plus cisplatin versus S-1 in metastatic gastric cancer: a randomised phase 3 study. *Lancet Oncol*, **10**, 1063–1069.

74. Narahara, H., Iishi, H., Imamura, H. *et al.* (2011) Randomized phase III study comparing the efficacy and safety of irinotecan plus S-1 with S-1 alone as first-line treatment for advanced gastric cancer (study GC0301/TOP-002). *Gastric Cancer*, **14**, 72–80.

75. Ohtsu, A., Shah, M.A., Van Cutsem, E. *et al.* (2011) Bevacizumab in combination with chemotherapy as first-line therapy in advanced gastric cancer: a randomized, double-blind, placebo-controlled phase III study. *J Clin Oncol*, **29**, 3968–3976.

76. Bang, Y.J., Van Cutsem, E., Feyereislova, A. *et al.* (2010) Trastuzumab in combination with chemotherapy versus chemotherapy alone for treatment of HER2-positive advanced gastric or gastro-oesophageal junction cancer

(ToGA): a phase 3, open-label, randomised controlled trial. *Lancet*, **376**, 687–697.

77. Shimoyama, R., Yasui, H., Boku, N. *et al.* (2009) Weekly paclitaxel for heavily treated advanced or recurrent gastric cancer refractory to fluorouracil, irinotecan, and cisplatin. *Gastric Cancer*, **12**, 206–211.

78. Thuss-Patience, P.C., Kretzschmar, A., Bichev, D. *et al.* (2011) Survival advantage for irinotecan versus best supportive care as second-line chemotherapy in gastric cancer—a randomised phase III study of the Arbeitsgemeinschaft Internistische Onkologie (AIO). *Eur J Cancer*, **47**, 2306–2314.

4 Small Intestinal Cancers

Nadir Arber and Menachem Moshkowitz

Tel Aviv Medical Center and Tel Aviv University, Tel Aviv, Israel

Key Points

- Small bowel tumors are extremely rare and account for only 2% of all gastrointestinal malignancies. Approximately one-third of the tumors are benign and two-thirds are malignant at the time of diagnosis.
- Adenocarcinoma is the most common malignancy accounting for 40% of primary small bowel neoplasms. Other tumors are neuroendocrine tumors (carcinoid), 20–40%; lymphomas, 14%; and sarcomas, 11–13%.
- Small bowel tumors are usually asymptomatic in the early stages, but eventually patients develop symptoms due to progression of the disease. The most frequent presenting symptoms are abdominal pain, nausea, vomiting, and intestinal obstruction.
- The diagnostic strategies for detecting small tumors include conventional noninvasive imaging modalities (small bowel barium series, enteroclysis, CT scan, and MRI,) as well as endoscopic modalities (push enteroscopy, double-balloon enteroscopy, and video-capsule endoscopy. The later newer techniques had improved the diagnostic accuracy of detecting small bowel tumors.

Key Web Links

http://www.macmillan.org.uk/Cancerinformation/Cancertypes/Smallbowel/Smallbowelcancer.aspx

Potential Pitfalls

- Small bowel cancers (SBCs) are often missed because they are not considered.
- SBC is increased in patients with Crohn's disease, celiac disease, adenoma, familial adenomatous polyposis, and Peutz-Jeghers syndrome.
- Patients who are obese and smoke cigarettes are recognized as risk factors for SBC.

Handbook of Gastrointestinal Cancer, First Edition. Edited by Janusz Jankowski and Ernest Hawk.
© 2013 John Wiley & Sons, Ltd. Published 2013 by John Wiley & Sons, Ltd.

Epidemiology

Small bowel cancers (SBCs) are extremely rare and account for only 0.4% of total cancer cases, and 2% of all gastrointestinal (GI) malignancies in the Western population.[1-4] Its global incidence is less than 1.0 per 100,000 population, and the mortality from SBC is even lower, accounting for only 0.2% of total cancer deaths in the Western population. The low incidence of SBC is interesting considering the fact that the small bowel comprises 75% of the length (about 6-m long and four times as long as the large intestine) and 90% of the absorptive mucosal surface area of the GI tract. Various theories have attempted to explain this resistance to carcinogenesis; among them are the short contact time between potential carcinogens, lower bacterial load, reduced intestinal concentrations of inherent potential carcinogens, protection of the stem cells that are buried deep in the mucosa, and the well-developed local immunoglobulin A (IgA)-mediated immune and lymphatic systems in the small intestine.[5] Data from American as well as British registries of long-term surveillance show increased rates of SBC incidence in the recent four decades (from 1.18 in 1973 to 2.27 per 100,000 population in 2004).[6] The incidence increased more than fourfold for carcinoid tumors (from 0.21 in 1973 to 0.93 in 2004) and less dramatic increases for adenocarcinomas (from 0.57 to 0.73) and lymphomas (from 0.22 to 0.44) and relatively stable for sarcomas (from 0.18 to 0.19). The increase occurred in both men and in women and in all ethnic groups, but was most pronounced among African American males.[7] The reason for the increase in incidence could be due to the increase in some risk factors such as the rising prevalence of obesity, and the improved imaging of the small bowel by various techniques.

Approximately two-thirds out of all small bowel tumors are malignant at the time of diagnosis.

SBC has four major histologic subtypes: adenocarcinoma, neuroendocrine tumor (carcinoid), lymphoma, and sarcoma. Adenocarcinoma is the most common malignancy accounting for 40% of small bowel tumors. The incidence of the other tumors has been reported as follows: carcinoids tumors, 20–40%; lymphomas, 14%; and sarcomas, 11–13%.

Adenocarcinoma of the small bowel

Adenocarcinoma is the most common primary malignancy of the small bowel, accounting for 40% of SBC in the Western world.[4] The reported average annual age-adjusted incidence rates in the Western population are 1.45 and 1.00, per 100,000, for males and females, respectively. Rates for American Africans were more than twice those of whites (1.29 vs. 0.63).[2] The mean age at diagnosis is 57 years (median 67 years). It occurs most frequently within the duodenum (49% of cases), particularly around the ampulla of Vater, and with decreasing frequency in the jejunum (21%) and ileum (15%).[8] One exception is in Crohn's disease–associated adenocarcinoma, where 70% are present in the ileum.[9]

Risk factors

The risk of small bowel carcinoma is increased in the setting of several diseases including Crohn's disease,[10] familial adenomatous polyposis (FAP),[11] hereditary nonpolyposis colorectal cancer (HNPCC) syndrome, Celiac disease, Peutz-Jeghers syndrome (PJS), and patients with small bowel adenomas.

Crohn's disease: Crohn's disease is characterized by transmural, granulomatous inflammation of the small and large bowel with a tendency to form fistulae. Crohn's disease is recognized as an important risk factor for cancer of the small intestine, with reported relative risks between 33 and 60.[12-18] Several factors have been reported to be associated with an increased risk of small bowel carcinoma in patients with Crohn's disease. These include extended duration of the disease, distal jejunal and ileal location, male sex, small bowel bypass loops, strictures, chronic fistulous disease, and young age at diagnosis.[19-21]

Celiac disease: Patients with celiac disease are at elevated risk for both T-cell non-Hodgkin's lymphoma (NHL) and for adenocarcinoma of the small intestine.[22-26]

The reported relative risk of adenocarcinoma of the small intestine in celiac disease patients is between 60 and 80.[27-29]

Most small intestinal carcinomas in celiac patients are located in the jejunum.

Small intestine adenomas: The prevalence of adenomas in the small intestine is much lower than their prevalence in the colon. However, just as in the colon, an adenoma in the small intestine appears to be a precursor of adenocarcinoma.[30-32] Most of the adenomas in the small bowel occur in the duodenum. A retrospective analysis of 192 villous adenomas of the duodenum found malignant changes in 42% at the time of presentation.[33] Villous histology, increasing polyp size, and a higher dysplastic grade have shown to be risk factors of neoplastic transformation from adenoma to carcinoma.[34]

Familial adenomatous polyposis (FAP): FAP is an autosomal-dominant genetic disorder caused by mutations in the APC gene on the long arm of chromosome 5.[35] Most patients diagnosed with FAP have multiple adenomas in the small bowel, usually in the duodenum,[36,37] and these patients are at increased risk of small intestinal cancer, especially duodenal cancer,[38-40] around the ampulla of Vater. The prevalence of duodenal adenomatosis in FAP patients is 50–90% with 3–5% of these patients progressing to duodenal cancer; however, periampullary adenomas seem to have a high risk of malignant transformation.[41]

Peutz-Jeghers syndrome: PJS is an autosomal-dominant condition due to a mutation in the *serine/threonine kinase 11* (*STK11*) gene on the short arm of chromosome 19, characterized by melanin spots on lips and buccal mucosa and multiple GI hamartomatous polyps.[42,43] Polyps in PJS subjects are usually found in the small intestine and are more common in the jejunum than the ileum, followed by the duodenum.[44] Patients with PJS are increased risk for both GI and non-GI cancers including breast and ovarian cancers in women; testicular tumors in males; and cancers of the pancreas, esophagus, stomach, and lung in both sexes.[45–48] PJS has been clearly demonstrated to be associated with an increased risk of small intestinal adenocarcinoma.[49] A meta-analysis of 210 PJS patients observed a statistically significant increase in relative risk for cancer of small bowel (RR, 520), stomach (RR, 213), colon (RR, 84), esophagus (RR, 57), pancreas (RR, 132), lung (RR, 17), breast (RR, 15.2), uterus (RR, 16.0), and ovary (RR, 27).[49]

Hereditary nonpolyposis colorectal cancer: HNPCC, or Lynch syndrome, is an autosomal-dominant disorder related to a germline mutation in one of several mismatch repair genes, including the *Mut S homologue 2* (*hMSH2*), MSH6, *Mut L homologue 1* (*hMLH1*), or PMS2.[50] HNPCC is associated with a substantially increased risk of cancers of the colorectum, endometrium, stomach, ovary, small intestine, urinary tract, and brain.[51–54] The relative risk of SBC in patients with HNPCC has been estimated to be more than 100 compared with the general population, with a lifetime risk of 1–7%.[55] The risk for SBC has been reported to be higher in *MLH1* mutation carriers than in *MSH2* mutation carriers[52] HNPCC-associated SBCs are mainly adenocarcinoma, occur at an earlier age, and appear to have a better prognosis than those occurring in the general population.[56,57]

Sporadic colorectal cancer: The demonstration of a geographical correlation between rates of SBC and colorectal cancer suggests a common etiology. Various studies have shown that the risk of SBC following primary colorectal cancer were elevated; also, in those diagnosed with primary SBC, there was a four- to fivefold risk of developing colorectal cancer.[58–63] These studies suggest etiological similarities between cancers of the small intestine and colorectal cancers but, to date, potential common carcinogenic agents have not been elucidated in analytic epidemiological studies.

Other cancers: The risk of SBC has been reported to be elevated in patients with a diagnosis of NHL and cancers of the prostate, female genitalia, lung, and skin, as well as others.[64–68] One study reported that SBC risk could be increased (although not statistically significant) in patients diagnosed with Merkel cell carcinoma of the skin.[69]

Environmental risk factors: Nutritional factors such as high intake of sugar, red meat, salt cured/smoked foods or low intake of fish, fruits, and vegetables and environmental factors such as radiation therapy have been associated with increased risk for SBC.[70] Increased risk of small bowel tumors have been found among obese persons and alcohol and tobacco users.[71] A recent report found that patients with an adenomatous component had a better survival than those without an adenomatous component, and that distal location of the tumor in the jejunum or ileum was associated with worse prognosis.[72]

Neuroendocrine tumors

This term is used for all endocrine tumors of the digestive system that derive from the diffuse intestinal neuroendocrine system.[73] Other synonyms are used by clinicians and pathologists for these tumors, including "carcinoid tumor," "APUD-oma," "neuroendocrine tumor," and "neuroendocrine carcinoma." The mucosa of the GI tract contains at least 15 different endocrine cell types producing hormonal peptides and/or biogenic amines.[74] Neuroendocrine tumors (NETs) can be subclassified into those with, and those without, a clinical syndrome and are accordingly termed "functionally active" and "functionally inactive" NET, respectively. Furthermore, NET can arise sporadically or as a result of genetic predisposition. NET is the second most common small bowel malignancy, representing approximately 25% of all primary SB tumors. Its average annual incidence rates per 100,000 population are 1.00 and 0.70 for men and women, respectively. These rates are higher for African Americans, and lower for Hispanics and Asians/Pacific Islanders (incidence rate ratios (IRRs) are 1.63, 0.64, and 0.29, respectively.[75]

NETs are more common in the ileum (mostly located within 60 cm of the ileocecal valve). These are slow-growing tumors, which first appear as submucosal nodules. Although the vast majority of these tumors occur sporadically, a subset of tumors are associated with inherited syndromes, among which multiple endocrine neoplasia type 1 (MEN1) is the most significant. The diagnostic strategies for imaging NETs include conventional noninvasive imaging modalities such as ultrasound, CT scan, MRI, capsule endoscopy (CE), and bone scanning, as well as invasive imaging modalities (angiography and selective venous sampling for hormonal gradients). Recently, somatostatin receptor scintigraphy (SRS) has gained a central role, whereas tomographic procedures such as CT and MRI serve for the completion of the oncologic workup.[76]

Lymphomas

The gut is the most common extralymphatic site, and up to 40% of the lymphomas arise in sites other than the lymph nodes.[77] Lymphomas, whether primary or secondary, account for 15–20% of all small bowel malignancies and 20–30% of all primary GI lymphomas. The ileum is the most common site (60–65%) followed by the jejunum (20–25%), duodenum (6–8%), and other GI sites (8–9%).[78] The age-adjusted incidence rates of GI lymphomas in the United States are low at 0.54 in males and 0.26 in females per 100,000.[2] Several patterns of SB lymphoma have been identified and include an infiltrating pattern that appears as wall thickening, an exophytic mass; these sometimes simulate an adenocarcinoma or GI stromal tumor, multifocal submucosal nodules within the SB, or a single mass lesion, which can lead to intussusception.

Four different histological types of lymphomas may be found in the small bowel:

1. *Celiac-associated T-cell high-grade lymphoma*: Enteropathy-associated T-cell lymphoma (EATL) is a rare form of high-grade, T-cell NHL of the upper small intestine that is associated with celiac disease.[79] In approximately 80% of refractory celiac disease cases, an abnormal clonal IEL (intraepithelial lymphocytes) cell population is diffusely present throughout the GI tract. These

cells are characterized by a low ratio of CD_8^+/CD_3^+ and TCR-γ gene rearrangement.[80]

2. *Burkitt-type lymphoma of the small intestine*: Burkitt's lymphoma is an aggressive type of B-cell lymphoma that has two major forms: endemic (African) and nonendemic (sporadic). The sporadic form usually involves abdominal organs, with the most common involvement of the distal ileum, cecum, or mesentery. Burkitt's lymphoma is a childhood tumor, but it is also observed in adult patients. It is characterized by a high rate of malignant cell proliferation (indicated by ki-67 expression) and by morphologic features that are distinct from diffuse large B-cell lymphoma. Burkitt's lymphoma can be seen in the setting of AIDS or chronic immunosuppression state.[81]

3. *Mucosa-associated lymphoid tissue lymphoma—MALToma*: MALToma was defined first as primary low-grade gastric B-cell lymphoma and immunoproliferative small intestinal disease (IPSID). Subsequently, the definition of MALToma was extended to include several other extranodal low-grade B-cell NHLs. The gastric form is the most common and best characterized MALToma. These tumors tend to stay localized in the mucosal wall without involvement of regional lymph nodes. Recently, this type of malignancy has been tied with bacterial infections and most important is gastric MALToma that can be cured, in early stages by simple antibiotic therapy aiming to eradicate *Helicobacter pylori*.[82]

4. *Immunoproliferative small intestinal disease*: IPSID, which is also named *Mediterranean lymphoma* or *alpha heavy chain disease*, is an unusual intestinal B-cell lymphoma that occurs usually in children and young adults of Mediterranean ancestry. This lymphoproliferative disease is characterized by "centrocyte-like" mucosal infiltration with plasma cells that secrete monotypic and truncated immunoglobulin, a heavy chain lacking of an associated light chain.[83] Treatment with antibiotics can lead to a remission, suggesting that the proliferative burst is due to an aberrant immunogenic response to bacterial infection. *Campylobacter jejuni* was shown to play a role in IPSID as *H. pylori* plays in gastric MALToma.[78]

Sarcomas

Small intestinal sarcomas constitute only 10–15% of the malignancies seen in the small intestine.[84,85] There are various benign and malignant mesenchymal tumors arising in the small intestine. The most common type of small intestinal sarcomas, representing more than 90% of sarcomas, is the gastrointestinal stromal tumors (GISTs).[86–88] Other types include leiomyomas, leiomyosarcomas, lipoma, angiosarcoma, and Kaposi's sarcoma. The reported average annual incidence rates of small intestinal sarcomas per 100,000 population are 0.24 and 0.17 for males and females, respectively, and have been found to be higher for Asians (IRR, 1.36; 95% CI, 1.13–1.62).[89,4]

Gastrointestinal stromal tumors

GISTs are the fourth most common malignant small bowel tumors (9%). These rare mesenchymal neoplasms derived probably from the interstitial cells of Cajal, and can occur anywhere along the GI tract, but are most common in the stomach (60–70%), followed by the small bowel (20–25%).[90] They are submucosal lesions, which most frequently grow endophytically in parallel with the lumen of the affected structure, but may also manifest as exophytic extraluminal excrescences. These highly vascular tumors have been reported ranging in size from 1 cm to as large as 40 cm in diameter. Ulceration of these lesions is common and intestinal bleeding is a frequent symptom. GISTs may invade adjacent organs directly or spread via peritoneal seeding. GISTs may be benign or malignant, and compared with gastric GISTs, small bowel GISTs tend to be more aggressive and have a worse prognosis. Metastases develop in nearly 50% of patients primarily via the hematogenous route, commonly involving the liver and peritoneum. GISTs smaller than 2 cm are generally considered benign with a very low risk of recurrence. About 5% of GIST cases are multiple, and increased incidence is seen in patients with neurofibromatosis type 1 (NF1). Gain-of-function mutations in exon 11 of the c-*kit* proto-oncogene are associated with most GISTs.[91]

Clinical features

Small bowel tumors are usually asymptomatic in the early stages, but eventually symptoms do develop due to disease progression. The rareness of these tumors and the subtle presenting symptoms may delay the diagnosis. The most frequent presenting symptoms are abdominal pain, nausea, vomiting, and intestinal obstruction. Half of the patients undergo emergency surgery for intestinal obstruction.[8] GISTs present more commonly with acute GI bleeding. Symptoms mainly depend on the size and location of the tumor, with lesions distal to the ligament of Treitz having a tendency to present with either obstruction or bleeding. The most common laboratory abnormality found is hypochromic microcytic anemia, and many of these patients present with a positive test for fecal occult blood. Direct hyperbilirubinemia and increased alkaline phosphatase are present usually in cases of duodenal tumors as a consequence of extrahepatic biliary obstruction.

Diagnosis

Early detection of small bowel neoplasms is desirable but challenging for both clinicians and radiologists. The detection of small intestinal tumors by traditional imaging modalities is often compromised by overlapping bowel loops and suboptimal bowel distention. There are some newer techniques described in the following sections that may improve the diagnostic accuracy of imaging.

Imaging modalities

Small Bowel Follow-Through (SBFT): This is the oldest barium study traditionally used for evaluation of the small bowel. There is a questionable role for this noninvasive test due to a reported wide range of sensitivities for tumor detection (30–90%).[92] This modality is rarely used now.

Enteroclysis: This procedure is based on the intubation of nasojejunal tube under fluoroscopic guidance and administration of barium sulphate suspension followed by 0.5% methylcellulose. Enteroclysis is considered superior than SBFT due to the exquisite mucosal detail that can be demonstrated and its higher yield and sensitivity, especially when evaluating patients with bleeding of obscure origin, but it is a more difficult examination for both the radiologist and the patient, requiring nasojejunal intubation and oral administration of large volumes of contrast material. The sensitivity of enteroclysis is as high as 95% with 90% correct estimation of the actual size of the tumor. Push enteroscopy (PE) is very useful for the evaluation of the first 100 cm of small bowel.[93]

Multidetector CT scan: This is also named multislice spiral computed tomography, produces high-resolution cross-sectional imaging of the abdomen and the small bowel. The lumen of the small bowel must be distended with orally administered contrast to demonstrate the wall thickening that characterizes small bowel tumors on CT. It allows multiplanar visualization of small bowel tumors and demonstrates signs of small bowel obstruction as well as the mural and extramural extent of small bowel malignancies.

Multidetector CT enteroclysis: This test shares the advantages of both conventional enteroclysis and cross-sectional imaging. This technique is more sensitive than conventional barium studies and less invasive than enteroscopy, and lesions as small as 5 mm can be identified. Studies have shown 100% sensitivity and 85–95% concordance with enteroscopy.[94]

MRI enterography: The advantages of MRI over CT include superb soft-tissue contrast, absence of radiation and iodine contrast exposure, and multiple contrast sources. MR enterolysis includes small bowel intubation and administration of a biphasic contrast agent. This protocol can provide anatomic demonstration of the normal intestinal wall, identification of wall thickening or timorous lesions, lesion characterization or evaluation of disease activity, and assessment of exoenteric/mesenteric disease extension.[95] In a large study that included 91 symptomatic patients with either suspected or established small bowel disease, 86 of the patients were correctly interpreted (diagnostic accuracy 95%), and a small bowel neoplasm was confirmed histopathologically (by endoscopy or surgery) in 32. The sensitivity, specificity, positive predictive value, and negative predictive value were 94%, 95%, 91%, and 97%, respectively.[96,97]

Positron emission tomography (PET): The role of PET in the initial diagnosis of small bowel malignant tumors is not yet established. However, there are indications for the utility of PET in monitoring response to treatment, manifested as change in metabolic activity of the tumor. (18) F-FDG PET is highly sensitive and specific for evaluation of the treatment response of nodal and extranodal diseases in patients with malignant lymphomas.[98]

Endoscopy: Endoscopy has the advantage of visualizing intestinal mucosa directly and, above all, of carrying out targeted biopsies. For many years, the small bowel, beyond the proximal jejunum, has remained an elusive anatomic location. Recently, novel endoscopic methods have been able to fully evaluate the entire small bowel. The new endoscopic methods include PE, video CE, double-balloon enteroscopy (DBE), and intraoperative enteroscopy.

PE: It permits evaluation of the proximal one-third of the small intestine, to a distance that is approximately 50–100 cm beyond the ligament of Treitz. The use of an overtube, back loaded onto the endoscope shaft, may help limit looping of the enteroscope within the stomach and facilitate deeper small bowel intubation. The diagnostic yield with PE is reported to increase with a greater depth of scope insertion. Data regarding the diagnostic yield of small bowel tumors and polyps using PE are limited to studies investigating PE in the context of obscure GI bleeding, and range from 1% to 5%.[99] A major advantage of PE over alternative radiological diagnostic modalities is the ability to obtain tissue, perform polypectomy or hemostasis if necessary, and mark lesion sites with India ink tattoo. PE, however, does not allow for the visualization of the entire small bowel, and several complications, including perforation and mucosal laceration, have been reported with the use of an overtube.

Video CE: This is a relatively new technology that is able to obtain endoscopic images from the entire small bowel.[100] CE is safe, easy, minimally invasive, patient-friendly, and has become a first-line tool in imaging and managing small bowel pathologies. The video capsule endoscope is a wireless capsule composed of a light source, lens, complementary metal oxide semiconductor imager, battery, and a wireless transmitter. The utility of CE has more than doubled the rate of detection of small bowel tumors from the precapsule endoscopy era of approximately 3% to today's 6–9% prevalence rate, when the procedure is done for obscure GI bleeding. Small bowel tumors found in such patients undergoing CE for evaluation of obscure GI bleeding are malignant in more than 50% of such cases.[101] The diagnostic yield of CE for various clinical indications has been shown to be comparable with DBE and superior to enteroclysis. The overall diagnostic yield of CE for small intestinal tumors varies in the literature, ranging from 2% to 9%.[102–104]

CE has some limitations as biopsy, therapy, or endoscopic marking (e.g., India ink tattooing) are possible. In addition, not all CE examinations make it to the cecum (complete small bowel exam occurs approximately 80% of the time), and in some patients, luminal debris and bubbles interfere with viewing. Capsule retention is the major, and for all practical purposes, the only complication of CE. The reported incidence of capsule retention ranges from 0% in healthy volunteers to up to 2% in obscure GI hemorrhage, and up to 21% in persons with suspected small bowel obstruction. The retention rate in patients with small bowel tumors may be as high as 10%.

DBE: This is a novel endoscopic insertion technique that uses a high-resolution, dedicated video endoscope that has a working length of 200 cm and two soft, latex balloons: one balloon is attached to the tip of the endoscope and the other to the distal end of a soft, flexible overtube. The balloons can be inflated and deflated using an air pump that is controlled by the endoscopist while monitoring air pressure. The balloons grip the wall of the bowel, thus allowing the endoscope to be advanced without looping. The procedure can be performed via an oral and/or transanal approach while under fluoroscopic guidance.

DBE has been shown to be able to visualize the entire length of the small bowel and allows for biopsy, marking of lesions for subsequent surgical resection (e.g., India ink tattoo), and therapeutics. In a study in patients with obscure bleeding, DBE was found to be accurate in demonstrating bleeding site in 115 (75.7%) patients, of which 45 (39.1%) were small bowel tumors.[105] DBE findings impacted patient management in 39 (86.6%) patients undergoing surgical resection of the tumor.

There are, however, limitations of DBE including concerns about the endoscopic learning curve, common need for endoscopy on two separate days (transoral and then transanal approaches), limitations in visualization of the entire small bowel, miss rates for subepithelial lesions due to insufflation issues, a time-consuming procedure that also requires a high level of ancillary staffing, increased moderate sedation requirements, and patient tolerance and preferences. In addition, although uncommon, the reported incidence of severe complications associated with DBE has ranged from 0% to 2.5% and has included pancreatitis, perforations, bleeding, abdominal pain, and fever.

Intraoperative enteroscopy: Exploratory laparotomy with intraoperative enteroscopy has been utilized since the 1980s and is an important diagnostic and potentially therapeutic endoscopic modality in suspected small bowel disease, including small bowel polyps and tumors.[106] It is considered to be the ultimate endoscopic evaluation of the small bowel. Reported complications associated with intraoperative enteroscopy include mucosal lacerations, perforations, prolonged ileus, abdominal abscess, and bowel ischemia.

Cancer management

Adenocarcinoma: Surgical resection of the primary tumor is the treatment of choice. The use of adjuvant therapy is increasing, although its role is still unclear. In metastatic disease, a palliative surgical resection of the primary tumor and palliative chemotherapeutic treatment are frequently needed in order to prevent or treat complications as bowel obstruction or bleeding. Newer regimens of chemotherapy and biological modalities may provide some clinical benefit. The options for clinical trials are limited because of the rarity of these tumors. Nearly all results are from retrospective studies. Fluoropyrimidines as the first-line and CPT-11 as the second-line chemotherapy yielded low response, although the adverse effects were mild. The FOLFOX (folinic acid, fluorouracil (5-FU), oxaliplatin

(Eloxatin)) and FOLFIRI (folinic acid, fluorouracil (5-FU), irinotecan) regimens are potential alternative strategies.[107]

SBAs are treated according to either a colorectal or a gastric cancer regimen. The molecular biology of a tumor is a pivotal determinant for therapy response. A recent paper confirmed our original observations that SBAs are more similar to colorectal than to gastric cancer. These molecular similarities provide added support for treatment of SBCs according to colorectal cancer regimens.[108]

Carcinoid tumors

Management of carcinoid tumors generally consists of resection of the tumor in localized disease, and control of carcinoid-related symptoms in the setting of unresectable or metastatic disease.[109] Prior to surgery, a thorough examination of the entire GI tract is indicated to rule out synchronous or metachronous noncarcinoid tumors (most likely adenocarcinomas) along the GI tract, but also in the lung, the prostate, cervix, and ovary.

In the setting of moderate-to-severe carcinoid symptoms, treatment with the somatostatin analogs octreotide and lanreotide is considered as the gold standard. In patients resistant to somatostatin analogs, addition of interferon alpha has shown to be effective in controlling carcinoid-related symptoms.[106] Hepatic artery embolization or chemoembolization should be reserved for patients with unresectable liver metastases without extrahepatic spread or for progressive disease and/or severe carcinoid symptoms not responding to somatostatin analogs or interferon.

Lymphoma

The majority of primary intestinal lymphomas can be cured by surgery alone (resection of the affected segment of small bowel together with its subjacent mesentery) in the case of low-grade histology. In some cases with localized low-grade lymphoma, especially in the elderly, watchful surveillance is sufficient. In more advanced stages, aggressive chemotherapy is the mainstay of treatment. Even in advanced stages, complete surgical resection is usually performed in order to alleviate symptoms of mass effect and to avoid complications during chemotherapeutic treatment. In Mediterranean lymphoma or IPSID, restricted to mucosa and/or submucosa, as well as MALToma confined to the gastric mucosa, remission can be induced by antibiotic treatment alone.

GIST and sarcoma

The surgical management of leiomyosarcomas and GISTs consists of adequate "en bloc" resection leaving the pseudocapsule intact to avoid intra-abdominal tumor spillage. Dense adhesions often hamper resection. In the presence of metastatic disease, a local resection of the primary tumor may be considered for control of bleeding or relief of obstruction. Imatinib mesylate, a small molecule tyrosine kinase inhibitor of KIT and platelet derived growth factor-α, and sunitinib, a broad-spectrum tyrosine kinase inhibitor, have been shown to be effective in metastatic disease. Recent randomized controlled trials demonstrated that with these new drugs, the median overall survival of advanced GIST has improved from approximately 2 years to more than 5 years.[110] A systematic review also suggested that *imatinib* used in the adjuvant setting improved recurrence-free survival of KIT-positive localized GIST.[111]

Prognosis

Recent data shows that without resection, the 5-year relative survival rates were 81% for neuroendocrine (primarily carcinoid) cancers, 28% for adenocarcinomas, 58% for sarcomas, and 64% for lymphomas,[75] while for patients who underwent resection, the 5-year observed survival rates were 64.6% for carcinoid tumors, 32.5% for adenocarcinomas, 39.9% for sarcomas, and 49.6% for lymphomas.[7] No significant changes in long-term survival rates for any of these four histological subtypes, but to GIST, have been demonstrated over the last two decades. Earlier tumor stages at diagnosis (stages I and II), small tumor size, and curative resection have been identified as favorable factor for overall survival, whereas poorly differentiated tumors, lymph node involvement, or metastasis as poor predicting prognosis.[112–116] For small intestinal lymphoma, the survival is largely determined by histological grade, stage, and respectability[112] with a higher survival for B-cell lymphoma than for T-cell lymphoma.[117] For small intestinal sarcomas, the prognosis is mainly dependent on the mitotic count, size, depth of invasion, and the presence of metastasis.[112] Age is suggested as a more powerful prognostic factor for carcinoid tumors compared with the other histology subtypes. In addition, being male and black is associated with a poorer prognosis.[7]

Prevention

The association of SBC with underlying conditions makes it possible to identify populations at risk and to develop screening programs. People with a family history of polyposis syndromes, such as PJS, FAP, and HNPCC who are genetically predisposed to develop SBC, should be included in surveillance programs and may benefit from regular screening. Surveillance and management of polyposis of the small intestine have been markedly improved by advances in videoendoscopic capsule and DBE, and despite the lack of supporting data, endoscopic surveillance with enteroscopy or capsule endoscopy every 1–2 years may be justifiable in high-risk individuals. Microsatellite instability testing or immunohistochemistry analysis of small bowel tumors may aid in patient selection.[118] People with celiac disease who are at higher risk of developing both adenocarcinoma and lymphoma of the small bowel need to maintain strictly a gluten-free diet. In patients with both Crohn's disease and celiac disease, awareness and recognition of new onset symptoms such as weight loss, diarrhea, or abdominal pain need immediate medical attention including imaging studies of the small bowel to rule out cancer.

Conclusions

Cancers of the small intestine are rare. They are composed of four major histological types (adenocarcinomas, NETs, lymphomas, and sarcomas). The incidence of small intestine cancer has increased over the past several decades, with a fourfold increase in NETs and less profound for adenocarcinoma and lymphoma and relatively stable for sarcomas. Risk of SBC is increased in patients with Crohn's disease, celiac disease, adenoma, FAP, and PJS. Obesity and cigarette smoking are recognized as risk factors for SBC and might provide the foundation for a prevention program aimed at reducing the incidence and mortality of cancers of the small intestine.

Case Study

A 57-year-old man with 21 years of Crohns' disease of the terminal ileum presents with mild unintentional weight loss of 5 kg. He is in complete remission for more than a decade and hence, had stopped any treatment. His initial bloods are within normal limit but to mild deficiency of vitamin B12. Repeat colonoscopy including biopsies from the terminal ileum is normal. Subsequent weight loss continues. An abdominal CT enterography scan showed thickened mid-ileum folds. A subsequent enteroscopy revealed a small mass (< 1 cm) in that area. Biopsies confirmed the diagnosis of adenocarcinoma.

References

1. Jemal, A., Siegel, R., Ward, E. *et al.* (2009 Cancer statistics, 2009. *CA Cancer J Clin*, **59**, 225–249.
2. Ries, L.A.G., Harkins, D., Krapcho, M. *et al.* (2006) *SEER Cancer Statistics Review, 1975–2003*. National Cancer Institute, Bethesda, MD.
3. Curado, M.P., Edwards, B., Shin, H.R. *et al.* (2007) *Cancer Incidence in Five Continents Vol. IX*, Vol. 160. IARC, IARC Scientific Publication, Lyon.
4. Neugut, A.I., Jacobson, J.S., Suh, S. *et al.* (1998) The epidemiology of cancer of the small bowel. *Cancer Epidemiol Biomarkers Prev*, **7(3)**, 243–251.
5. Ciresi, D.L., Scholten D.J. (1995) The continuing clinical dilemma of primary tumors of the small intestine. *Am Surg*, **61(8)**, 698–702; discussion 702–703.
6. Pan, S.Y., Morrison, H. (2011) Epidemiology of cancer of the small intestine. *World J Gastrointest Oncol*, **3(3)**, 33–42.
7. Bilimoria, K.Y., Bentrem, D.J., Wayne, J.D. *et al.* (2009) Small bowel cancer in the United States: changes in epidemiology, treatment, and survival over the last 20 years. *Ann Surg*, **249**, 63–71.
8. Dabaja, B.S., Suki, D., Pro, B. *et al.* (2004) Adenocarcinoma of the small bowel: presentation, prognostic factors, and outcome of 217 patients. *Cancer*, **101(3)**, 518–526.

9. Michelassi, F., Testa, G., Pomidor, W.J. *et al.* (1993) Adenocarcinoma complicating Crohn's disease. *Dis Colon Rectum*, **36**(7), 654–661.

10. Kaerlev, L., Teglbjaerg, P.S., Sabroe, S. *et al.* (2001) Medical risk factors for small-bowel adenocarcinoma with focus on Crohn disease: a European population-based case-control study. *Scand J Gastroenterol*, **36**(6), 641–646.

11. Offerhaus, G.J., Giardiello, F.M., Krush, A.J. *et al.* (1992) The risk of upper gastrointestinal cancer in familial adenomatous polyposis. *Gastroenterology*, **102**(6), 1980–1982.

12. Feldstein, R.C., Sood, S., Katz S. (2008) Small bowel adenocarcinoma in Crohn's disease. *Inflamm Bowel Dis*, **14**, 1154–1157.

13. Von Roon, A.C., Reese, G., Teare, J. *et al.* (2007) The risk of cancer in patients with Crohn's disease. *Dis Colon Rectum*, **50**, 839–855.

14. Dossett, L.A., White, L.M., Welch, D.C. *et al.* (2007) Small bowel adenocarcinoma complicating Crohn's disease: case series and review of the literature. *Am Surg*, **73**, 1181–1187.

15. Kodaira, C., Osawa, S., Mochizuki, C. *et al.* (2009) A case of small bowel adenocarcinoma in a patient with Crohn's disease detected by PET/CT and double-balloon enteroscopy. *World J Gastroenterol*, **15**, 1774–1778.

16. Kronberger, I.E., Graziadei, I.W., Vogel W. (2006) Small bowel adenocarcinoma in Crohn's disease: a case report and review of literature. *World J Gastroenterol*, **12**, 1317–1320.

17. Solem, C.A., Harmsen, W.S., Zinsmeister, A.R. *et al.* (2004) Small intestinal adenocarcinoma in Crohn's disease: a case control study. *Inflamm Bowel Dis*, **10**, 32–35.

18. Canavan, C., Abrams, K.R., Mayberry, J. (2006) Meta-analysis: colorectal and small bowel cancer risk in patients with Crohn's disease. *Aliment Pharmacol Ther*, **23**, 1097–1104.

19. Chen, C.C., Neugut, A.I., Rotterdam H. (1994) Risk factors for adenocarcinomas and malignant carcinoids of the small intestine: preliminary findings. *Cancer Epidemiol Biomarkers Prev*, **3**, 205–207.

20. Lashner, B.A. (1992) Risk factors for small bowel cancer in Crohn's disease. *Dig Dis Sci*, **37**, 1179–1184.

21. Bernstein, C.N., Blanchard, J.F., Kliewer, E. *et al.* (2001) Cancer risk in patients with inflammatory bowel disease: a population-based study. *Cancer*, **91**, 854–862.

22. Peters, U., Askling, J., Gridley, G. *et al.* (2003) Causes of death in patients with celiac disease in a population-based Swedish cohort. *Arch Intern Med*, **163**, 1566–1572.

23. Green, P.H., Fleischauer, A.T., Bhagat, G. *et al.* (2003) Risk of malignancy in patients with celiac disease. *Am J Med*, **115**, 191–195.

24. Howdle, P.D., Jalal, P.K., Holmes, G.K. *et al.* (2003) Primary small-bowel malignancy in the UK and its association with coeliac disease. *QJM*, **96**, 345–353.

25. Catassi, C., Fabiani, E., Corrao, G. *et al.* (2002) Risk of non-Hodgkin lymphoma in celiac disease. *JAMA*, **287**, 1413–1419.

26. Green, P.H., Cellier, C. (2007) Celiac disease. *N Engl J Med*, **357**, 1731–1744.

27. Green, P.H.R, Stavropoulos, S.N., Panagi, S.G. *et al.* (2001) Characteristics of adult celiac disease in the USA: results of a national survey. *Am J Gastroenterol*, **96**, 126–131.

28. Swinson, C.M., Slavin, G., Coles, E.C. *et al.* (1983) Coeliac disease and malignancy. *Lancet*, **1**, 111–115.

29. Askling, J., Linet, M., Gridley, G. *et al.* (2002) Cancer incidence in a population-based cohort of individuals hospitalized with celiac disease or dermatitis herpetiformis. *Gastroenterology*, **123**, 1428–1435.

30. Sellner, F. (1987) Hypothesis on the existence of an adenoma-carcinoma sequence in the small intestine. *Z Gastroenterol*, **25**, 151–165.

31. Sellner, F. (1990) Investigations on the significance of the adenoma-carcinoma sequence in the small bowel. *Cancer*, **66**, 702–715.

32. Bjork, K.J., Davis, C.J., Nagorney, D.M., Mucha, P. Jr. (1990) Duodenal villous tumors. *Arch Surg*, **125**, 961–965.

33. Witteman, B.J., Janssens, A.R., Griffioen, G., Lamers, C.B. (1993) Villous tumours of the duodenum. An analysis of the literature with emphasis on malignant transformation. *Neth J Med*, **42(1–2)**, 5–11.

34. Gill, S.S., Heuman, D.M., Mihas A.A. (2001) Small intestinal neoplasms. *J Clin Gastroenterol*, **33**, 267–282.

35. Groden, J., Thliveris, A., Samowitz, W. *et al.* (1991) Identification and characterization of the familial adenomatous polyposis coli gene. *Cell*, **66**, 589–600.

36. Arrigoni, A., Ponz de Leon, M., Rossini, F.P. *et al.* (1996) High prevalence of adenomas and microadenomas of the duodenal papilla and periampullary region in patients with familial adenomatous polyposis. *Eur J Gastroenterol Hepatol*, **8**, 1201–1206.

37. Alexander, J.R., Andrews, J.M., Buchi, K.N. *et al.* (1989) High prevalence of adenomatous polyps of the duodenal papilla in familial adenomatous polyposis. *Dig Dis Sci*, **34**, 167–170.

38. Lepistö, A., Kiviluoto, T., Halttunen, J. *et al.* (2009) Surveillance and treatment of duodenal adenomatosis in familial adenomatous polyposis. *Endoscopy*, **41**, 504–509.

39. Wieman, T.J., Taber, S.W., Reed, D.N. Jr. *et al.* (2003) Upper gastrointestinal cancer risk in familial adenomatous polyposis. *J Ky Med Assoc*, **101**, 142–145.

40. Björk, J., Akerbrant, H., Iselius, L. *et al.* (2001) Periampullary adenomas and adenocarcinomas in familial adenomatous polyposis: cumulative risks and APC gene mutations. *Gastroenterology*, **121**, 1127–1135.

41. Kadmon, M., Tandara, A., Herfarth, C. (2001) Duodenal adenomatosis in familial adenomatous polyposis coli. A review of the literature and results from the Heidelberg Polyposis Register. *Int J Colorectal Dis*, **16**, 63–75.

42. Launonen, V. (2005) Mutations in the human LKB1/STK11 gene. *Hum Mutat*, **26**, 291–297.

43. Sanchez-Cespedes, M. (2007) A role for LKB1 gene in human cancer beyond the Peutz-Jeghers syndrome. *Oncogene*, **26**, 7825–7832.

44. McGarrity, T.J., Amos, C. (2006) Peutz-Jeghers syndrome: clinicopathology and molecular alterations. *Cell Mol Life Sci*, **63**, 2135–2144.

45. Boardman, L.A., Thibodeau, S.N., Schaid, D.J. *et al.* (1998) Increased risk for cancer in patients with the Peutz-Jeghers syndrome. *Ann Intern Med*, **128**, 896–899.

46. Hearle, N., Schumacher, V., Menko, F.H. *et al.* (2006) Frequency and spectrum of cancers in the Peutz-Jeghers syndrome. *Clin Cancer Res*, **12**, 3209–3215.

47. Mehenni, H., Resta, N., Park, J.G. *et al.* (2006) Cancer risks in LKB1 germline mutation carriers. *Gut*, **55**, 984–990.

48. Ji, H., Ramsey, M.R., Hayes, D.N. *et al.* (2007) LKB1 modulates lung cancer differentiation and metastasis. *Nature*, **448**, 807–810.

49. Giardiello, F.M., Brensinger, J.D., Tersmette, A.C. *et al.* (2000) Very high risk of cancer in familial Peutz-Jeghers syndrome. *Gastroenterology*, **119**, 1447–1453.
50. Chung, D.C., Rustgi, A.K. (2003) The hereditary nonpolyposis colorectal cancer syndrome: genetics and clinical implications. *Ann Intern Med*, **138**, 560–570.
51. Lynch, H.T., Smyrk, T.C., Lynch, P.M. *et al.* (1989) Adenocarcinoma of the small bowel in lynch syndrome II. *Cancer*, **64**, 2178–2183.
52. Vasen, H.F., Wijnen, J.T., Menko, F.H. *et al.* (1996) Cancer risk in families with hereditary nonpolyposis colorectal cancer diagnosed by mutation analysis. *Gastroenterology*, **110**, 1020–1027.
53. Aarnio, M., Sankila, R., Pukkala, E. *et al.* (1999) Cancer risk in mutation carriers of DNA-mismatch-repair genes. *Int J Cancer*, **81**, 214–218.
54. Parc, Y., Boisson, C., Thomas, G., Olschwang, S. (2003) Cancer risk in 348 French MSH2 or MLH1 gene carriers. *J Med Genet*, **40**, 208–213.
55. Vasen, H.F., Stormorken, A., Menko, F.H. *et al.* (2001) MSH2 mutation carriers are at higher risk of cancer than MLH1 mutation carriers: a study of hereditary nonpolyposis colorectal cancer families. *J Clin Oncol*, **19**, 4074–4080.
56. Rodriguez-Bigas, M.A., Vasen, H.F., Lynch, H.T. *et al.* (1998) Characteristics of small bowel carcinoma in hereditary nonpolyposis colorectal carcinoma. International Collaborative Group on HNPCC. *Cancer*, **83**, 240–244.
57. Schulmann, K., Brasch, F.E., Kunstmann, E. *et al.* (2005) HNPCC-associated small bowel cancer: clinical and molecular characteristics. *Gastroenterology*, **128**, 590–599.
58. Neugut, A.I., Santos, J. (1993) The association between cancers of the small and large bowel. *Cancer Epidemiol Biomarkers Prev*, **2**, 551–553.
59. Murray, M.A., Zimmerman, M.J., Ee, H.C. (2004) Sporadic duodenal adenoma is associated with colorectal neoplasia. *Gut*, **53**, 261–265.
60. Lagarde, S., Dauphin, M., Delmas, C. *et al.* (2009) Increased risk of colonic neoplasia in patients with sporadic duodenal adenoma. *Gastroenterol Clin Biol*, **33**, 441–445.
61. Evans, H.S., Møller, H., Robinson, D. *et al.* (2002) The risk of subsequent primary cancers after colorectal cancer in southeast England. *Gut*, **50**, 647–652.
62. Scélo, G., Boffetta, P., Hemminki, K. *et al.* (2006) Associations between small intestine cancer and other primary cancers: an international population-based study. *Int J Cancer*, **118**, 189–196.
63. Tichansky, D.S., Cagir, B., Borrazzo, E. *et al.* (2002) Risk of second cancers in patients with colorectal carcinoids. *Dis Colon Rectum*, **45**, 91–97.
64. Brennan, P., Scélo, G., Hemminki, K. *et al.* (2005) Second primary cancers among 109 000 cases of non-Hodgkin's lymphoma. *Br J Cancer*, **93**, 159–166.
65. Ripley, D., Weinerman, B.H. (1997) Increased incidence of second malignancies associated with small bowel adenocarcinoma. *Can J Gastroenterol*, **11**, 65–68.
66. Alexander, J.W., Altemeier, W.A. (1968) Association of primary neoplasms of the small intestine with other neoplastic growths. *Ann Surg*, **167**, 958–964.
67. Beales, I.L., Scott, H.J. (1994) Adenocarcinoma of the duodenum with a duodeno-colic fistula occurring after childhood Wilms' cancer. *Postgrad Med J*, **70**, 933–936.

68. Chaturvedi, A.K., Engels, E.A., Gilbert, E.S. *et al.* (2007) Second cancers among 104,760 survivors of cervical cancer: evaluation of long-term risk. *J Natl Cancer Inst*, **99**, 1634–1643.

69. Howard, R.A., Dores, G.M., Curtis, R.E. *et al.* (2006) Merkel cell carcinoma and multiple primary cancers. *Cancer Epidemiol Biomarkers Prev*, **15**, 1545–1549.

70. Wu, A.H., Yu, M.C., Mack, T.M. (1997) Smoking, alcohol use, dietary factors and risk of small intestinal adenocarcinoma. *Int J Cancer*, **70(5)**, 512–517.

71. Negri, E., Bosetti, C., La Vecchia, C. *et al.* (1999) Risk factors for adenocarcinoma of the small intestine. *Int J Cancer*, **82(2)**, 171–174.

72. Chang, H.K., Yu, E., Kim, J. (2010) Adenocarcinoma of the small intestine: a multi-institutional study of 197 surgically resected cases. *Hum Pathol*, **41(8)**, 1087–1096.

73. Polak, J.M. (ed). (1993) *Diagnostic Histopathology of Neuroendocrine Tumours*. Churchill-Livingstone, Edinburgh.

74. Rindi, G., Capella, C., Solcia, E. (1999) Pathobiology and classification of digestive endocrine tumors. In: M. Mignon, J.F. Colombel (eds), *Recent Advances in the Pathophysiology of Inflammatory Bowel Disease and Digestive Endocrine Tumors*, pp. 177–191. John Libbey Eurotext, Montrouge.

75. Qubaiah, O., Devesa, S.S., Platz, C.E. *et al.* (2010) Small intestinal cancer: a population-based study of incidence and survival patterns in the United States, 1992 to 2006. *Cancer Epidemiol Biomarkers Prev*, **19**, 1908–1918.

76. Lebtahi, R., Cadiot, G., Sarda, L. *et al.* (1997) Clinical impact of somatostatin receptor scintigraphy in the management of patients with neuroendocrine gastroenteropancreatic tumors. *J Nucl Med*, **38**, 853–858.

77. Crump, M., Gospodarowicz, M., Shepherd, F.A. (1999) Lymphoma of the gastrointestinal tract. *Semin Oncol*, **26(3)**, 324–337.

78. Schottenfeld, D., Beebe-Dimmer, J.L., Vigneau, F.D. (2009) The epidemiology and pathogenesis of neoplasia in the small intestine. *Ann Epidemiol*, **19**, 58–69.

79. Catassi, C., Bearzi, I., Holmes, G.K. (2005) Association of celiac disease and intestinal lymphomas and other cancers. *Gastroenterology*, **128(4, Suppl 1)**, S79–S86.

80. Verkarre, V., Romana, S.P., Cellier, C. *et al.* (2003) Recurrent partial trisomy 1q22-q44 in clonal intraepithelial lymphocytes in refractory celiac sprue. *Gastroenterology*, **125(1)**, 40–46.

81. Bishop, P.C., Rao, V.K., Wilson, W.H. (2000) Burkitt's lymphoma: molecular pathogenesis and treatment. *Cancer Invest*, **18**, 574–583.

82. Isaacson, P., Wright, D.H. (1983) Malignant lymphoma of mucosa-associated lymphoid tissue. A distinctive type of B-cell lymphoma. *Cancer*, **52(8)**, 1410–1416.

83. Salem, P.A., Estephan, F.F. (2005) Immunoproliferative small intestinal disease: current concepts. *Cancer J*, **11(5)**, 374–382.

84. Lecuit, M., Abachin, E., Martin, A., *et al.* (2004) Immunoproliferative small intestinal disease associated with *Campylobacter jejuni*. *N Engl J Med*, **350(3)**, 239–248.

85. Howe, J.R., Karnell, L.H., Scott-Conner, C. (2001) Small bowel sarcoma: analysis of survival from the National Cancer Data Base. *Ann Surg Oncol*, **8**, 496–508.

86. Katz, S.C., DeMatteo, R.P. (2008) Gastrointestinal stromal tumors and leiomyosarcomas. *J Surg Oncol*, **97**, 350–359.

87. Miettinen, M., Kopczynski, J., Makhlouf, H.R. *et al.* (2003) Gastrointestinal stromal tumors, intramural leiomyomas, and leiomyosarcomas in the duodenum: a clinicopathologic, immunohistochemical, and molecular genetic study of 167 cases. *Am J Surg Pathol*, **27**, 625–641.

88. Vij, M., Agrawal, V., Kumar, A., Pandey, R. (2010) Gastrointestinal stromal tumors: a clinicopathological and immunohistochemical study of 121 cases. *Indian J Gastroenterol*, **29**, 231–236.

89. Gustafsson, B.I., Siddique, L., Chan, A. *et al.* (2008) Uncommon cancers of the small intestine, appendix and colon: an analysis of SEER 1973-2004, and current diagnosis and therapy. *Int J Oncol*, **33**, 1121–1131.

90. Pidhorecky, I., Cheney, R.T., Kraybill, W.G. *et al.* (2000) Gastrointestinal stromal tumors: current diagnosis, biologic behavior, and management. *Ann Surg Oncol*, **7(9)**, 705–712.

91. Hirota, S., Isozaki, K., Moriyama, Y. *et al.* (1998) Gain-of-function mutations of c-kit in human gastrointestinal stromal tumors. *Science*, **279(5350)**, 577–580.

92. Korman, M.U. (2002) Radiologic evaluation and staging of small intestine neoplasms. *Eur J Radiol*, **42(3)**, 193–205.

93. Bessette, J.R, Maglinte, D.D., Kelvin, F.M. *et al.* (1989) Primary malignant tumors in the small bowel: a comparison of the small-bowel enema and conventional follow-through examination. *Am J Roentgenol*, **153**, 741–744.

94. Horton, K.M., Fishman, E.K. (2004) Multidetector-row computed tomography and 3-dimensional computed tomography imaging of small bowel neoplasms: current concept in diagnosis. *J Comput Assist Tomogr*, **28(1)**, 106–116.

95. Semelka, R.C., John, G., Kelekis, N.L. *et al.* (1996) Small bowel neoplastic disease: demonstration by MRI. *J Magn Reson Imaging*, **6(6)**, 855–860.

96. Van Weyenberg, S.J., Meijerink, M.R., Jacobs, M.A. *et al.* (2010) MR enteroclysis in the diagnosis of small-bowel neoplasms. *Radiology*, **254**, 765.

97. Masselli, G., Polettini, E., Casciani, E. *et al.* (2009) Small-bowel neoplasms: prospective evaluation of MR enteroclysis. *Radiology*, **251**, 743.

98. Kumar, R., Xiu, Y., Potenta, S. *et al.* (2004) 18F-FDG PET for evaluation of the treatment response in patients with gastrointestinal tract lymphomas. *J Nucl Med*, **45(11)**, 1796–1803.

99. Chak, A., Koehler, M.K., Sundaram, S.N. *et al.* (1998) Diagnostic and therapeutic impact of push enteroscopy: analysis of factors associated with positive findings. *Gastrointest Endosc*, **47**, 18–22.

100. Triester, S.L., Leighton, J.A., Grigoris, L.I. *et al.* (2005) A meta-analysis of the yield of capsule endoscopy compared to other diagnostic modalities in patients with obscure gastrointestinal bleeding. *Am J Gastroenterol*, **100**, 2407–2418.

101. Pennazio, M., Rondonotti, E., de Franchis, R. (2008) Capsule endoscopy in neoplastic diseases. *World J Gastroenterol*, **14(34)**, 5245–5253.

102. Cobrin, G.M., Pittman, R.H., Lewis, B.S. (2006) Increased diagnostic yield of small bowel tumors with capsule endoscopy. *Cancer*, **107**, 22–27.

103. Bailey, A.A., Debinski, H.S., Appleyard, M.N. *et al.* (2006) Diagnosis and outcome of small bowel tumors found by capsule endoscopy: a three-center Australian experience. *Am J Gastroenterol*, **101**, 2237–2243.

104. Rondonotti, E., Pennazio, M., Toth, E. *et al.* (2008) Small-bowel neoplasms in patients undergoing video capsule endoscopy: a multicenter European study. *Endoscopy*, **40**, 488–495.

105. Sun, B., Rajan, E., Cheng, S. *et al.* (2006) Diagnostic yield and therapeutic impact of double-balloon enteroscopy in a large cohort of patients with obscure gastrointestinal bleeding. *Am J Gastroenterol*, **101(9)**, 2011–2015.

106. Matsumoto, T., Esaki, M., Yanaru-Fujisawa, R. *et al.* (2008) Small-intestinal involvement in familial adenomatous polyposis: evaluation by double-balloon endoscopy and intraoperative enteroscopy. *Gastrointest Endosc*, **68**, 911–919.

107. Suenaga, M., Mizunuma, N., Chin, K. *et al.* (2009) Chemotherapy for small-bowel adenocarcinoma at a single institution. *Surg Today*, **39**, 27–31.

108. Kulke, M.H., Mayer, R.J. (1999) Carcinoid tumors. *N Engl J Med*, **340**, 858–868.

109. Haan, J.C., Buffart, T.E., Eijk, P.P. *et al.* (2012) Small bowel adenocarcinoma copy number profiles are more closely related to colorectal than to gastric cancers. *Ann Oncol*, **23**, 367–374.

110. Modlin, I.M., Lye, K.D., Kidd, M. (2003) A 5-decade analysis of 13,715 carcinoid tumors. *Cancer*, **97(4)**, 934–959.

111. George, S., Trent, J.C. (2011) The role of imatinib plasma level testing in gastrointestinal stromal tumor. *Cancer Chemother Pharmacol*, **67(Suppl 1)**, S45–S50.

112. Essat, M., Cooper, K. (2011) Imatinib as adjuvant therapy for gastrointestinal stromal tumors: a systematic review. *Int J Cancer*, **128**, 2202–2214.

113. Hamilton, S.R., Aaltonen L.A. (2000) *World Health Organization Classification of Tumors. Pathology and Genetics of Tumors of the Digestive System*, pp. 69–92, Chapter 4; IARC Press, Lyon.

114. Wu, T.J., Yeh, C.N., Chao, T.C., Jan, Y.Y., Chen M.F. (2006) Prognostic factors of primary small bowel adenocarcinoma: univariate and multivariate analysis. *World J Surg*, **30**, 391–398.

115. Veyrières, M., Baillet, P., Hay, J.M. *et al.* (1997) Factors influencing long-term survival in 100 cases of small intestine primary adenocarcinoma. *Am J Surg*, **173**, 237–239.

116. Talamonti, M.S., Goetz, L.H., Rao, S. *et al.* (2002) Primary cancers of the small bowel: analysis of prognostic factors and results of surgical management. *Arch Surg*, **137**, 564–570.

117. Yin, L., Chen, C.Q., Peng, C.H. *et al.* (2007) Primary small-bowel non-Hodgkin's lymphoma: a study of clinical features, pathology, management and prognosis. *J Int Med Res*, **35**, 406–415.

118. Terauchi, S., Snowberger, N., Demarco, D. (2006) Double-balloon endoscopy and Peutz–Jeghers syndrome: a new look at an old disease. *Proc (Bayl Univ Med Cent)*, **19**, 335–337.

5 Colorectal Cancer

Shahab Ahmed and Cathy Eng

The University of Texas MD Anderson Cancer Center, Houston, TX, USA

Key Points

- Colorectal cancer is the third leading cause of cancer death for men and women combined, and incidences and mortalities are higher in individuals older than 50 years. A sedentary lifestyle and regular high intake of red meat maybe associated with increased risks of developing colorectal cancer (CRC).
- Patients diagnosed with ulcerative colitis have higher risk of developing CRC than those without known risk factors. Almost all individuals diagnosed with familial adenomatous polyposis will develop CRC without a prophylactic colectomy by age 40.
- Early detection is lifesaving. Every person with no family history of CRC should be screened with colonoscopy at the age of 50 years and 10 years earlier if there is a positive family history.
- Endoscopic ultrasound is the gold standard to stage rectal cancer.
- Neoadjuvant chemoradiation for stages II and III rectal cancer demonstrates better outcomes on disease-free recurrence.
- For patients undergoing curative resection of CRC, overall survival rates vary between 55% and 75%, with most recurrences seen in the first 2 years of follow-up.
- Surgical resection should be considered for resectable isolated liver or pulmonary metastases.
- Fluoropyrimidine is still the mainstay chemotherapeutic agent. Addition of cetuximab to the conventional chemotherapeutics shows favorable outcomes for K-RAS wild-type patients, across all lines of therapy.
- Monitoring carcinoembryonic antigen level is recommended during treatment for evaluation of disease recurrence or metastasis.

Key Web Links

http://www.cancer.gov
Provides accurate, up-to-date, comprehensive cancer information from the US government's principal agency for cancer research.

Handbook of Gastrointestinal Cancer, First Edition. Edited by Janusz Jankowski and Ernest Hawk.
© 2013 John Wiley & Sons, Ltd. Published 2013 by John Wiley & Sons, Ltd.

http://www.cancer.org
American Cancer Society—Supports research, patient services, early detection, treatment, and education.

http://www.asco.org
American Society of Clinical Oncology—Provides practice guidelines, research resources, education and training, and public policy.

http://www.nccn.org
National Comprehensive Cancer Network—Provides clinical practice guidelines on oncology.

http://www.cdc.gov/cancer/colorectal
CDC (Centers for Disease Control and Prevention)—Promotes colorectal (colon) prevention by building partnerships, encouraging screening, supporting education and training, and conducting surveillance.

http://seer.cancer.gov
Surveillance Epidemiology and End Results by National Cancer Institute (NCI)—Provides information on cancer statistics.

Potential Pitfalls

- The potential negative physical and psychological effects associated with a false-positive colonoscopy include anxiety induced by fear of being diagnosed with colorectal cancer.
- Permanent stoma is a major quality-of-life concern in the management of colorectal cancer postoperatively.
- Pre- or postoperative radiation may result in genitourinary and sexual dysfunction.
- Providing the appropriate remedy for chronic malignant pain is the most important challenge in managing the end-stage colorectal cancer patient.
- Finally, colorectal cancer requires multidisciplinary interaction between gastrointestinal medical oncology, surgical oncology, radiation oncology, and pathology to execute a sustainable and favorable outcome.

Introduction

The diagnosis and treatment of cancer has a long history stretching back to early human civilization. Hippocrates (460–370 BC), the father of medicine, first used the word "Karkinos" (the Greek word for crab) to describe the difference between benign and malignant tumors.[5] Ancient Chinese civilizations used special herbs to treat the symptoms associated with colorectal cancer (CRC) for decades.[6]

CRC remains one of the most challenging malignancies to treat. Historically, CRC care has always been costly. The US national cost of CRC care in 2010 (including the initial care year after diagnosis, continuing care, and last year of life care) was $14.14 billion.[7]

Breakdown of CRC care cost:
- Risk assessment
- Primary prevention
- Screening/detection
- Diagnosis
- Treatment
- Recurrence surveillance
- End-of-life care

According to the American Cancer Society's "Colorectal Cancer Facts and Figures 2011–2013," CRC is the third most commonly diagnosed cancer and the third leading cause of cancer death in both men and women. Globally, more than 1.2 million new cases and 608,700 deaths occurred in 2008.[8] According to the American Cancer Society (ACS), 141,210 people were diagnosed with CRC and 49,380 people died of the disease in the United States in 2011.

From 2003 to 2007, the median ages at diagnosis and death of CRC were 70 and 75 years of age, respectively.[9] According to the SEER (Surveillance, Epidemiology, and End Results) database, lifetime risk in men for developing CRC is 1 in 19 (5.2%) and in women is 1 in 20 (5.0%).

Incidence
In general, about 90% of new cases occur in individuals 50 years and older (15 times more than in age between 20 and 49, according to SEER), and the incidence is 35% higher in men than in women and racially highest in African Americans.[10] CRC incidence rates have been declining in the United States since the 1980s.[9] Since 1998, rates have been declining by 3.0% per year in men and by 2.3% per year in women.[11] Moreover, for that period of time, rates have declined among men and women in every major racial/ethnic group except for American Indian/Alaskan Native women (Figure 5.2).[11] But CRC incidence rates are rapidly increasing in Spain and in a number of Eastern Asian and Eastern European counties.[12,13] Table 5.1 shows the percent of US men and women developing CRC over 10- and 20-year intervals.

Mortality
About 94% of deaths from CRC occur in individuals 50 years and older, and the mortality is 40% higher in men than in women and racially highest in African Americans.[10] Figure 5.1 shows the mortality and incidence graph of CRC for different age groups. Since 1998, the overall mortality rates in the United States have decreased by 2.8% per year in men and 2.6% per year in women, and have been generally decreasing in both sexes in every major racial/ethnic group except for American Indian/Alaska Native men and women (Figure 5.2).[11]

Research funding
CRC is an active area of scientific research. The National Cancer Institute's (NCI) reports show a gradual increase in the US national CRC research

Table 5.1 Percent of US men and women who develop colorectal cancer over 10- and 20-year intervals according to their current age during 2005–2007.

Population	Current age	10 years	20 years
US men	50	0.70	2.04
	60	1.46	3.43
	70	2.34	3.96
US women	50	0.53	1.53
	60	1.05	2.64
	70	1.78	3.44

Notes: The above table illustrates that 1.46% of men who are now 60 years old will get colorectal cancer some time during the next 10 years. That is, 1–2 out of every 100 men who are 60 years old today will get colorectal cancer by the age of 70.
Data according to CDC.[14]

funding since 2006 (FY 2006: $244.1 million, FY 2007: $258.4 million, FY 2008: $273.7 million, and FY 2009: $308.6 million (including funding from The American Recovery and Reinvestment Act 2009 signed by President Obama, and funding by ACS for more than $80 million)[10]).

Cancer distribution
- Cecum: 16%.
- Ascending colon: 7%.
- Hepatic flexure: 3%.
- Transverse colon: 6%.
- Splenic flexure: 2%.
- Descending colon: 4%.
- Sigmoid colon: 31%.
- Rectum: 31%.

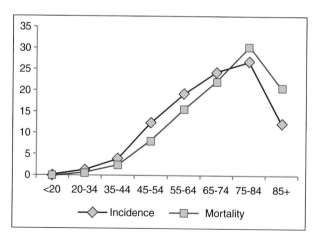

Figure 5.1 Colorectal cancer mortality and incidence in different age groups from 2003 to 2007 in the United States. (Data according to SEER.[9])

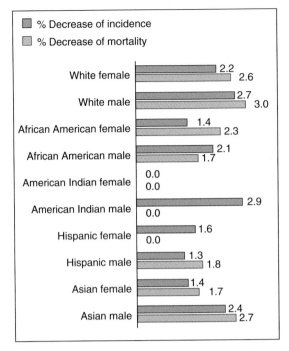

■ % Decrease of incidence
■ % Decrease of mortality

Figure 5.2 Colorectal cancer mortality and incidence trends from 1997 to 2006 in the United States. (Data according to Center for Disease Control (CDC).[14])

The development of CRC depends on two distinct pathways, both characterized by genetic instability: microsatellite instability and chromosome instability.[15] The first pathway involves oncogenes (KRAS, BRAF, MYC, etc.) and tumor-suppressor genes (TP53, APC, etc.), which directly regulate cell birth and cell death.[16] In the second pathway, stability genes (hMSH26, hMLH1, hPMS2, etc.) are involved that do not directly regulate cell birth or death but rather control the mutation rate of other genes, including growth controlling genes.

Molecular types[17]
CIMP, CpG island methylated phenotype; MSS, microsatellite stable; MSI, microsatellite instable:
1. Group 1: MSS positive/CIMP negative.
2. Group 2: MSI positive/CIMP positive.
3. Group 3: MSS positive/CIMP positive.
4. Group 4: MSS negative/CIMP negative.

Nonmodifiable risk factors
Age and hereditary factors are the most important nonmodifiable risk factors.

The lifetime risk of developing colorectal adenomas is nearly 19% in the US population and nearly 95% of sporadic CRCs develop from these adenomas.[18] After histological type, size and duration are the next

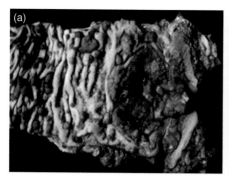
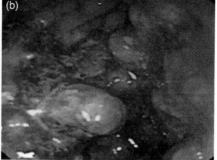

Figure 5.3 View of familial adenomatous polyposis (a) specimen and (b) colonoscopic.

important indicators of risk of developing CRC. A polyp of 1 cm in diameter has a one in six (17%) chance of developing into a cancer over 10 years.[19] For already cancerous polyps, the most important prognostic factor is the depth of invasion.

Genetic patterns of CRC
- Sporadic: 60–85%.
- Familial: 10–30%.
- Hereditary nonpolyposis colon cancer (HNPCC): 5%.
- Familial adenomatous polyposis (FAP): 1%.
- Autosomal dominant inheritance other than FAP and HNPCC: <1%.

FAP
FAP is an autosomal dominant disorder of APC gene mutations that affects 1 in 1000 births,[19] characterized by hundreds to thousands of polyps (Figure 5.3) arising within the colorectal region. Each polyp has the potential to become malignant as early as age 20 and by age 40; almost all people with this disorder will develop CRC without a prophylactic colectomy. About 25% of FAP patients do not have positive family history, and they should be tested for biallelic MYH mutation.[20]

Subtypes of FAP
- Gardner's syndrome: polyposis, epidermoid cysts, osteoma.
- Turcot's syndrome: polyposis, CNS tumors (medulloblastoma).
- Other extracolonic manifestations: dental abnormalities, congenital hypertrophy of the retinal pigmented epithelium (CHRPE), pancreatic and thyroid tumors, etc.

HNPCC/lynch syndrome
HNPCC is the most common inherited type of CRC. It is an autosomal dominant disorder caused by a mutation in one of the mismatch repair genes (hMLH1, hMSH2, hMSH6, or PMS2) that are responsible for proofreading DNA during replication and thus maintaining genomic stability.[19] HNPCC is associated with an 80% lifetime risk of CRC with the majority occurring on the right side of the colon.[19]

Amsterdam criteria II for diagnosis of HNPCC

- *Three* or more family members with HNPCC-related cancers, one of whom is a first-degree relative of the other two.
- *Two* successive affected generations.
- *One* or more of the HNPCC-related cancers diagnosed under age 50 years.
- *FAP* has been excluded.

MSI

Microsatellites are DNA sequences, usually consisting of one to five nucleotide repeats. MSI refers to a gain or loss in the number of repeats in DNA in a tumor, compared with the number of repeats in the same region in nontumor DNA from the same individual. MSI is recognized by observing multiple bands on electrophoresis of PCR products using tumor DNA, where fewer bands are seen using PCR products of nontumor DNA. The multiplicity of bands results from the failure to correct transcription errors. Errors occur most likely in regions of short repeated sequences (microsatellites), which may induce slippage of DNA polymerase, resulting in insertion or deletion in the repeated units. The tumor is termed MSI-high (MSI-H) if two or more of the five microsatellite sequences (BAT25, BAT26, D2S123, D5S346, and D17S250) recommended by the NCI have been mutated; it is termed MSI-low (MSI-L) if only one sequence has been mutated.[21]

MYH-associated polyposis

MYH-associated polyposis (MAP) is an autosomal recessive inherited disease. Mutations of the MYH gene (caretaker) are thought to lead to somatic mutation of APC (gatekeeper).[20] Usually the patients do not have a positive family history. There is a twofold increase in the incidence of CRC among patients with MAP, compared with the general population.[22] Most patients are ≥45 years of age at the time of diagnosis, with 10–100 polyps.[20]

Peutz–Jeghers syndrome

Peutz–Jeghers syndrome (PJS) is an autosomal dominant disease that presents with hamartomatous polyps and mucocutaneous melanin pigmentations. Lifetime risk for CRC development is 39%.[20] Currently only mutations in STK11 (LKB1) have been identified as cause for PJS.

Juvenile polyposis syndrome

Juvenile polyposis syndrome (JPS) is an autosomal dominant disease that presents with hamartomatous polyps. Lifetime risk for developing CRC is 20–60% and the median age of diagnosis is 35–40 years.[20] The genes known to be associated with JPS are BMPR1A and SMAD4.

Inflammatory bowel disease

First portrayed by both Crohn and Rosenberg in 1925 in a report,[23,24] the increased risk of CRC in patients with ulcerative colitis (UC) and Crohn's disease (CD) has long been recognized.[18,19,23,25] The risk of CRC with associated

UC is twofold higher[26,27] compared with the normal population, and CRC is observed in 5.5–13.5% of all patients with UC and 0.4–0.8% of patients with CD.[26] Based on long-term follow-up in a subset of studies included in the meta-analysis, Eaden's group estimated that the cumulative risk of CRC in UC patients to be 1.6% at 10 years, 8.3% at 20 years, and 18.4% at 30 years. Lesions are often found proximal to the splenic flexure and are of mucinous type.[27] The pathology of developing CRC in inflammatory bowel disease (IBD) patients begins with no dysplasia, progressing to indefinite dysplasia, low-grade dysplasia (10% risk of CRC[20]), high-grade dysplasia (30–40% risk of CRC[20]), and finally to carcinoma. The incidence of KRAS mutations has been found to be reduced in UC-associated CRC.[28-30] BRAF mutations have been reported in 9% of IBD-associated CRC.[28,31]

The tumor microenvironment includes cells (fibroblasts, endothelia cells, and infiltrating immune cells), molecules, and blood vessels that surround and feed a tumor cell.[31] Figure 5.4 shows the progressive increase of vascular endothelial growth factor (VEGF) that effects the growth of CRC. Figure 5.5 depicts how tumor microenvironment interplays in the development of CRC.

Metabolic environment and neoangiogenesis

Due to intermittent blood flow in a tumor and resultant hypoxia, there is a propensity for increased free radical production. Reperfusion injury may also apply additional selection pressure on cancer cells.[35] Hypoxia and low pH alter the regulation of various angiogenic growth factors including VEGF, Ang2, PDGF, TGF, COX1-2, iNOS, endothelin-1, -2, HGF, IL-8, tissue factor, PAI1, and thrombospondin-1, -2.[35,36]

Epithelial–mesenchymal transition

Cancer cell detachment from the primary site is one of the key initial events required for metastasis to occur. It is closely associated with epithelial–mesenchymal transition (EMT), which is a morphogenetic

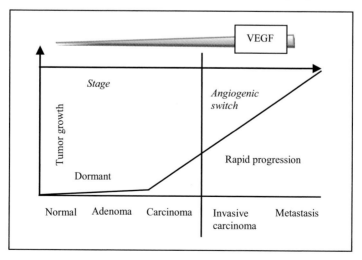

Figure 5.4 Angiogenesis and colorectal cancer. VEGF, vascular endothelial growth factor.[32-34]

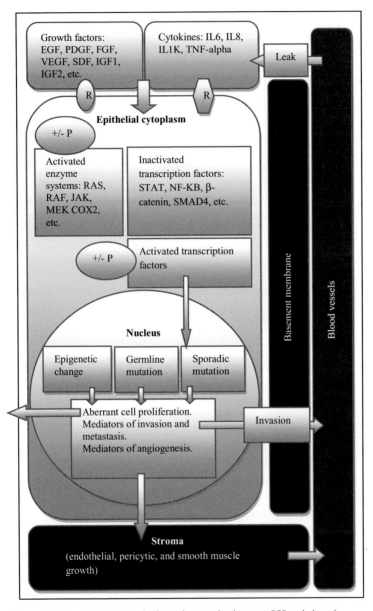

Figure 5.5 Microenvironment and colorectal cancer development. EGF, endodermal growth factor; PDGF, platelet-derived growth factor; FGF, fibroblast growth factor; VEGF, vascular endothelial growth factor; SDF, stromal cell-derived factor; IGF, insulin-like growth factor; TNF, tumor necrosis factor; STAT, signal transducer and activator of transcription; IL, interleukin; +/– P, phosphorylation or dephosphorylation; R, receptor.

process where epithelial cells lose their characteristics and gain mesenchymal properties during embryogenesis.[37] One of the major elements that characterizes EMT of carcinoma cells is the loss of E-cadherin-mediated cell–cell adhesion.[38,39]

Epigenetics

Epigenetics is defined as heritable changes in gene expression that are not due to any alteration in the DNA sequence.[40] The repertoire of epigenetic marks includes modifications to histone proteins, methylation (hypo/hyper) of DNA, and the phenomenon of RNA inheritance.[41] Although the genetic code provides the blueprint for all cellular elements, the epigenetic code controls elaboration of the blueprint; individuals have a single genome but many "epigenomes."[41] CpG island methylation is a common epigenetic event in colorectal neoplasia with hMLH1 promoter methylation representing a classic example of this phenomenon.[32,40,41] Disruption of the function of a tumor-suppressor gene, as defined by Knudson, requires a complete loss of function of both copies of the involved gene. When caused solely by genetic changes due to germline or somatic mutation of the coding genes, this is called the first hit.[42] The second hit generally involves somatic loss of the chromosomal region containing the other copy of the gene, or loss of heterozygosity (LOH). Hence, epigenetic changes may occur in normal cells, but may also prime the mucosa for cancer progression. However, unlike genetic changes in cancer, theses epigenetic changes are potentially reversible.[40]

The Wnt signaling pathway plays a key role during embryonic development[43] as well as in CRC development.[32] The Wnt families of proteins are involved in cell–cell signaling and adhesion during embryonic development. This includes the formation of the embryonic axes to end-stage organ development by regulation of β-catenin intracellular location and function.[32] Lack of regulation of the Wnt/β-catenin pathway is observed in CRC.[32]

The morphologic adenocarcinoma sequence was recognized at least 40 years ago and several studies, including those of Vogelstein's group (Figure 5.6) and National Polyp Study, suggest that CRC results from sequential accumulation of genetic and molecular alterations.[44] Although the earliest identifiable lesion in CRC formation is the aberrant crypt focus,[45,46] there are currently two proposed morphological pathways of spontaneous microadenoma development. First is the "bottom-up" theory where a stem cell situated in a niche in the crypt base acquires a second mutation and subsequently expands stochastically, producing neoplastic daughter cells. These cells migrate upward to colonize the entire crypt and form a clonal monocryptal adenoma that eventually further replicates and undergoes crypt fission.[47] Second is the "top-down" theory where an initial stem cell mutation occurs in the epithelial mucosa located between two crypt orifices with subsequent stem cell division producing a mutant clone that expands laterally and downward into the crypt displacing the normal epithelial cells.[47] Based on early investigations of non-FAP adenomas, about 50% of samples showed LOH for APC in the upper portion of the crypts with nuclear localization of β-catenin, verifying the loss of a gene in the Wnt pathway, most likely APC.[47] Ultimately, the product of the APC-Crypt fission sequence, along with other gene alterations (as outlined in Figure 5.6),

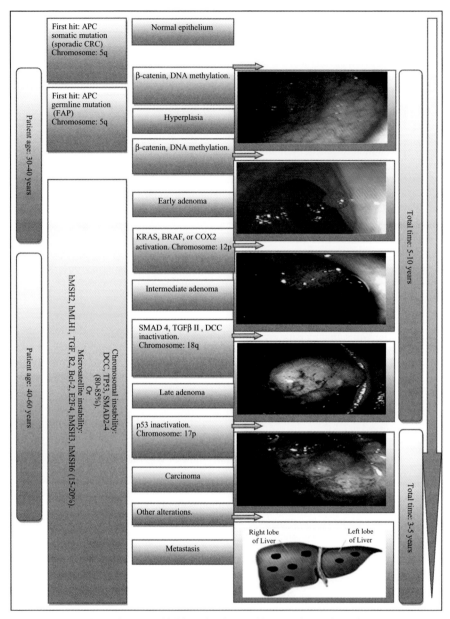

Figure 5.6 Vogelstein's model. (Photos by Chris Macklin, Consultant Colorectal Surgeon, Mid Yorkshire Hospitals NHS Trust, UK.)

acquires malignant characteristics, penetrates the muscular layer that lies underneath the lamina propria, and becomes an invasive carcinoma.[45,46]

Histological variants of colorectal cancer

Pure adenocarcinoma is mostly occurred in histological variant of CRC followed by mucinous and signet-ring type (Table 5.2).

Table 5.2 Major histological variants of CRC.

	Pure adenocarcinoma	Adenocarcinoma variant: Mucinous (≥50% mucin)[48]	Adenocarcinoma variant: Signet-ring
Incidence/100,000	46.6	5.5	0.6
Annual percent change	Decreasing	Stable	Increasing
Location, %	29 ® vs. 71 ©	18 ® vs. 82 ©	21 ® vs. 79 ©
Age of onset (years)	70.3 ± 12.7	70.3±13.2[49]	65.9±16.6[49,50]
Stage of diagnosis (III/IV), %	49.5	52.8	80.9
Grade (high), %	17.5	20.9	73.5
Metastasis[51]	Liver/lung > peritoneum/ ovary	Peritoneum/ovary > liver/lung	Peritoneum/ovary > liver/ lung
5-year survival	Better than signet-ring	Better than signet-ring	Worst[49,52]

®, rectal; ©, colon

Screening tests are necessary to detect the predisease conditions that lack clinical features (primary prevention). Screening tests can also find early stage colon cancer (secondary prevention).[14,53] The cost-effectiveness of CRC screening is estimated to be approximately $40,000 per year of life gained.[54] Unfortunately, less than half of Americans are up to date in terms of CRC screening.[55]

The American College of Gastroenterology (ACG) continues to recommend that screening begins at the age of 50 years in persons with average risk (without a family history of CRC, personal history of adenomas, or familial syndromes associated with CRC), except for African Americans who should begin at the age of 45 years.[56,57] The current evidence also supports a decision by clinicians with individual patients possessing an extreme smoking history or obesity to begin screening at an age earlier than 50 years and perhaps as early as 45 years.[57]

According to the AGC, the screening tests are subgrouped into (A) cancer prevention tests and (B) cancer detection tests.[58]

Cancer prevention tests: These tests have the potential to image both cancer and polyps. Colonoscopy is the gold standard.[57] Double contrast barium enema, flexible sigmoidoscopy, and CT colonography (virtual CT) are also under this category.[59]

Cancer detection tests: These tests have a low sensitivity for polyps and typically a lower sensitivity for cancer. Annual fecal immunochemical test to detect occult bleeding is the test of choice.[57] Fecal occult blood test and stool DNA test are also in this category.[59] Colonoscopy should be done if any of these are positive.

Physical

Digital rectal exam

Less than 10% of CRCs are located within the 7–8 cm reach of the examining finger. Stool obtained during a digital rectal exam (DRE) is inadequate to screen for the presence of blood, and there is no evidence that DRE reduces mortality from CRC and thus it is not indicated as a screening test for the prevention or early detection of CRC.[54]

Available screening tests are discussed in detail in Table 5.3. This table has been largely based on "The CRICO/RMF Colorectal Screening Algorithm" publication.[56]

Table 5.3 Available screening tests.

Tests	Evidence	Advantage/s	Disadvantage/s
Annual FOBT (low-to-moderate sensitivity) *Likelihood of negative test*[53]: If cancer present: 15–20% If advanced polyps: 50–80%	Large randomized controlled trials demonstrate a decrease in CRC mortality	Easy, safe, and convenient	Standard FOBT requires dietary restrictions, multiple samples, and must be repeated annually
Flexible sigmoidoscopy (moderate sensitivity and specificity) *Likelihood of negative test*[53]: If advanced polyps: 30–65%	Studies suggest a decrease in CRC mortality of about 60% overall and 70% from distal CRC. The risk of perforation is less than 1 in 1000.	Takes about 10 minutes to perform and usually well tolerated without sedation. Most patients can drive home alone or return to work following the procedure	Requires bowel preparations. Only reaches 60 cm (misses all right-sided lesions)
FOBT and flexible sigmoidoscopy (moderate sensitivity and specificity)	In a large prospective trial, the addition of FOBT to one-time flexible sigmoidoscopy increased detection of advanced adenomas and CRC from 70% to 76%	Combination of annual FOBT plus flexible sigmoidoscopy every 5 years may provide a small additional benefit over flexible sigmoidoscopy alone	Includes the disadvantages of either test alone, plus the need to comply with two tests
Colonoscopy (high sensitivity and specificity) Likelihood of negative test[53]: If advanced polyps: 2–12%	Case controlled study shows a 53–72% reduction in the incidence of CRC. In US studies, the overall risk of perforation was approximately 2 in 1000, but lower if polypectomy was not performed	Enables direct visualization of the entire colon when evidence via landmarks indicates the cecum was reached. Allows removal of polyps at the same time as the initial diagnostic exam, and the procedure is typically well tolerated	Requires bowel preparation. The exam takes about 30 minutes plus recovery time. The patients need to be escorted home and are advised not to go back to work the same day

(continued)

Table 5.3 *Continued*

Tests	Evidence	Advantage/s	Disadvantage/s
CT colonography (virtual CT) (high sensitivity and specificity)	In a study of asymptomatic adults, CT colonographic screening identified 90% of patients with CRC or adenomas 10 mm or larger in diameter[60]	Safe, fast (10–15 minute), noninvasive imaging of the entire colon. Sedation is not required; patients may drive home or return to work the same day	Requires bowel preparation[53] Can miss small and flat adenomas
Likelihood of negative test[53]: If cancer present: Uncertain If advanced polyps: 10–20			
Fecal DNA (sDNA) (low-to-moderate sensitivity and specificity)	Better than FOBT for detecting invasive colorectal cancer and large adenomas	Safe, noninvasive, performed at home. A stool DNA test that focused on three markers: KRAS mutations, APC mutations, and methylation of the vimentin gene	May not be widely available
Double contrast barium enema (DCBE)	In a study in Italy, DCBE was responsible for an increase in detection rates of cancer or adenoma of 2.3/1000 or 3.8/1000, respectively[61]	Safe, does not require sedation. Can usually view the entire colon	Requires bowel preparation, takes 30–45 minutes. DCBE is being used less frequently for screening[54]

A CRC screening and diagnosis algorithm is outlined in Table 5.4 (based on CRICO/RMF, ACG, and US Preventive Services Task Force (USPSTF)).

Imaging

Imaging is vital in CRC management. Not only is it important for diagnosis and guiding biopsies but it is also crucial in assessing extent of disease progression and thus determining treatment.[63] Figure 5.7 describes the imaging studies available to stage CRC.

X-ray

The disadvantage of this technique is that all structures are projected in one plane, and although there is good contrast between air, soft tissue, and bone, the inherent soft-tissue contrast is too low to allow differentiation of various soft-tissue structures (e.g., a tumor in muscle or a metastasis in

Table 5.4 CRC screening and diagnostic algorithm.[56,57,62]

Symptom/s negative	Family or personal history positive	Family or personal history negative	**Age <50 years:** African American: Colonoscopy at 45 years, if negative repeat every 10 years. Non-African American: start colonoscopy at 50 years, if negative repeat every 10 years.
			Age 50–75 years: colonoscopy at 50 years, if negative repeat every 10 years.
			Age >75 years: no CRC screening recommended.
		Non-FAP/HNPCC	*Family history:* One first degree with CRC or advanced adenoma (adenoma >1 cm in size, with high-grade dysplasia or villous elements) diagnosed at age ≥60 years: colonoscopy at 50 years, if negative repeat every 10 years.One first degree with CRC or advanced adenoma diagnosed at age <60 years or two first degrees with CRC or advanced adenoma: Colonoscopy at 40 years or 10 years before the age when the youngest affected relative was diagnosed, repeat every 5 years. *Personal history of adenoma:* Evidence for adenoma: repeat colonoscopy every 5 years *IBD:* Pancolitis: colonoscopy after ≥8 years and repeat every 1–2 years Left-sided colitis: colonoscopy after ≥15 years and repeat every 1–2 years
		FAP/HNPCC	*FAP:* Patients with classic FAP (>100 adenomas) should be advised to pursue genetic counseling and genetic testing, if they have siblings or children who could potentially benefit from this testing Patients with known FAP or who at risk of FAP based on family history (genetic testing has not been performed) should undergo annual flexible sigmoidoscopy or colonoscopy (starting at age 10–12 years), as appropriate, until such time as colectomy is deemed by physician and patient as the best treatmentPatients with retained rectum after subtotal colectomy should undergo flexible sigmoidoscopy every 6–12 months Patients with classic FAP, in whom genetic testing is negative, should undergo genetic testing for biallelic MYH mutations. Patients with 10–100 adenomas can be considered for genetic testing for attenuated FAP and if negative, MYH-associated polyposis *HNPCC:* Patients who meet the Bethesda criteria should undergo microsatellite instability testing of their tumor or a family member's tumor and/or tumor immunohistochemical staining for mismatch repair proteins. Patients with positive tests can be offered genetic testing. Those with positive genetic testing, or those at risk when genetic testing is unsuccessful in an affected proband, should undergo colonoscopy every 2 years beginning at age 20–25 years, until age 40 years. Subsequent colonoscopy every year thereafter
Symptom/s positive			Any symptoms/findings highly associated with CRC (rectal bleeding, anemia, obstructing lesions on abdominal imaging, etc.) along with consideration of age and sex: colonoscopy. If positive, consider staging workup if necessary for possible surgical evaluation.

Notes: Any positive colonoscopy for CRC should proceed to staging workup. For screening purpose, alternate CRC prevention or detection tests could be performed if any contraindications or patient's refusal to colonoscopy: flexible sigmoidoscopy every 5–10 years, CT colonography every 5 years; annual Hemoccult SENSA, stool DNA testing every 3 years.

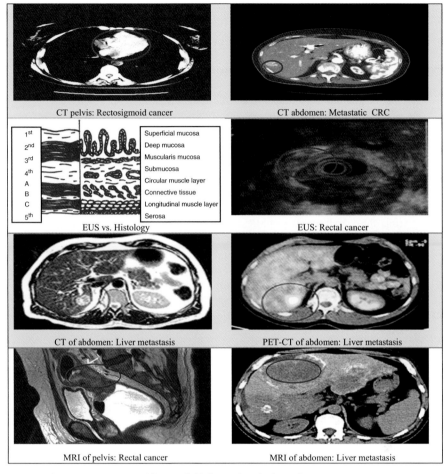

Figure 5.7 Imaging modalities available for staging of colorectal cancer.

the liver).[63] Given that conventional x-ray images show limited contrast, they are only of value if the tumor absorbs substantially more or less of the x-ray beam than surrounding tissues, consequently distinguishing tumor from surrounding tissue is only possible in lung and bone cancer, not in CRC.[63]

CT

CT imaging has good spatial and contrast resolution: all tissues can be visualized three dimensionally in an investigator-independent and highly reproducible way.[63] Although earlier studies stated the accuracy ranging between 85% and 90%, larger studies showed that the accuracy was more in 50–70% range, varying directly with the stage of the tumor.[64] Results from a multi-institutional study reported 74% accuracy of CT assessment of wall invasion and a sensitivity of 48% in evaluating lymph node metastases. CT demonstrated 85% accuracy and 97% specificity in detecting liver metastases.[65]

MRI

Advantages of MRI include the combination of high resolution and high soft-tissue contrast, the possibility to obtain direct images in any plane, and the potential for enhancing specific imaging characteristics by the use of MR-contrast agents.[63] The visibility of these contrast agents is 1000-fold higher than with iodine x-ray contrast agents that in turn enhance the tumor visibility considerably.[63] Disadvantages of MRI are (1) long examination time, significantly longer than a CT scan and (2) lack of uniform technique, though by using general protocols and the same type of MR scanner, reproducibility can be achieved.[63] MRI has revolutionized the management of more advanced rectal cancer. With the use of external coils, the overall accuracy of MRI for the T staging (depth of tumor) of rectal cancer varies from 65% to 86%, with considerable interobserver variability (recent studies reported 86–100%).[66] Nodal metastases (N staging) were better depicted.[66,67] In meta-analysis of pooled sensitivity and specificity of MRI for predicting circumferential margin involvement, they were reported to be 94% and 85%, respectively.[68]

EUS

Endoscopic ultrasound (EUS) has become the gold standard procedure for staging rectal carcinoma.[69–71] EUS enables one to distinguish layers within the rectal wall[72]; it appears to be an accurate method for detecting depth of tumor penetration and perirectal spread.[73,74] The accuracy of T staging for rectal carcinoma has been reported up to 80–96%.[64,72] The assessment of nodal involvement is less accurate than T staging with accuracies around 75%.[72,75] The major disadvantages are (1) it is unable to outline the M staging and (2) it tends to overstage cancers.[72,75]

Indications for EUS in rectal cancer[75]
- Large cancers: to determine candidacy for preoperative radiation/chemotherapy.
- Small cancers: to determine candidacy for transanal excision.

Potential impact of EUS staging on rectal cancer management[75]
- uT1: transanal local resection.
- uT2: radical resection ± postoperative radiation.
- uT3–4 or uN1: preoperative chemoradiation before radical resection.

FDG-PET

FDG is a glucose analog and its uptake reflects cellular metabolism, which is increased in many tumors.[63] But it is also accumulated in activated inflammatory cells such as granulocytes and macrophages, thus making the differentiation between tumor and normal tissue response difficult.[63] The lack of anatomic detail has been solved by the introduction of

Table 5.5 Treatment options for CRC.[77]

Stage	Colon	Rectal
Stage I T1-2N0M0	Definitive surgical resection	Same as colon
Stage II T3-4bN0M0	Definitive surgical resection ± adjuvant chemotherapy	Preoperative chemoradiation + definitive surgical resection + adjuvant chemotherapy
Stage III any T, N1-N2a-b, M0	Definitive surgical resection + adjuvant chemotherapy	Preoperative combined chemoradiation + definitive surgical resection + adjuvant chemotherapy
Stage IV M1a-b with any T or N	Preoperative chemotherapy ± radiation therapy ± palliative/ definitive primary vs. metastatic surgical resection	Same as colon

AJCC7: T4a, penetrates through the surface of the visceral peritoneum; T4b, directly invades or adheres to other organs or structures; N2a, 4–6 nodes; N2b, >6 nodes; M1a, confined to one organ or sites; M1b, to >1 organs/site or to the peritoneum.

integrated PET-CT scanners.[63] Compared with CT staging alone, PET-CT is significantly more accurate in defining TNM stage (difference 22%; 95% CI 9–36%; $p = 0.003$),[76] and has been shown to yield a cost savings of $2761 per patient,[64] and to avoid exploratory surgery in 6.1% of patients.

The treatment intent for CRC could be curative or noncurative (palliative, symptomatic relief, etc.). The available modalities are surgery, chemotherapy, radiotherapy, and chemoradiotherapy (Table 5.5).

Surgery is the only cure for CRC. Eighty percent of patients present without detectable metastases. For colon cancer, surgery is usually the first step, whereas for rectal cancer, a preoperative MRI or EUS is required to determine whether the patient clinically has stage II or III disease, in which case neoadjuvant chemoradiation is offered off study.[78]

The principles of surgery for CRC include en bloc resection to achieve a complete resection with negative margins, lymphadenectomy to the level of the primary feeding vessel, and removal of at least 12 regional lymph nodes.[79] By definition, regional lymph nodes include those nodes along the vascular arcades of the marginal artery and those adjacent to the colon/rectum along its mesocolic/rectal (upper third) border. Involved nodes outside the primary node-draining basin and extraregional lymph nodes are staged as metastatic disease.[80] During surgery, the abdomen should be explored to rule out metastasis to the peritoneum, distant lymph nodes, or other visceral organs. Approximately 10% of CRC patients have invasion of adjacent organs or inflammatory adhesions involving neighboring structures. According to the guidelines of the National Comprehensive Cancer Network (NCCN), NCI, and the American Society of Colon and Rectal Surgeons, the appropriate surgical management for CRCs that grow through the bowel wall into adjacent structures or organs should include multivisceral resection with a negative margin of the adjacent structure(s).[80]

Data suggests that laparoscopic colectomy can be a safe[81] alternative to open colectomy without compromising long-term outcomes.[82,83] For rectal cancer, a wide anatomical resection of the mesorectum with ideal bowel margins at least 2 cm distally and 5 cm proximally, as well as clear radial margins, is optimal.[79] Concerns about achieving negative lateral and circumferential margins have been addressed by the wider acceptance of total mesorectal excision for rectal cancers. The mesorectum is the initial site of spread for rectal cancer, making its complete removal in a single anatomic block an important feature of rectal surgery.[84]

For patients undergoing curative resection of CRC, overall survival (OS) rates vary between 55% and 75%, with most recurrences seen in the first 2 years of follow-up.[85] For node-negative patients, survival with surgery alone mimics that of general population's.[86] Surgery is also curative in 25–40% of highly selected patients who develop resectable metastases in the liver and lung.[87,88]

Procedures
For colon cancer[80]:
- Right hemicolectomy: for tumors of the cecum, ascending colon, and hepatic flexure.
- Extended right hemicolectomy: for tumors of proximal, mid, and distal transverse colon.
- Transverse colectomy: for tumors of mid transverse colon.
- Left hemicolectomy: for tumors of distal transverse, descending, and proximal sigmoid colon.
- Sigmoid colectomy: for tumors of sigmoid colon.
- Subtotal and total colectomy: for synchronous tumors of right and left side.

For rectal cancer:
- Transanal excision: for early, small, and clinically lymph node negative tumor.
- LAR: for proximal and mid rectal tumor.
- Abdominoperineal resection: for distal rectal tumors. Permanent colostomy needed as anal sphincter cannot be preserved.

Sentinel node mapping
According to the sentinel lymph node (SLN) hypothesis, tumor cells migrating from a primary tumor colonize one or a few lymph nodes (first few in the chain) before involving other lymph nodes.[80] Injection of vital blue dye with or without radiolabeled colloid around the area of the tumor permits identification of an SLN in the majority of the patients, and its status accurately predicts the status of the remaining regional lymph nodes. It has been established that SLN mapping has altered the surgical management of breast cancer; however, this is not the case in CRC. SLN mapping carries a false-negative rate of approximately 10% in larger studies, but will also potentially upstage a proportion of patients from node negative to positive following the detection of micrometastases; hence, the prognostic implication of these micrometastases requires further evaluation.[89]

Medical therapy

The role of medical treatment is usually as adjuvant to the definitive treatment of primary and resectable metastases, or as palliative in case of metastatic disease. In general, adjuvant chemo is not indicated for all stage II CRC[90-92]; this is according to the Cancer Care Ontario Program in Evidence-Based Care, an expert panel convened by the American Society of Clinical Oncology (ASCO) and the NCCN.[84] Pooled analyses and meta-analyses have shown a 2–4% improvement in OS for patients with adjuvant single agent fluorouracil (5-FU) based therapy compared with observation.[87,93-95] But it may be considered for high-risk stage II that includes any of the following[84,90] (also according to the study ECOG INT-0035 (Table 5.6)):

Table 5.6 Key adjuvant clinical trials.

Study	N	End points	Stage included	Conclusions
INT-0035	929	OS	III	5F-FU/levamisole superior to observation[96]
NSABP C-04	2078	DFS, OS	Dukes B/C	5-FU/LV superior to 5-FU/levamisole[97]
INT-0089	3759	DFS	II or III	Equivalency of 6 and 12 months treatment cycles of high-dose vs. low-dose LV[98]
QUASAR	3238	OS	II	5-FU/LV superior to observation (improves stage II survival by 3.1%)[99]
GERCOR C96	905	DFS	Dukes B2/C	Equivalency of LVFU2 and monthly 5-FU/LV[100]
X-ACT	1987	DFS	III	Capecitabine equivalency with 5-FU/LV bolus; less toxic[101]
NSABP C-06	1553	DFS	II or III	Equivalency of UFT/LV and 5-FU/LV (UFT not approved in the United States)[102]
MOSAIC	2246	DFS	II or III	Superiority of FOLFOX4 to LVFU2 in terms of 5-year DFS and 6-year OS for stage III[103]
NSABP C-07	1407	DFS	II or III	Bolus 5-FU/LV + oxaliplatin (FLOX) superior to 5-FU/LV[104]
CALGB 89803	1264	OS	III	No bolus IFL in stage III adjuvant CRC[105]
PETACC-3	3278	DFS	II or III	LVFU2 + CPT-11 not superior to LVFU2[106]
NSABP C-08	2710	DFS	II or III	Bevacizumab for 1 year with mFOLFOX 6 does not significantly prolong DFS in stages II and III colon cancer[1]
AVANT	2867	DFS, OS	III	Bevacizumab does not prolong DFS or OS when added to either FOLFOX4 or XELOX in patients with stage III colon cancer[2]
NCCTG N0147	1760	DFS, OS	III	The addition of cetuximab to mFOLFOX6 is of no benefit for patients with resected stage III wild-type KRAS colon cancer[3]

Source: Based on the consensus report of the International Society of Gastrointestinal Oncology 2007 on adjuvant therapy for stages II and III colon cancer, and on data from www.clinicaltrials.gov (Goldberg *et al.*[107]) CALGB, cancer and leukemia group B; CPT-11, irinotecan; GERCOR, group D 'Etude et de Recherché en Onco-Radiothérapic; PETACC, Pan-European Trial in Adjuvant Colon Cancer; QUASAR, quick and simple and reliable; AVANT, Avastin in adjuvant therapy; NCCTG, North Central Cancer Treatment Group; UFT, uracil/tegafur; X-Act, Xeloda in adjuvant colon cancer therapy.

Table 5.7 Available regimens.

Regimen	Description
Roswell Park (NSABP)	5-FU + leucovorin, IV; cycle every 8 weeks for 4 cycles. No longer in use
Mayo Clinic (NCCTG)	5-FU + leucovorin, IV; cycle every 4 weeks for 6 cycles. No longer in use
LV25FU (de Gramont)	High-dose LV as a 2-h infusion followed by 5-FU as an intravenous bolus plus a 22-h continuous infusion, 2 days for 2 weeks
FOLFIRI (Doulliard)	5-FU+ leucovorin + irinotecan, IV; cycle every 14 days
FOLFOX 4, 6, 7	5-FU + leucovorin + oxaliplatin, IV; cycle every 14 days
FOLFOXIRI	5-FU + leucovorin + oxaliplatin + irinotecan, IV; cycle every 14 days
IFL (Saltz)	Irinotecan + 5-FU + leucovorin, IV: cycle every 6 weeks
Capecitabine	PO; cycle every 21 days
CAPIRI	Capecitabine + irinotecan; cycle every 21 days
CAPOX	Capecitabine + oxaliplatin; cycle every 21 days
Irinotecan	Cycle every 6 weeks or 21 days

- T4 primary tumor.
- Poorly differentiated histology.
- Lymphovascular invasion.
- Perineural invasion.
- Bowel obstruction or perforation.
- Less than 12 regional lymph nodes in the surgical specimen.
- Positive surgical margins.
- MSS.

Commonly used combination chemotherapy regimens are discussed in Table 5.7.

Fluoropyrimidine

Before 2000, 5-FU was the only cytotoxic chemotherapy for CRC.[87] It acts through the inhibition of thymidylate synthetase (TS), the rate-limiting enzyme in pyrimidine nucleotide synthesis. Adjuvant 5-FU as a single agent had no survival benefit compared with surgery alone.[108] Since the late 1980s, it has been administered with leucovorin (LV), a reduced folate that stabilizes the binding of fluorouracil to TS.

According to the NCCTG trial, after a median follow-up of 8 years, patients treated with 5-FU/levamisole had a 31% reduction in recurrence for patients with stage III disease.[109–112] Adjuvant 5-FU/ levamisole reduced the risk of recurrence by 41% and death by 33%, compared with surgery alone for stage III disease.[113]

In 1990, an NCI consensus conference recommended 5-FU-based adjuvant therapy as the standard of care for patients with resected

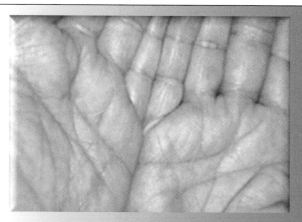

Figure 5.8 5-FU toxicity: hand–foot syndrome.

stage III disease.[114] The major side effects are dependent on the method of administration. When given as a bolus dose for 5 consecutive days for 4–5 weeks (Mayo Clinic), neutropenia and stomatitis are common. Diarrhea is more frequent with weekly bolus doses (Roswell Park). Regimens involving intravenous infusion associate with less hematological and gastrointestinal toxicity, but palmar-planter erythrodysesthesia ("hand–foot syndrome") is more common[115,116] (Figure 5.8).

Capecitabine (Xeloda©)
Capecitabine is a prodrug that undergoes three-stage enzymatic conversion to 5-FU after being absorbed intact through the gastrointestinal mucosa:
    Capecitabine ————————-> 5′-deoxy-5-fluorocytidine ————
——> 5′-deoxy-5-fluorouridine —————> 5-FU. Capecitabine was found to be therapeutically equivalent to bolus 5-FU/LV (Mayo Clinic) as first-line therapy in metastatic CRC (mCRC).[117] In the adjuvant treatment of 1987 patients with stage III disease, capecitabine was also shown to be similarly effective when compared with the Mayo Clinic regimen of bolus 5-FU/LV.[101]

The side effect profile of capecitabine is similar to that found with protracted infusion of 5-FU. Hand–foot syndrome is a prominent toxicity, and other adverse reactions include diarrhea, nausea, vomiting, and bone marrow suppression.[101,118]

Oxaliplatin
Oxaliplatin is a diaminocyclohexane platinum compound that forms bulky DNA adducts and induces cellular apoptosis.[119,120] It downregulates TS [121] and thus acts synergistically when used with 5-FU.[119]

Oxaliplatin was evaluated in mCRC in two phase III clinical trials, which demonstrated that the addition of oxaliplatin to infusional fluorouracil and LV increased response rate (RR) and

DFS, with a trend to OS.[122] In the Multicenter International Study of Oxaliplatin/5-FU/Leucovorin in the Treatment of Colon Cancer (MOSAIC) study (Table 5.6), adjuvant FOLFOX4 demonstrated prolonged OS for patients with stage III colon cancer compared with patients receiving 5-FU/LV without oxaliplatin.[103] The 6-year OS of patients with stage III colon cancer was 72.9% in the patients receiving FOLFOX and 68.9% in the patients receiving 5-FU/LV (hazard ratio (HR, 0.80; 95% confidence interval (CI), 0.65–0.97, $p = 0.023$).[103]

In the NSABP study (C-07, Table 5.6), comparison of the Roswell Park regimen with or without oxaliplatin (FLOX), after a median follow-up of 34 months, the probability of 3-year DFS was significantly improved in patients who received oxaliplatin (76.5% vs. 71.6%, $p = 0.004$)[84] but at the cost of increased diarrhea and gastrointestinal distress.

In a randomized phase III trial, the addition of oxaliplatin to FOLFIRI showed that FOLFOXIRI (5-FU, leucovorin, oxaliplatin, and irinotecan) had improved RR, DFS, and OS compared with FOLFIRI with an increased, but manageable, toxicity in patients with metastatic colon cancer.[123] But to the contrary, in a phase III trial according to British Journal of Cancer (BJC), data showed that in chemo-naïve patients of mCRC, the FOLFOXIRI regimen failed to demonstrate any superiority to the FOLFIRI regimen.[124]

Mainly two types of neuropathy are generally observed with oxaliplatin: (1) transient dysesthesias, manifested as numbness or tingling of the distal extremities, oral or perioral regions, exacerbated by exposure to cold temperature, and (2) sensory neuropathy (Figure 5.9), dose dependent, presented with persistent peripheral dysesthesias and paresthesias that remain between cycles of therapy, usually decreasing following end of treatment.[122] The latter may be dose limiting:

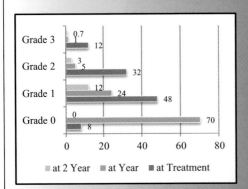

Figure 5.9 Oxaliplatin-induced peripheral sensory neuropathy (PSN) in percentile according to the MOSAIC study. 0, no change or no symptoms; 1, mild paresthesias, loss of deep tendon reflex; 2, mild or moderate objective sensory loss, moderate paresthesias; 3, severe objective sensory loss or paresthesias that interferes with function.[103,125]

Irinotecan

Irinotecan is a systemic derivative of the natural alkaloid camptothecin and inhibits topoisomerase I, an enzyme that catalyzes breakage and rejoining of DNA strands during DNA replication.[126,127] According to two studies for mCRC, median OS was extended by 2–3 months with a similar or improved quality of life in the irinotecan group versus either best supportive care or continuous infusion of 5-FU.[128–130] Patients also tended to have fewer tumor-related symptoms.[128]

However, in the adjuvant setting, irinotecan has no role. Trials such as the Cancer and Leukemia Group B (CALGB 89803, Table 5.6) study using IFL (irinotecan/5-FU/LV), the Pan European Trials in Adjuvant Colon Cancer 3 (PETACC3, Table 5.6) using infusional 5-FU and LV with or without irinotecan did not demonstrate any OS or DFS benefit.[84] Furthermore, the role of adjuvant FOLFIRI following hepatic resection was also negative in the metastatic setting. Hence, irinotecan appears to be most effective with macroscopic disease. Diarrhea, myelosuppression, and alopecia are the most commonly observed side effects with the use of irinotecan.[131–134]

Cancer therapy has entered a new era; biologically targeted therapies are now commonly used as part of the standard therapy for CRC[135] (Figure 5.10). Moreover, specificity of these agents renders them capability of individually targeting the inherent abnormalities of cancer cells, thus potentially resulting in less toxicity than traditional nonselective cytotoxic modalities.[137,138]

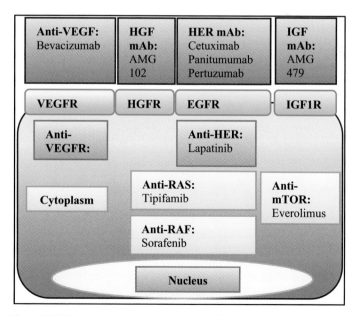

Figure 5.10 Targeting agents previously or currently being evaluated in trials for colorectal cancer.[136]

Cetuximab/Panitumumab

The Food and Drug Administration has approved cetuximab as the second-line therapy for previously treated mCRC patients, whereas panitumumab is approved as a single agent as the third-line therapy for mCRC patients.[139,140]

Cetuximab is a chimeric (human mouse) IgG1 antibody indicated for mCRC in irinotecan-refractory disease, either alone or in combination with irinotecan.[141] As monotherapy, approximately 10% of patients will have an antitumor response,[134,142] and 20% will respond to a combination of irinotecan and cetuximab.[142,143] In the Crystal study (NCT00154102), the addition of cetuximab was associated with an improved progression-free survival (PFS) (HR = 0.85; 95% CI, 0.72–0.99, p = 0.048 by a stratified log-rank test), but not OS in stage IV patients.[144] But in the adjuvant setting, unfortunately, like in the phase III NCCTG N0147 study of mFOLFOX (modified FOLFOX) ± cetuximab, the addition of cetuximab demonstrated no role[3] (Table 5.6).

Panitumumab is a fully human IgG2 monoclonal antibody with single-agent antitumor activity comparable with cetuximab in mCRC.[145] According to a randomized phase III trial, panitumumab significantly increased DFS over best supportive care only (13.8 weeks vs. 8.5 weeks), but did not prove any significant change in OS for mCRC.[146]

The most common side effects of cetuximab are dermatological, including acne-like rash (Figure 5.11), xerosis, and fissures of the skin.[134,147]

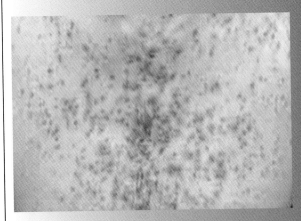

Figure 5.11 Cetuximab toxicity: acne-like rash.

Bevacizumab

Bevacizumab is a humanized monoclonal antibody directed against the VEGF family. In a randomized phase III trial, patients who received IFL plus bevacizumab survived a median of 20.3 months, while those on IFL plus placebo had a median survival of 15.6 months; the median PFS was 10.6 months in the bevacizumab group compared with 6.2 months in the other group: the RR was improved by 10%.[148] In ECOG 3200

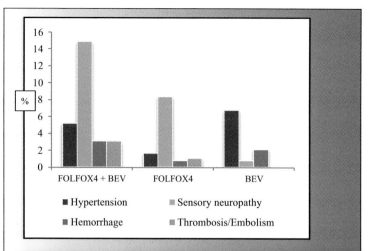

Figure 5.12 Bevacizumab-induced side effects according to the E3200 study (showing here only Grade 3).

study, patients with mCRC previously treated with 5-FU and irinotecan, the combination of FOLFOX and bevacizumab also demonstrated a statistically significant improvement in DFS and OS when compared with FOLFOX alone.[149] Similar to cetuximab, bevacizumab has no role in the adjuvant setting (NSABP C-08[1] and AVANT[2]).

Reversible hypertension and proteinuria are the two common side effects of bevacizumab. The other important adverse effects include hemorrhage, sensory neuropathy, and thromboembolism (Figure 5.12).[149]

The concept of personalized therapy

Systemic chemotherapy has long been the only effective modality for mCRC. In most patients with unresectable mCRC, whether such combination therapies should be used as first-line treatment or as a second-line treatment after 5-FU treatment failure remains unclear.[150] According to CAIRO (capecitabine, irinotecan, and oxaliplatin in advanced colorectal cancer) and FOCUS (fluorouracil, oxaliplatin, and CPT-11 (irinotecan): use and sequencing) studies, there was no improvement in OS with combination or sequential approaches.[151] Moreover, patient therapeutic management could be driven by individual variability in toxicity and efficacy of chemotherapeutic agents.[152] Therefore, identifying biomarkers that could help select the most appropriate regimen for each patient could be useful.

Proposed single agent treatment markers[153,154]

- 5-FU: expression of TS, dihydropyrimidine dehydrogenase (DPD), thymidine phosphorylase, high level leads to resistance.
- Capecitabine: same as 5-FU.

- Oxaliplatin: expression of x-ray cross-complementing factor 1 (XRCC1), and excision repair cross-complementing group 1 (ERCC1), high levels lead to poor prognosis.
- Bevacizumab: not identified.[155]
- Cetuximab: KRAS mutation (codon 12); only wild-type KRAS has response.[155–157]
- Panitumumab: same as cetuximab.[158]

KRAS mutation

In 2009, ASCO offered a "provisional clinical opinion," the statement that "all patients with metastatic colon cancer should have their tumors tested for KRAS mutations."[159]

KRAS is a gene, the human homolog of the Kirsten rat sarcoma-2 virus oncogene, which is linked with cellular signaling pathways, including those involving epidermal growth factor receptor (EGFR) itself.[160] KRAS acts as a molecular on/off switch for the recruitment and activation of proteins necessary for the propagation of growth factor and other receptor signals, such as B-RAF and PI 3-kinase.[161] KRAS gene mutations (codons 12, 13, and 61) have been widely studied as markers for cancer prognosis. These mutations are particularly found in codons in about 35–50% of CRCs, and population-based studies have suggested that the mutations might be associated with some tumor phenotypes.[162] KRAS mutation predicts unresponsiveness to EGFR-targeted monoclonal antibodies (cetuximab or panitumumab) in previously treated patients or in the first-line therapy (studies presented in the 2008 ASCO annual meeting: Phase III CRYSTAL and CAIRO 2 trials and Phase II OPUS trial; compared outcomes in patients treated with standard chemotherapy regimens such as FOLFIRI, CAPOX-bevacizumab, and FOLFOX[163–165]) of mCRCs.[161] In the NCIC study, in patients with wild-type KRAS tumors, treatment with cetuximab as compared with supportive care alone significantly improved OS and PFS, whereas among patients with mutated KRAS tumors, there was no significant difference between those who were treated with cetuximab and those who received supportive care alone, with respect to OS or PFS.[156] However, providing EGFR inhibition in a KRAS WT patient only identifies the potential of response, but does not guarantee response. It has been found that the cost of KRAS testing incident cases (estimated $13 million a year in the United States, $452/patient) is much less than the cost of giving drugs predicted to be of no benefit to the recipient who are KRAS mutants.[166] By and large, KRAS-based treatment selection is likely to result in cost savings across all lines of therapy.[166,167]

Advancements in genetic testing known as gene expression tests help support the continued development of the personalized care concept.

Gene Expression Test

There are three gene expression tests for CRC that have been or being studied up to date: Oncotype DX® by Genomic Health®, ColoPrint® by Agendia®, and OncoDefender™-CRC by Everist Genomics®.

Four development studies (surgery (Sx) alone; NSABP C-01/C-02 and CSF study; Sx + 5-FU/LV; and NSABP C-04/C-06) were performed to select the genes for prediction of recurrence for stage II CRC.[168]

Oncotype DX®

The Oncotype DX colon cancer recurrence score for stage II cancer is calculated from the quantitated expression of seven recurrence genes and five reference genes in the tumor tissue and is expressed as an individual score ranging from 0 to 100.[169] In the QUASAR validation study, the recurrence risk increased with increasing recurrence scores, with an average recurrence risk at 3 years of 12%, 18%, and 22% in the predefined low, intermediate, and high recurrence risk groups, respectively.[168,169] The study further defined a continuous individualized recurrence risk at 3 years ranging from a low risk of 9–11% to a high risk of 25–27%.

Recurrent assessment and treatment plan for Oncotype DX have been considered as follows[170] (MMR, mismatch repair):

- T3 and MMR deficient (low risk): consider observation.
- T3 and MMR present (standard risk): consider Oncotype DX.
- T4 and MMR present (high risk): consider chemotherapy.

ColoPrint®

ColoPrint test uses fresh tissue that is more advantageous than Oncotype DX. Moreover, it analyzes on 18 genes compared with 12 genes in Oncotype DX. It identifies patients as either high-risk group or low-risk group. In the first validation study, ColoPrint was superior to the ASCO criteria in assessing the risk of cancer recurrence without prescreening for MSI.[171] According to the second validation study, 80.5% of high-risk group were free of 5-year distant metastases compared with 94.9% of low-risk group.[172] A more detailed comparison between ColoPrint and clinical parameters will be available in the PARSC (Prospective Study for the Assessment of Recurrence in Stage II CC Patients using ColoPrint) clinical trial.[173]

But the disadvantage for both Oncotype DX and ColoPrint is that they do not predict benefit from chemotherapy.[174]

OncoDefender™-CRC

OncoDefender evaluates the expression levels of five specific genes (identified by Everist genomics as predictor of recurrence) using formalin fixed paraffin embedded CRC tissues.

It is the only molecular prognostic test capable of accurately predicting the risk of recurrence in previously surgically treated stage I/II colon cancer and stage I rectal cancer (sensitivity, specificity, and accuracy: 69%, 88%, and 79%, respectively, for stage I CRC; 70%, 55%, and 61%, respectively, for stage II colon cancer).[175]

Radiation alone has a limited role in mCRC treatment. It is often utilized for patients with locally advanced rectal cancer. Radiation may be necessary for palliation of certain metastases in locations such as the local recurrence to the sacrum, brain, etc.

In Europe, short-course preoperative radiation therapy (SCPRT) is delivered on a neoadjuvant basis, 5 Grays daily over 5 days. SCPRT is appealing in that a reduction in the time required for delivery of RT may result in a superior outcome. This is because the brief treatment time combats the effects of accelerated cellular repopulation, a phenomenon displayed by malignant cells exposed to RT. Concerns regarding the routine use of SCPRT include the omission of radiosensitizing chemotherapy,[176] inclusion of all stages and increased late toxicity.[177] Despite downsizing (mean diameter 4.5 cm vs. 4 cm, $p < 0.0001$), no significant downstaging effect is found, and it is not recommended if there is intention to preserve the sphincter.[177]

Patients with clinical stage II or stage III rectal cancer who received radiation (45–50 Grays in 25–28 fractions of 1.8 Grays over a period of 5.5 weeks) and chemotherapy (5-FU or Capecitabine) before surgery had fewer problems afterward and a lower risk that their cancer would recur in the rectum, compared with patients who had radiation and chemotherapy after surgery.[178,179] The neoadjuvant setting also showed an increase in the percentage of sphincter sparing procedures, reduced toxicities during therapy, and increased adherence to the adjuvant chemotherapy.[180] If given postoperatively, diarrhea and local strictures at the anastomotic site are more prevalent, and it is apparently due to radiation treatment effect.[78]

Figure 5.13 outlines the different approaches to treat CRC.

AJCC7 recommendations

The pathologic response to preoperative adjuvant treatment should be recorded according to the CAP (College of American Pathologists) guidelines for recording the tumor regression grade, because neoadjuvant chemoradiation in rectal cancer is often associated with significant tumor response and down staging. Specimens from patients receiving neoadjuvant chemoradiation should be carefully examined at the primary site, in regional nodes and for peritumoral satellite nodes or deposits in the rest of the specimen. Those patients with minimal or no residual disease after therapy may have a better prognosis than gross residual disease.

Tumor regression grade (pathological):
- Grade 0 (complete response): no viable cancer cells.
- Grade 1 (moderate response): single cells or small group of cancer cells.
- Grade 2 (minimal response): residual cancer outgrown by fibrosis.
- Grade 3 (poor response): minimal or no tumor kill, extensive residual cancer.

ECOG performance status:
- 0: fully active, able to carry on all predisease performance without restriction.

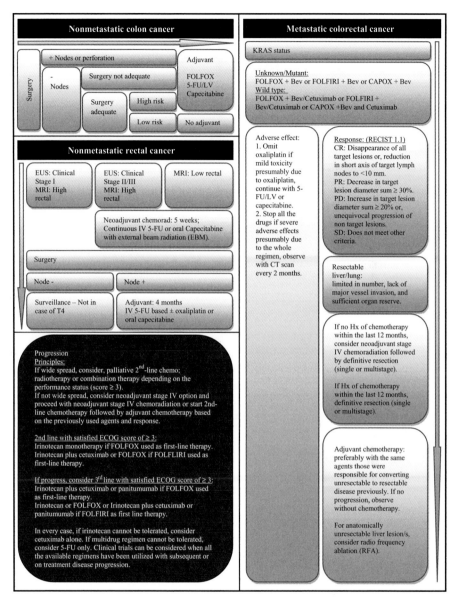

Nonmetastatic colon cancer

Surgery	+ Nodes or perforation		Adjuvant
	- Nodes	Surgery not adequate	FOLFOX 5-FU/LV Capecitabine
		Surgery adequate / High risk	
		Low risk	No adjuvant

Nonmetastatic rectal cancer

| EUS: Clinical Stage I MRI: High rectal | EUS: Clinical Stage II/III MRI: High rectal | MRI: Low rectal |

Neoadjuvant chemorad: 5 weeks; Continuous IV 5-FU or oral Capecitabine with external beam radiation (EBM).

Surgery

| Node - | Node + |

| Surveillance – Not in case of T4 | Adjuvant: 4 months IV 5-FU based ± oxaliplatin or oral capecitabine |

Progression
Principles:
If wide spread, consider, palliative 2nd-line chemo; radiotherapy or combination therapy depending on the performance status (score ≥ 3).
If not wide spread, consider neoadjuvant stage IV option and proceed with neoadjuvant stage IV chemoradiation or start 2nd-line chemotherapy followed by adjuvant chemotherapy based on the previously used agents and response.

2nd line with satisfied ECOG score of ≥ 3:
Irinotecan monotherapy if FOLFOX used as first-line therapy.
Irinotecan plus cetuximab or FOLFOX if FOLFLIRI used as first-line therapy.

If progress, consider 3rd line with satisfied ECOG score of ≥ 3:
Irinotecan plus cetuximab or panitumumab if FOLFOX used as first-line therapy.
Irinotecan or FOLFOX or Irinotecan plus cetuximab or panitumumab if FOLFIRI as first line therapy.

In every case, if irinotecan cannot be tolerated, consider cetuximab alone. If multidrug regimen cannot be tolerated, consider 5-FU only. Clinical trials can be considered when all the available regimens have been utilized with subsequent or on treatment disease progression.

Metastatic colorectal cancer

KRAS status

Unknown/Mutant:
FOLFOX + Bev or FOLFIRI + Bev or CAPOX + Bev
Wild type:
FOLFOX + Bev/Cetuximab or FOLFIRI + Bev/Cetuximab or CAPOX +Bev and Cetuximab

Adverse effect:
1. Omit oxaliplatin if mild toxicity presumably due to oxaliplatin, continue with 5-FU/LV or capecitabine.
2. Stop all the drugs if severe adverse effects presumably due to the whole regimen, observe with CT scan every 2 months.

Response: (RECIST 1.1)
CR: Disappearance of all target lesions or, reduction in short axis of target lymph nodes to <10 mm.
PR: Decrease in target lesion diameter sum ≥ 30%.
PD: Increase in target lesion diameter sum ≥ 20% or, unequivocal progression of non target lesions.
SD: Does not meet other criteria.

Resectable liver/lung:
limited in number, lack of major vessel invasion, and sufficient organ reserve.

If no Hx of chemotherapy within the last 12 months, consider neoadjuvant stage IV chemoradiation followed by definitive resection (single or multistage).

If Hx of chemotherapy within the last 12 months, definitive resection (single or multistage).

Adjuvant chemotherapy: preferably with the same agents those were responsible for converting unresectable to resectable disease previously. If no progression, observe without chemotherapy.

For anatomically unresectable liver lesion/s, consider radio frequency ablation (RFA).

Figure 5.13 Different treatment approaches for colorectal cancer.[59,87,155,181–193,107]

- 1: restricted in physically strenuous activity but ambulatory and able to carry out work of a light or sedentary nature.
- 2: ambulatory and capable of all self-care but unable to carry out any work activities; up and about more than 50% of waking hours.
- 3: capable of only limited self-care, confined to bed or chair, more than 50% of waking hours.

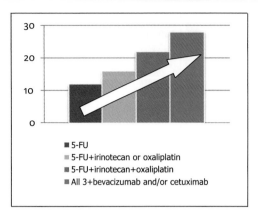

Figure 5.14 Median survival in months with mCRC.[77]

- 4: completely disabled; cannot carry on any self-care; totally confined to bed or chair.

Metastatic disease

Surgical resection should be considered for resectable isolated liver or pulmonary metastasis. After complete resection (R0) of metastases (liver or lung), the 5-year survival reaches 25–65%.[184–186] Radiofrequency ablation (5-year survival rate: 14–55%[194]) in combination with systemic treatment has also come under recent consideration.[184,186]

Surgery can be performed safely after 4 weeks from the last cycle of chemotherapy plus or minus cetuximab, and 5–8 weeks following chemotherapy plus bevacizumab.[155] Figure 5.14 portrays that the use of multiple chemo agents increases survival in CRC. Although prior trials have shown that surgery followed by hepatic arterial infusion of floxuridine alternating with systemic fluorouracil improves survival rates (OS 86–88% for combined vs. 76% for systemic alone, over 2 years),[195,196] in cases of unresectable liver metastasis, the benefit to OS is unclear.[197] Hence, HAI has largely fallen out of favor. For absolutely unresectable metastases (synchronous or metachronous), the goal of treatment is usually palliative, some patients may tolerate third-line chemotherapy or clinical trials.

Prognostic factors

Staging is the most accurate predictor of initial survival for CRC patients. Five-year stage-specific survivals for stages I, II, II, and IV are 100%, 68%, 44%, and 2%, respectively ($p < 0.001$).[198]

According to the AJCC7, there are new prognostic factors that are clinically important in addition to CEA level. These include tumor deposits (the number of satellite tumor deposits discontinuous from the leading edge of the carcinoma and that lack of evidence of residual lymph node); a regression grade (discussed in detail previously) that enables the pathologic response to neoadjuvant therapy to be graded; the circumferential margin (measured in mm from the edge of tumor to the nearest dissected margin of the surgical resection (R0, negative overall; R1, margins positive microscopically; R2, margins positive macroscopically)); MSI, an important but controversial prognostic factor especially for colon cancer; and perineural invasion (histologic evidence of invasion of regional nerves) that may have a similar prognosis as lymphovascular invasion. Additionally, demographic factors (already discussed earlier) and performance status (ECOG 2 and above) is a poor prognostic factor should be considered.[199]). Weight loss of more than 5–10% during the previous 3 months is a negative prognostic factor.[199]

Pretreatment hemoglobin <11 g/dL, ALP ≥300, LDH >1.5 times upper normal limit are considered negative prognostic factors for survival in mCRC.[200]

Patients with a high or increasing level (>5 mg/mL) of CEA have a poor prognosis.[201] CEA is most sensitive for hepatic or retroperitoneal metastasis and relatively insensitive for local, pulmonary, or peritoneal involvement.[202] In a molecular study, it was postulated that CEA had significantly protected human HT29 colon cancer cells from undergoing apoptosis under various conditions, including confluent growth, UV light, IFN-gamma treatment, and treatment with 5-FU.[203] CRCs with MSI-H have a significantly better prognosis.[204]

The number of circulating tumor cells (≥3/7.5 mL of blood) is an independent predictor of PFS and OS in mCRCs.[205] CXCR4 gene expression in primary CRC demonstrated significant association with recurrence, survival, and liver metastasis.[206]

After initial diagnosis, history and clinical exams should be performed every 3–6 months for the first 3 years, and every 6 months during years 4 and 5; subsequent surveillance is at the discretion of the physician.[207,208] Observation guidance for no evidence of disease is discussed in Table 5.8.

Colonoscopy

Among patients with no colorectal neoplasia on initial screening colonoscopy, the 5-year risk of CRC is extremely low.[209] Following the surgical definitive treatment, a colonoscopy is recommended after 3 years (but in clinical practice, it is done 1 year following the surgery, then if

Table 5.8 Key observation for no evidence of disease according to ASCO 2005 update on Colorectal Cancer Surveillance.[207]

Year	CEA (months)	CT (months)
1	3	3
2	3	3
3	6	6
4	6	6
5	6	6

normal, after 3 years). If normal after 3 years, once every 5 years thereafter is the AGI guideline.[207] ESMO recommends a colonoscopy at year 1 and then every 3 years thereafter as well as more frequent sigmoidoscopies.

CEA

ASCO recommends clinical follow-up every 3–6 months for the first 3 years, and subsequent follow-up every 6 months until at least 5 years postresection for patients with stage II and stage III CRCs.[201,207,208] An elevated CEA, if confirmed by retesting, warrants further evaluation for metastatic disease, but does not justify the institution of adjuvant therapy or systemic therapy for presumed metastatic disease.[201] CEA elevations within a week or two following chemotherapy should be interpreted with caution. Monitoring CEA level is recommended every 1–3 months during treatment for evaluation of disease recurrence or metastasis.[210]

CT

For node-positive tumors at surgery, ASCO recommends annual CT of the chest and abdomen for 3 years extended to include the pelvis in rectal cancer patients.[207,211]

In a randomized trial on the surveillance of 530 patients during adjuvant treatment for stage II or III disease, it was found that patients who were unable to undergo curative surgery were best detected by CT (26.5%) or CEA (17.8%) compared with symptoms (3.1%).[212] CEA in combination with CT is a valuable component of postoperative follow-up, especially if aggressive resection of metastatic disease can be performed.[201]

Modifiable risk factors have been estimated to be responsible for 39–71% of CRCs.[213,214] According to the Harvard Report on Cancer Prevention Volume 4, the associated risk factors for CRC and their strength of association are displayed in Table 5.9.

Some evidence also supports that a sedentary lifestyle maybe associated with an increased risk of developing CRC.[224–226] Exercise might reduce the risk for colon cancer by reducing the risk of developing precancerous polyps.[227] The ACS also recommends at least 30 minutes of moderate activity on 5 days or more per week, and says that 45–60 minutes of intentional physical activity is preferable. High levels of physical activity decrease the risk of colon cancer among men and women by possibly as much as 50%.[228]

Current recommendations for the prevention of colorectal cancer are as follows[10]:
- Get screened regularly.
- Maintain a healthy weight throughout life.
- Adopt a physically active lifestyle.
- Consume a healthy diet with an emphasis on plant sources, specifically.
- Choose foods and beverages in amounts that help achieve and maintain a healthy weight:
  - Eat five or more servings of a variety of vegetables and fruits each day.
  - Choose whole grains in preference to processed (refined) grains.
  - Limit your consumption of processed and red meats.
- If you drink alcoholic beverages, limit consumption.

Table 5.9 Association of risk factors for CRC.[215]

Strength of evidence	Strength of association	Relative risk (RR) and correlation	
Definitive	Family history, 10, nm	1.8	++
Chance, bias, and confounding can be ruled out with reasonable confidence in this association	Obesity[18,216-218] (>27 vs. <21), m	1.5	++
	Screening (FOBT or sigmoidoscopy vs. none), m	0.5	--
	Aspirin (15 years of regular use), m (acts through the β-catenin pathway to inhibit the progression of colon cancer)[219]	0.7	--
	IBD (>10 years), nm	1.5	++
	Folate, m	0.5	--
Probable	Vegetables,[217,218] m	0.7	-
Chance, bias, and confounding cannot be ruled out with reasonable confidence.	Alcohol[18,216-218,220] (>1 drink/day vs. 0), m	1.4	+
	Height (6" increment), nm	1.3	+
	Physical activity[217,218] (≥3 h/week vs. none), m	0.6	--
	Estrogen replacement[221] (≥5 years vs. none), m	0.8	-
	Oral contraceptive use (≥5 years vs. none), m	0.7	-
	Red meat,[217,218] m (due to presence of heme iron, heterocyclic amines, and polycyclic hydrocarbons)[178,222,223]	1.5	++
Possible	Fruits,[217,218] m	0.8	-
Available studies are of insufficient quality for this association	Fiber, m	0.7	-
	Saturated fat, m	1.4	+
	Smoking[217,218] (≥25 cigarettes/day vs. none), m	1.5	++

Source: Based on Harvard Report on Cancer Prevention Volume 4: Harvard Cancer Risk Index[215] with permission.

m, modifiable; nm, non-modifiable; +. positive; –, negative.

Recent issues

According to a meta-analysis of 15 studies of 2,593,935 participants, diabetes was associated with increased risk of CRC, compared with no diabetes (RR = 1.30, 95% CI = 1.20–1.44).[217,229]

Statins do not reduce the risk of CRC during treatment for hypercholesterolemia.[230] Epidemiologic evidence consistently suggests that dairy intake is protective against CRC.[231] Calcium supplements have shown to reduce the risk of adenomatous polyps, not CRCs.[32,231,232] Calcium can sequester bile and fatty acids and inhibit epithelial proliferation by modulating protein kinase C activity, stabilizing membranes, and/or modifying KRAS mutations.[54]

Vitamin D, whose biological effects are mediated by the vitamin D receptor (VDR), has been postulated to play a role in CRC prevention.[233] Its function is linked to the inhibition of cancer cell growth and stimulation of cellular differentiation, and thus VDR is presumed to be an important target for CRC prevention and therapy.[233] In an epidemiological observational study, it was found that CRC cancer risk was 67% lower in women in the highest quintile of vitamin D intake over time.[128]

COX2 activity is generally low in normal proliferative epithelial cells, but overexpressed in a number of cancers, including colon and breast carcinomas.[32] COX2 inhibitors demonstrated a 28% reduction in colorectal adenomas over 6 months among patients with FAP receiving 400 mg twice a day.[234] Additionally, agent-induced reductions in proliferation and increases in apoptosis in adenomas were observed in patients who used COX2 inhibitors for the same duration.[235]

According to the Women's Health Initiative Estrogen Plus Progestin Clinical trial, an approximately 40% lower risk for CRC was noted in the treatment group, as compared with the placebo group. Interestingly, among hysterectomized women treated with estrogen alone, the study did not show a lower risk of CRC.[236] Mechanisms by which HRT may reduce risk of CRC include direct or indirect reductions in secondary bile acids production and inhibition of insulin-like growth factor 1, which stimulates cell proliferation.[237]

Quality-of-life issues

Although nonstoma patients fare better than do stoma patients, they also suffer from physical impairments induced by sphincter saving procedures.[238] These impairments may become more prevalent as ultralow anastomosis is more frequently observed, resulting in bowel and sexual dysfunction and related psychologic distress.[238–240] Evidence shows that anterior resection and nonstoma patients, despite suffering micturition and defecation problems, had better quality-of-life scores than abdominoperineal extirpation patients (based on European Organization for Research and Treatment of Cancer (EORTC) generic and rectal-specific cancer questionnaires).[240]

A major quality-of-life concern includes the prevention of a life-threatening complication such as deep venous thrombosis, which is usually followed by pulmonary embolism. However, the most important challenge when treating end-stage CRC patients is providing the appropriate remedy for chronic malignant pain.[205]

Consent issues

Screening strategy should be based on patient preferences, medical contraindications, patient adherence, and available resources. Clinicians must inform the patients about the benefits and potential harm associated with each option before selecting a screening strategy. For CRC screening, of particular concern is increased anxiety experienced as a result of false-positive results.[241] The potential negative physical and psychological effects associated with a false-positive test include anxiety induced by fear of being diagnosed with CRC, physical effects of the performance of invasive diagnostic procedures such as colonoscopy, and the diagnosis of nonlethal lesions.[241]

Awareness

The most challenging personal obstacles to screening are as follows (www.ccawreness.com):

1. It's too personal to talk about.
2. I don't understand how the test works.
3. I'll get tested if I start feeling bad.

4. I'm scared they'll find something.
5. I'm not old enough to get colon cancer.

However, the responses to these concerns are very simple (www.ccawreness.com):

1. Colon cancer is 90% preventable with early and regular screening.
2. Screening can stop cancer before it starts by catching polyps before they become cancerous.
3. When caught early, colon cancer is more easily treated and can be cured.

Finally, these solutions would be easier to implement if individuals (www.ccawareness.com) (1) commit to be screened, (2) take action now, and (3) talk to their loved ones.

March is "National Colorectal Cancer Awareness Month" in the United States and in Europe (ECCAM). Studies showed that workplace CRC awareness programs can potentially mitigate both patient and physician barriers to screening.[242] To this end, MD Anderson Cancer Center has been arranging the annual "Sprint for Colorectal Oncology Prevention and Education (SCOPE5K)" since 2005 to enhance awareness and education in our city and communities.

Case Studies

Case 1

A 60-year-old patient underwent screening colonoscopy outside 5 years ago according to his primary care physician's recommendation. The colonoscopy report demonstrated a 2.5-cm sessile polypoid mass in the ascending colon that was partially removed. The rest of the ascending, transverse, descending, and sigmoid colons were unremarkable. The pathology report of an ascending colon mass revealed invasive moderate-to-poorly differentiated adenocarcinoma arising in a tubular adenoma. A staging computed tomography (CT) demonstrated a low-density lesion in the right lower lobe of the liver (see the figure below; left), which was subsequently found to be cyst by intraoperative ultrasound (see the figure below; right). His preoperative carcinoembryonic antigen (CEA) was less than 1.

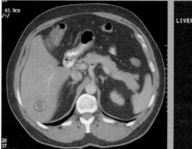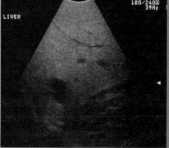

After being consulted at MD Anderson Cancer Center, the patient underwent right colon segmental resection with extended lymphadenectomy and intraoperative ultrasound, and cholecystectomy in early 2007. The pathology reported a poorly differentiated adenocarcinoma infiltrating into deep submucosa and abutting but not extending to the muscularis propria with 4 out of 19 lymph nodes positive. The surgical margins were clear. Thus, the patient was finally staged as T2N2M0 (American Joint Committee on Cancer 7 (AJCC7): IIIB). Subsequently, the patient received 12 cycles of adjuvant FOLFOX with the last 2 cycles with only 5-fluorouracil (5-FU) due to toxicity and neuropathy. Biologic therapy in conjunction with chemotherapy has not been determined to provide additional benefit for disease-free survival (DFS) (National Surgical Adjuvant Breast Bowel Project (NSABP) C-08,[1] Avastin in adjuvant therapy (AVANT),[2] and North Central Cancer Treatment Group (NCCTG)[3] N0147) in stage II or stage III patients. The patient was reevaluated in 2011 by magnetic resonance imaging (MRI) of the abdomen/pelvis with no definitive sign of recurrence.

Case 2

A 42-year-old male had an abdominal CT and a colonoscopy at an outside hospital in 2010 due to abdominal pain and blood in stool. The CT revealed abnormalities in the sigmoid colon as well as in the liver (indeterminate). The colonoscopy was completed with findings of a nonobstructing sigmoid cancer. His preoperative CEA was 6.5. Subsequently, the patient had a low anterior resection (LAR) with T3N2b (AJCC7) moderate-to-poorly differentiated adenocarcinoma with 12 out of 20 lymph nodes positive. The surgical margins were free of tumor. KRAS mutation analysis by PCR was positive for the KRAS mutation at codon 12. Postoperative PET showed metastatic nodal lesions. The patient proceeded to receive six cycles of FOLFOX/bevacizumab with evident decrease in some of the mediastinal lymph nodes. But due to a hypersensitivity reaction to oxaliplatin, his regimen was ultimately changed to FOLFIRI/Bevacizumab in late 2010. He continued the regimen for 10 cycles with PET/CT done on early 2011 and showed treatment response (the BRiTE study demonstrates continuation of bevacizumab beyond initial disease progression may improve median overall survival[4]). His CEA also came down to 2 (see the figure below).

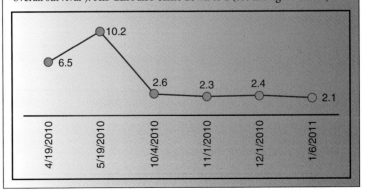

Acknowledgments

The authors would like to thank Courtney Barnes, Shontornia Collins, and Jonathan Phillips, GI Medical Oncology, Colorectal Database, MD Anderson Cancer Center.

References

1. Allegra, C. (2011) Phase III Trial Assessing Bevacizumab in Stages II and III Carcinoma of the Colon: Results of NSABP Protocol C-08. *J Clin Oncol*, **29(1)**, 11–16.
2. De Gramont, A. (2011) AVANT: Results from a randomized, three-arm multinational phase III study to investigate bevacizumab with either XELOX or FOLFOX4 versus FOLFOX4 alone as adjuvant treatment for colon cancer. *J Clin Oncol*, **29(Suppl 4)**, abstract 362.
3. Alberts, S.R., Sargent, D.J., Smyrk, T.C. *et al.* (2010) Adjuvant mFOLFOX6 with or without cetuximab (Cmab) in KRAS wild-type (WT) patients (pts) with resected stage III colon cancer (CC): Results from NCCTG Intergroup Phase III Trial N0147. *J Clin Oncol*, **28**, 18s.
4. Grothey, A., Sugrue, M.M., Purdie, D.M. *et al.* (2008) Bevacizumab beyond first progression is associated with prolonged overall survival in metastatic colorectal cancer: results from a large observational cohort study (BRiTE). *J Clin Oncol*, **26**, 5326–5334.
5. MedicineWorld.Org, medicineworld.org.
6. Jackson, M. (2010) The History of colorectal cancer, eHow. http://carcinomadecolon2010.blogspot.com/2010/06/history-of-colorectal-cancer_14.html
7. Mariotto, A.B., Yabroff, K.R., Shao, Y. *et al.* (2010) Projections of the cost of cancer care in the United States: 2010–2020. *J Natl Cancer Inst*, **103**, 117–28
8. Jemal, A. (2011) Global cancer statistics. *CA Cancer J Clin*, **61**, 69–90.
9. NCI (2007) *Cancer of the Colon and Rectum—SEER Stat Fact Sheets, Surveillance Epidemiology and End Results*. National Cancer Institute, Bethesda, MD.
10. American Cancer Society (ACS) (2011) *Colorectal Cancer Facts & Figures 2011–2013*. ACS.
11. Kohler, B.A., Ward, E., McCarthy, B.J., *et al.* (2011) Annual report to the nation on the status of cancer, 1975–2007, featuring tumors of the brain and other nervous system. *J Natl Cancer Inst*, **103**, 1–23.
12. Center, M.M., Jemal, A., Smith, R.A., Ward, E. (2009) Worldwide variations in colorectal cancer. *CA Cancer J Clin*, **59(6)**, 366–378
13. Center, M.M., Jemal, A., Ward, E. (2009) International trends in colorectal cancer incidence rates. *Cancer Epidemiol Biomarkers Prev*, **18(6)**, 1688–1694.
14. CDC (2009) *Colorectal Cancer Screening, Center for Disease Control and Prevention*, Basic Fact Sheet.
15. Simone, C., Resta, N., Bagella, L., *et al.* (2001) Cyclin E and chromosome instability in colorectal cancer cell lines. *J Clin Pathol: Mol Pathol*, **55(3)**, 200–203.
16. Vogelstein, B. (2008) *The Molecular Basis of Colorectal Cancer and Its Implications for Patients*. Howard Hughes Medical Institute, Maryland.
17. Jass, J.R., Do, K.A., Simms, L.A., *et al.* (1998) Morphology of sporadic colorectal cancer with DNA replication errors. *Gut*, **42**, 673–9

18. Haggar, F.A., Boushey, R.P. (2009) Colorectal cancer epidemiology: incidence, mortality, survival, and risk factors. *Clin Colon Rectal Surg*, **22**, 191–197.

19. Bhalla, V., Bhalla, A. (2009) Risk factors for colorectal cancer. *Oncology News*, **4(3)**, 84–85.

20. Wiggett, W., Becker, J. (2008) *Premalignant Conditions of the Colon*, University of Pretoria.

21. Kurzawski, G., Suchy, J., Debniak, T., *et al.* (2004) Importance of Microsatellite Instability (MSI) in colorectal cancer: MSI as a diagnostic tool. *Ann Oncol*, **15(Suppl 4)**, iv283–iv284.

22. Jones, N., Vogt, S., Nielsen, C. *et al.* (2009) Increased colorectal cancer incidence in obligate carriers of heterozygous mutations in MUTYH. *Gastroenterology*, **137(2)**, 489–494.

23. Potack, J., Itzkowitz S (2008) Colorectal Cancer in Inflammatory Bowel Disease. *Gut and Liver*, **2**, 61–73.

24. Ekbom, A., Helmick, C., Zack, M., *et al.* (1990) Ulcerative Colitis and Colorectal Cancer: A population based study. *N Engl J Med*, **323**, 1228–1233.

25. Klampfer, L. (2011) Cytokines, inflammation and colon cancer, *Curr Cancer Drug Targets*, **11(4)**, 451–464.

26. Pohl, C., Hombach, A., Kruis W (2000) Chronic Inflammatory bowel disease and cancer. *Hepatogastroenterology*, **47**, 57–70.

27. Hardy, R.G., Meltzer, S.J., Jankowski, J.A. (2000) ABC of colorectal cancer. Molecular basis for risk factors. *BMJ*, **321**, 886–889.

28. Svrcek, M., El-Bchiri, J., Chalastanis, A., *et al.* (2007) Specific clinical and biological features characterize inflammatory bowel disease-associated colorectal cancers showing microsatellite instability. *J Clin Oncol*, **25**, 4231–4238.

29. Lyda, M.H., Noffsinger, A., Belli, J., *et al.* (2000) Microsatellite instability and K-ras mutations in patients with ulcerative colitis. *Hum Pathol*, **31**, 665–671.

30. Umetani, N., Sasaki, S., Watanabe, T., *et al.* (1999) Genetic alterations in ulcerative colitis-associated neoplasia focusing on APC, K-ras gene and microsatellite instability. *Jpn J Cancer Res*, **90**, 1081–1087.

31. Hedgehog signaling in the tumor microenvironment, www.biooncology.com.

32. Ruddon, R.W. (2007) *Cancer Biology*, 4th ed. Oxford University Press, New York.

33. Guba, M., Seeliger, H., Kleespies, A., *et al.* (2004) Vascular endothelial growth factor in colorectal cancer. *Int J Colorectal Dis*, **19**, 510–517.

34. VEGF expression in colorectal cancer by stage, www.biooncology.com.

35. Fukumura, D., Jain, R.K. (2007) Tumor microenvironment abnormalities: causes, consequences, and strategies to normalize. *J Cell Biochem*, **101**, 937–949.

36. Lin, Q., Yun, Z. (2010) Impact of the hypoxic tumor microenvironment on the regulation of cancer stem cell characteristics. *Cancer Biol Ther*, **9**, 946–956.

37. Berx, G., Raspe, E., Christofori, G., *et al.* (2007) Pre-EMTing metastasis? Recapitulation of morphogenetic processes in cancer. *Clin Exp Metastasis*, **24**, 587–597.

38. Gout, S., Huot J (2008) Role of cancer microenvironment in metastasis: focus on colon cancer. *Cancer Microenviron*, **1**, 69–83.

39. Cavallaro, U., Christofori, G. (2004) Cell adhesion and signalling by cadherins and Ig-CAMs in cancer. *Nat Rev Cancer*, **4**, 118–132.

40. Nystroem, M., Mutagen, M. (2009) Diet and epigenetics in colon cancer. *World J Gastroenteric*, **15**, 257–263.

41. Wong, J., Hawkins, N.J., Ward, R. (2007) Colorectal cancer: a model for epigenetic tumorigenesis. *Gut*, **56**, 140–148.

42. Herman, J., Bailyn, S. (2003) Gene silencing in cancer in association with promoter hypermethylation. *N Engl J Med*, **349**, 2042–2054.

43. Benz, M., Clovers, H. (2000) Linking colorectal cancer to Wnt signaling. *Cell*, **103**, 311–320.

44. Winawer, S.J., Zauber, A.G., Ho, M,N., *et al.* (1993) Prevention of colorectal cancer by colonoscopic polypectomy. The National Polyp Study Workgroup. *N Engl J Med*, **329**, 1977–1981.

45. Grady, W.M., Markowitz, S.D. (2002) Genetic and epigenetic alterations in colon cancer. *Annu Rev Genomics Hum Genet*, **3**, 101–128.

46. van den Brink, G.R., Offerhaus, G.J. (2007) The morphogenetic code and colon cancer development. *Cancer Cell*, **11**, 109–117.

47. Brittan, M., Wright, N.A. (2004) Stem cell in gastrointestinal structure and neoplastic development. *Gut*, **53**, 899–910.

48. Green, J.B., Timmcke, A.E., Mitchell, W.T., *et al.* (1993) Mucinous carcinoma–just another colon cancer? *Dis Colon Rectum*, **36**, 49–54.

49. Sung, C.O., Seo, J.W., Kim, K.M., *et al.* (2008) Clinical significance of signet-ring cells in colorectal mucinous adenocarcinoma. *Mod Pathol*, **21**, 1533–1541.

50. Secco, G.B., Fardelli, R., Campora, E., *et al.* (1994) Primary mucinous adenocarcinomas and signet-ring cell carcinomas of colon and rectum. *Oncology*, **51**, 30–34.

51. Pande, R., Sunga, A., Levea, C., *et al.* (2008) Significance of signet-ring cells in patients with colorectal cancer. *Dis Colon Rectum*, **51**, 50–55.

52. Makino, T., Tsujinaka, T., Mishima, H., *et al.* (2006) Primary signet-ring cell carcinoma of the colon and rectum: report of eight cases and review of 154 Japanese cases. *Hepatogastroenterology*, **53**, 845–849.

53. Lieberman, D.A. (2009) Clinical practice. Screening for colorectal cancer. *N Engl J Med*, **361**, 1179–1187.

54. Hawk, E.T., Levin, B. (2005) Colorectal cancer prevention. *J Clin Oncol*, **23**, 378–391.

55. Lloyd, S.C. (2011) Compliance, capacity, and quality in colonoscopy screening for CRC: a novel solution. *J Clin Oncol*, **29**.

56. Atlas, S.J. (2004) Colorectal cancer screening algorithm -a decision support tool, in Medical H (ed.), *CRICO/RMF.* http://www.rmf.harvard.edu/Clinician-Resources/Guidelines-Algorithms/2010/~/media/Files/_Global/KC/PDFs/RMFCRC.pdf

57. Rex, D.K., Johnson, D.A., Anderson, J.C., *et al.* (2009) American College of Gastroenterology guidelines for colorectal cancer screening 2009 [corrected]. *Am J Gastroenterol*, **104**, 739–50.

58. Griffith, J.M., Lewis, C.L., Brenner, A.R., *et al.* (2008) The effect of offering different numbers of colorectal cancer screening test options in a decision aid: a pilot randomized trial. *BMC Med Inform Decis Mak*, **8**, 4.

59. Learn About Cancer: Colorectal Cancer Early Detection, American Cancer Society, 2008.

60. Johnson, C.D., Chen, M.H., Toledano, A.Y., *et al.* (2008) Accuracy of CT colonography for detection of large adenomas and cancers. *N Engl J Med*, **359**, 1207–1217.

61. Ciatto, S., Castiglione G (2002) Role of double-contrast barium enema in colorectal cancer screening based on fecal occult blood. *Tumori*, **88**, 95–98.

62. Rex, D.K. (2009) American college of gastroenterology guidelines for colorectal cancer screening 2008. *Am J Gastroenterol*, **104**, 739–750.

63. Barentsz, J., Takahashi, S., Oyen, W., *et al.* (2006) Commonly used imaging techniques for diagnosis and staging. *J Clin Oncol*, **24**, 3234–3244.

64. Dewhurst, C., Rosen, M.P., Blake, M.A., *et al.* (1996) Pretreatment staging of colorectal cancer, American college of radiology. http://www.acr.org/~/media/ACR/Documents/AppCriteria/Diagnostic/PretreatmentStagingColorectalCancer.pdf

65. Zerhouni, E.A., Rutter, C., Hamilton, S.R., *et al.* (1996) CT and MR imaging in the staging of colorectal carcinoma: report of the Radiology Diagnostic Oncology Group II. *Radiology*, **200**, 443–451.

66. Iafrate, F., Laghi, A., Paolantonio, P., *et al.* (2006) Preoperative staging of rectal cancer with MR Imaging: correlation with surgical and histopathologic findings. *Radiographics*, **26**, 701–714.

67. Low, R.N., McCue, M., Barone, R., *et al.* (2003) MR staging of primary colorectal carcinoma: comparison with surgical and histopathologic findings. *Abdom Imaging*, **28**, 784–793.

68. Purkayastha, S., Tekkis, P.P., Athanasiou, T., *et al.* (2007) Diagnostic precision of magnetic resonance imaging for preoperative prediction of the circumferential margin involvement in patients with rectal cancer. *Colorectal Dis*, **9**, 402–411.

69. Rifkin, M.D., Ehrlich, S.M., Marks, G. (1989) Staging of rectal carcinoma: prospective comparison of endorectal US and CT. *Radiology*, **170**, 319–322.

70. Rifkin, M.D., Wechsler, R.J. (1986) A comparison of computed tomography and endorectal ultrasound in staging rectal cancer. *Int J Colorectal Dis*, **1**, 219–223.

71. Snady, H., Merrick, M.A. (1998) Improving the treatment of colorectal cancer: the role of EUS. *Cancer Invest*, **16**, 572–581.

72. Siddiqui, A.A., Fayiga, Y., Huerta, S. (2006) The role of endoscopic ultrasound in the evaluation of rectal cancer. *Int Semin Surg Oncol*, **3**, 36.

73. Boyce, G.A., Sivak, M.V. Jr., Lavery, I.C., *et al.* (1992) Endoscopic ultrasound in the pre-operative staging of rectal carcinoma. *Gastrointest Endosc*, **38**, 468–471.

74. Jochem, R.J., Reading, C.C., Dozois, R.R., *et al.* (1990) Endorectal ultrasonographic staging of rectal carcinoma. *Mayo Clin Proc*, **65**, 1571–1577.

75. Savides, T.J., Master, S.S. (2002) EUS in rectal cancer. *Gastrointest Endosc*, **56**, S12–S18.

76. Veit-Haibach, P., Kuehle, C.A., Beyer, T., *et al.* (2006) Diagnostic accuracy of colorectal cancer staging with whole-body PET/CT colonography. *JAMA*, **296**, 2590–2600.

77. Meyerhardt, J. (2007) *Colorectal Cancer: Dana-Farber Cancer Institute Handbook*, 1st ed, Mosby.

78. Sauer, R., Becker, H., Hohenberger, W., *et al.* (2004) Preoperative versus postoperative chemoradiotherapy for rectal cancer. *N Engl J Med*, **351**, 1731–1740.

79. Nelson, H., Petrelli, N., Carlin, A., *et al.* (2001) Guidelines 2000 for colon and rectal cancer surgery. *J Natl Cancer Inst*, **93**, 583–596.

80. Rodriguez-Bigas, M. (2010) Surgical oncologic principles for the resection of colon cancer, in K. Tanabe (ed.), *UpToDate*. http://www.uptodate.com/contents/surgical-oncologic-principles-for-the-resection-of-colon-cancer?source=see_link&anchor=H125358938#H125358938

81. Bonjer, H.J., Hop, W.C., Nelson, H., *et al.* (2007) Laparoscopically assisted vs open colectomy for colon cancer: a meta-analysis. *Arch Surg*, **142**, 298–303.

82. (2004) A comparison of laparoscopically assisted and open colectomy for colon cancer. *N Engl J Med*, **350**, 2050–2059.

83. Fleshman, J., Sargent, D.J., Green, E., *et al.* (2007) Laparoscopic colectomy for cancer is not inferior to open surgery based on 5-year data from the COST Study Group trial. *Ann Surg*, **246**, 655–662; discussion 662–664.

84. Wolpin, B.M., Meyerhardt, J.A., Mamon, H.J., *et al.* (2007) Adjuvant treatment of colorectal cancer. *CA Cancer J Clin*, **57**, 168–185.

85. O'Connell, M.J., Campbell, M.E., Goldberg, R.M., *et al.* (2008) Survival following recurrence in stage II and III colon cancer: findings from the ACCENT data set. *J Clin Oncol*, **26**, 2336–2341.

86. Newland, R.C., Dent, O.F., Chapuis, P.H., *et al.* (1995) Survival after curative resection of lymph node negative colorectal carcinoma. A prospective study of 910 patients. *Cancer*, **76**, 564–571.

87. NCI (2010) Colon Cancer Treatment (PDQ). National Cancer Institute, Bethesda, MD.

88. Khatri, V.P., Petrelli, N.J., Belghiti, J. (2005) Extending the frontiers of surgical therapy for hepatic colorectal metastases: is there a limit? *J Clin Oncol*, **23**, 8490–8499.

89. Mulsow, J., Winter, D.C., O'Keane, C., *et al.* (2003) Sentinel lymph node mapping in colorectal cancer (Br J Surg 2003; 90: 659–667). *Br J Surg*, **90**, 1452.

90. Nguyen, T., Pham, D. (2009) Adjuvant Chemotherapy for Colon Cancer. *Northeast Florida Medicine*, **60**, 20–21.

91. Figueredo, A., Charette, M.L., Maroun, J., *et al.* (2004) Adjuvant therapy for stage II colon cancer: a systematic review from the Cancer Care Ontario Program in evidence-based care's gastrointestinal cancer disease site group. *J Clin Oncol*, **22**, 3395–3407.

92. Buyse, M., Piedbois, P. (2001) Should Dukes' B patients receive adjuvant therapy? A statistical perspective. *Semin Oncol*, **28**, 20–24.

93. Efficacy of adjuvant fluorouracil and folinic acid in B2 colon cancer. International Multicentre Pooled Analysis of B2 Colon Cancer Trials (IMPACT B2) Investigators. *J Clin Oncol*, **17**, 1356–1363, 1999.

94. Gill, S., Loprinzi, C.L., Sargent, D.J., *et al.* (2004) Pooled analysis of fluorouracil-based adjuvant therapy for stage II and III colon cancer: who benefits and by how much? *J Clin Oncol*, **22**, 1797–1806.

95. Mamounas, E., Wieand, S., Wolmark, N., *et al.* (1999) Comparative efficacy of adjuvant chemotherapy in patients with Dukes' B versus Dukes' C colon cancer: results from four National Surgical Adjuvant Breast and Bowel Project adjuvant studies (C-01, C-02, C-03, and C-04). *J Clin Oncol*, **17**, 1349–1355.

96. Moertel, C.G., Fleming, T.R., Macdonald, J.S., *et al.* (1995) Intergroup study of fluorouracil plus levamisole as adjuvant therapy for stage II/Dukes' B2 colon cancer. *J Clin Oncol*, **13**, 2936–2943.

97. Wolmark, N., Rockette, H., Mamounas, E., *et al.* (1999) Clinical trial to assess the relative efficacy of fluorouracil and leucovorin, fluorouracil and levamisole, and fluorouracil, leucovorin, and levamisole in patients with Dukes' B and C carcinoma of the colon: results from National Surgical Adjuvant Breast and Bowel Project C-04. *J Clin Oncol*, **17**, 3553–3559.

98. Haller, D.G., Catalano, P.J., Macdonald, J.S., *et al.* (2005) Phase III study of fluorouracil, leucovorin, and levamisole in high-risk stage II

and III colon cancer: final report of Intergroup 0089. *J Clin Oncol*, **23**, 8671–8678.

99. Gray, R.G., Barnwell, J., Hills, R., McConkey, C., Williams, N., Kerr, D. (2004) QUASAR: A randomized study of adjuvant chemotherapy (CT) vs observation including 3238 colorectal cancer patients. *J Clin Oncol*, **22(Suppl 14)**, 3501.

100. Andre, T., Quinaux, E., Louvet, C. *et al.* (2005) Updated results at 6 year of the GERCOR C96.1 phase III study comparing LVFU2 to monthly 5-FU-Leucovorin (mFufol) as adjuvant treatment for Dukes B2 and C colon cancer patients. *J Clin Oncol*, **23(Suppl)**, 3522.

101. Twelves, C., Wong, A., Nowacki, M.P., *et al.* (2005) Capecitabine as adjuvant treatment for stage III colon cancer. *N Engl J Med*, **352**, 2696–2704.

102. Wolmark, N., Wieand, S., Lembersky, B., Colangelo, L., Smith, R., Pazdur, R. (2004) A phase III trial comparing oral UFT to FULV in stage II and III carcinoma of the colon: results of NSABP C-06. *J Clin Oncol*, **22(14S, Suppl)**, 3508.

103. Andre, T., Boni, C., Navarro, M., *et al.* (2009) Improved overall survival with oxaliplatin, fluorouracil, and leucovorin as adjuvant treatment in stage II or III colon cancer in the MOSAIC trial. *J Clin Oncol*, **27**, 3109–3116.

104. Kuebler, J.P., Wieand, H.S., O'Connell, M.J., *et al.* (2007) Oxaliplatin combined with weekly bolus fluorouracil and leucovorin as surgical adjuvant chemotherapy for stage II and III colon cancer: results from NSABP C-07. *J Clin Oncol*, **25**, 2198–1204.

105. Saltz, B., Niedzwiecki, D., Hollis, D. *et al.* (2004) Irinotecan plus fluorouracil/leucovorin (IFL) versus fluorouracil/leucovorin alone (FL) in stage III colon cancer (intergroup trial CALGB C89803). *J Clin Oncol*, **22(14S, Suppl)**, 3500.

106. Van Cutsem, E., Labianca, R., Hossfeld, D. *et al.* (2005) Randomized phase III trial comparing infused irinotecan/5-fluorouracil (5-FU)/folinic acid (IF) versus 5-FU/FA (F) in stage III colon cancer patients (pts). (PETACC3). *J Clin Oncol*, **23(16S, Suppl)**, 8.

107. Goldberg, R.M., Rothenberg, M.L., Van Cutsem, E., *et al.* (2007) The continuum of care: a paradigm for the management of metastatic colorectal cancer. *Oncologist*, **12**, 38–50.

108. Buyse, M., Zeleniuch-Jacquotte, A., Chalmers, T.C. (1988) Adjuvant therapy of colorectal cancer. Why we still don't know. *JAMA*, **259**, 3571–3578.

109. Bedikian, A.Y., Valdivieso, M., Mavligit, G.M., *et al.* (1978) Sequential chemoimmunotherapy of colorectal cancer: evaluation of methotrexate, Baker's Antifol and levamisole. *Cancer*, **42**, 2169–2176.

110. Buroker, T.R., Moertel, C.G., Fleming, T.R., *et al.* (1985) A controlled evaluation of recent approaches to biochemical modulation or enhancement of 5-fluorouracil therapy in colorectal carcinoma. *J Clin Oncol*, **3**, 1624–1631.

111. Windle, R., Bell, P.R.,, Shaw, D. (1987) Five year results of a randomized trial of adjuvant 5-fluorouracil and levamisole in colorectal cancer. *Br J Surg*, **74**, 569–572.

112. Laurie, J.A., Moertel, C.G., Fleming, T.R., *et al.* (1989) Surgical adjuvant therapy of large-bowel carcinoma: an evaluation of levamisole and the combination of levamisole and fluorouracil. The North Central Cancer Treatment Group and the Mayo Clinic. *J Clin Oncol*, **7**, 1447–1456.

113. Moertel, C.G., Fleming, T.R., Macdonald, J.S., *et al.* (1990) Levamisole and fluorouracil for adjuvant therapy of resected colon carcinoma. *N Engl J Med*, **322**, 352–358.

114. NIH Consensus Conference. Adjuvant therapy for patients with colon and rectal cancer. *JAMA*, **264**, 1444–1450, 1990.

115. de Gramont, A., Bosset, J.F., Milan, C., *et al.* (1997) Randomized trial comparing monthly low-dose leucovorin and fluorouracil bolus with bimonthly high-dose leucovorin and fluorouracil bolus plus continuous infusion for advanced colorectal cancer: a French intergroup study. *J Clin Oncol*, **15**, 808–815.

116. Weh, H.J., Wilke, H.J., Dierlamm, J., *et al.* (1994) Weekly therapy with folinic acid (FA) and high-dose 5-fluorouracil (5-FU) 24-hour infusion in pretreated patients with metastatic colorectal carcinoma. A multicenter study by the Association of Medical Oncology of the German Cancer Society (AIO). *Ann Oncol*, **5**, 233–237.

117. Van Cutsem, E., Twelves, C., Cassidy, J., *et al.* (2001) Oral capecitabine compared with intravenous fluorouracil plus leucovorin in patients with metastatic colorectal cancer: results of a large phase III study. *J Clin Oncol*, **19**, 4097–4106.

118. Mayer, R.J. (2001) Oral versus intravenous fluoropyrimidines for advanced colorectal cancer: by either route, it's all the same. *J Clin Oncol*, **19**, 4093–4096.

119. Raymond, E., Faivre, S., Woynarowski, J.M., *et al.* (1998) Oxaliplatin: mechanism of action and antineoplastic activity. *Semin Oncol*, **25**, 4–12.

120. Raymond, E., Chaney, S.G., Taamma, A., *et al.* (1998) Oxaliplatin: a review of preclinical and clinical studies. *Ann Oncol*, **9**, 1053–1071.

121. Raymond, E., Faivre, S., Chaney, S., *et al.* () Cellular and molecular pharmacology of oxaliplatin. *Mol Cancer Ther*, **1**, 227–235.

122. de Gramont, A., Figer, A., Seymour, M., *et al.* (2000) Leucovorin and fluorouracil with or without oxaliplatin as first-line treatment in advanced colorectal cancer. *J Clin Oncol*, **18**, 2938–2947.

123. Falcone, A., Ricci, S., Brunetti, I., *et al.* (2007) Phase III trial of infusional fluorouracil, leucovorin, oxaliplatin, and irinotecan (FOLFOXIRI) compared with infusional fluorouracil, leucovorin, and irinotecan (FOLFIRI) as first-line treatment for metastatic colorectal cancer: the Gruppo Oncologico Nord Ovest. *J Clin Oncol*, **25**, 1670–1676.

124. Souglakos, J., Androulakis, N., Syrigos, K., *et al.* (2006) FOLFOXIRI (folinic acid, 5-fluorouracil, oxaliplatin and irinotecan) vs FOLFIRI (folinic acid, 5-fluorouracil and irinotecan) as first-line treatment in metastatic colorectal cancer (MCC): a multicentre randomised phase III trial from the Hellenic Oncology Research Group (HORG). *Br J Cancer*, **94**, 798–805.

125. Urban, D. (2011) Oxaliplatin induced neuropathy, *Oncology Review Daily*.

126. Iyer, L., Ratain, M.J. (1998) Clinical pharmacology of camptothecins. *Cancer Chemother Pharmacol*, **42(Suppl)**, S31–S43.

127. Bleiberg, H. (1999) CPT-11 in gastrointestinal cancer. *Eur J Cancer*, **35**, 371–379.

128. Cunningham, D., Pyrhonen, S., James, R.D., *et al.* (1998) Randomised trial of irinotecan plus supportive care versus supportive care alone after fluorouracil failure for patients with metastatic colorectal cancer. *Lancet*, **352**, 1413–1418.

129. Rougier, P., Van Cutsem, E., Bajetta, E., *et al.* (1998) Randomised trial of irinotecan versus fluorouracil by continuous infusion after fluorouracil failure in patients with metastatic colorectal cancer. *Lancet*, **352**, 1407–1412.

130. O'Connell, M.J. (2009) Oxaliplatin or irinotecan as adjuvant therapy for colon cancer: the results are in. *J Clin Oncol*, **27**, 3082–3084.

131. Iyer, L., Das, S., Janisch, L., *et al.* (2002) UGT1A1*28 polymorphism as a determinant of irinotecan disposition and toxicity. *Pharmacogenomics J*, **2**, 43–47.

132. Ando, Y., Saka, H., Asai, G., *et al.* (1998) UGT1A1 genotypes and glucuronidation of SN-38, the active metabolite of irinotecan. *Ann Oncol*, **9**, 845–847.

133. Innocenti, F., Undevia, S.D., Iyer, L., *et al.* (2004) Genetic variants in the UDP-glucuronosyltransferase 1A1 gene predict the risk of severe neutropenia of irinotecan. *J Clin Oncol*, **22**, 1382–1388.

134. Cunningham, D., Humblet, Y., Siena, S., *et al.* (2004) Cetuximab monotherapy and cetuximab plus irinotecan in irinotecan-refractory metastatic colorectal cancer. *N Engl J Med*, **351**, 337–345.

135. Messersmith, W.A., Ahnen DJ (2008) Targeting EGFR in colorectal cancer. *N Engl J Med*, **359**, 1834–1836.

136. Normanno, N., Tejpar, S., Ciardiello, F. (2010) Re: Biomarkers predicting clinical outcome of epidermal growth factor receptor-targeted therapy in metastatic colorectal cancer. *J Natl Cancer Inst*, **102**, 573; author reply 573–575.

137. de Bono, J.S., Rowinsky, E.K. (2002) Therapeutics targeting signal transduction for patients with colorectal carcinoma. *Br Med Bull*, **64**, 227–254.

138. Ortega, J., Vigil, C.E., Chodkiewicz, C. (2010) Current progress in targeted therapy for colorectal cancer. *Cancer Control*, **17**, 7–15.

139. Giusti, R.M., Shastri, K., Pilaro, A.M., *et al.* (2008) U.S. Food and Drug Administration approval: panitumumab for epidermal growth factor receptor-expressing metastatic colorectal carcinoma with progression following fluoropyrimidine-, oxaliplatin-, and irinotecan-containing chemotherapy regimens. *Clin Cancer Res*, **14**, 1296–1302.

140. Sepulveda, A.R. (2010) Molecular Diagnosis for Colorectal Cancer Patients.

141. Cohen, S.J., Cohen, R.B., Meropol, N.J. (2005) Targeting signal transduction pathways in colorectal cancer–more than skin deep. *J Clin Oncol*, **23**, 5374–5385.

142. Saltz, L.B., Meropol, N.J., Loehrer, P.J. Sr., *et al.* (2004) Phase II trial of cetuximab in patients with refractory colorectal cancer that expresses the epidermal growth factor receptor. *J Clin Oncol*, **22**, 1201–1208.

143. Saltz, L., Rubin, M., Hochster, H., *et al.* (2001) Cetuximab (IMC-C225) plus Irinotecan (CPT-11) is active in CPT-11-Refractory Colorectal Cancer (CRC) that Expresses Epidermal Growth Factor Receptor (EGFR). *Proc Am Soc Clin Oncol*, **20**, abstract 7.

144. Van Cutsem, E. , Kohne, C.H., Hitre, E., *et al.* (2009) Cetuximab and chemotherapy as initial treatment for metastatic colorectal cancer. *N Engl J Med*, **360**, 1408–1417.

145. Hecht, J., Patnaik, A., Malik, I., *et al.* (2004) ABX-EGF monotherapy in patients with metastatic colorectal cancer (mCRC): an updated analysis. *J Clin Oncol*, **22(Suppl)**, abstract 3511.

146. Van Cutsem, E., Peeters, M., Siena, S., *et al.* (2007) Open-label phase III trial of panitumumab plus best supportive care compared with best supportive care alone in patients with chemotherapy-refractory metastatic colorectal cancer. *J Clin Oncol*, **25**, 1658–1664.

147. Segaert, S., Van Cutsem, E. (2005) Clinical signs, pathophysiology and management of skin toxicity during therapy with epidermal growth factor receptor inhibitors. *Ann Oncol*, **16**, 1425–1433.

148. Hurwitz, H., Fehrenbacher, L., Novotny, W., *et al.* (2004) Bevacizumab plus irinotecan, fluorouracil, and leucovorin for metastatic colorectal cancer. *N Engl J Med*, **350**, 2335–2342.

149. Giantonio, B.J., Catalano, P.J., Meropol, N.J., *et al.* (2007) Bevacizumab in combination with oxaliplatin, fluorouracil, and leucovorin (FOLFOX4) for previously treated metastatic colorectal cancer: results from the Eastern Cooperative Oncology Group Study E3200. *J Clin Oncol*, **25**, 1539–1544.

150. Seymour, M.T., Maughan, T.S., Ledermann, J.A., *et al.* (2007) Different strategies of sequential and combination chemotherapy for patients with poor prognosis advanced colorectal cancer (MRC FOCUS): a randomised controlled trial. *Lancet*, **370**, 143–152.

151. Shah, U. (2008) Sequential versus combination therapy in the treatment of patients with advanced colorectal cancer. *Clin Colorectal Cancer*, **7(5)**, 315–320.

152. Boige, V., Mendiboure, J., Pignon, J.P., *et al.* (2010) Pharmacogenetic assessment of toxicity and outcome in patients with metastatic colorectal cancer treated with LV5FU2, FOLFOX, and FOLFIRI: FFCD 2000–05. *J Clin Oncol*, **28**, 2556–2564.

153. Hamilton, S.R. (2008) Targeted therapy of cancer: new roles for pathologists in colorectal cancer. *Mod Pathol*, **21(Suppl 2)**, S23–S30.

154. Allen, W.L., Johnston, P.G. (2005) Role of genomic markers in colorectal cancer treatment. *J Clin Oncol*, **23**, 4545–4552.

155. Van Cutsem, E. , Nordlinger, B., Cervantes, A. (2010) Advanced colorectal cancer: ESMO Clinical Practice Guidelines for treatment. *Ann Oncol*, **21(Suppl 5)**, v93–v97.

156. Karapetis, C.S., Khambata-Ford, S., Jonker, D.J., *et al.* (2008) K-ras mutations and benefit from cetuximab in advanced colorectal cancer. *N Engl J Med*, **359**, 1757–1765.

157. Lievre, A., Bachet, J.B., Boige, V., *et al.* (2008) KRAS mutations as an independent prognostic factor in patients with advanced colorectal cancer treated with cetuximab. *J Clin Oncol*, **26**, 374–379.

158. Amado, R.G., Wolf, M., Peeters, M., *et al.* (2008) Wild-type KRAS is required for panitumumab efficacy in patients with metastatic colorectal cancer. *J Clin Oncol*, **26**, 1626–1634.

159. Allegra, C.J., Jessup, J.M., Somerfield, M.R., *et al.* (2009) American Society of Clinical Oncology provisional clinical opinion: testing for KRAS gene mutations in patients with metastatic colorectal carcinoma to predict response to anti-epidermal growth factor receptor monoclonal antibody therapy. *J Clin Oncol*, **27**, 2091–2096.

160. Sharp, D. (2009) Personalized Therapy Arrives for Patients with Colorectal Cancer, Sciencewatch. *Sciencewatch*.com, *Thomson Reuters*.

161. Chang, D.Z., Kumar, V., Ma, Y., *et al.* (2009) Individualized therapies in colorectal cancer: KRAS as a marker for response to EGFR-targeted therapy. *J Hematol Oncol*, **2**, 18.

162. Park, J.H., Kim, I.J., Kang, H.C., *et al.* (2004) Oligonucleotide microarray-based mutation detection of the K-ras gene in colorectal cancers with use of competitive DNA hybridization. *Clin Chem*, **50**, 1688–1691.

163. Bokemeyer, C., Bondarenko, I., hartmann, J.T., *et al.* (2008) KRAS status and efficacy of first-line treatment of patients with metastatic colorectal cancer (mCRC) with FOLFOX with or without cetuximab: The OPUS experience. *J Clin Oncol*, **26**, abstract 4000.

164. Van Cutsem, E., Lang, I., D'Haens, G., *et al.* (2008) KRAS status and efficacy in the first-line treatment of patients with metastatic colorectal cancer (mCRC) treated with FOLFIRI with or without cetuximab: The CRYSTAL experience. *Journal of Clinical Oncology*, **26**, abstract 2.

165. Cervantes, A., Macarulla, T., Martinelli, E., *et al.* (2008) Correlation of KRAS status (wild type [wt] vs. mutant [mt]) with efficacy to first-line cetuximab in a study of cetuximab single agent followed by cetuximab + FOLFIRI in patients (pts) with metastatic colorectal cancer (mCRC). *J Clin Oncol*, **26**, abstract 4129.

166. Shankaran, V., Bentrem, D., Mulcahy, M.F., *et al.* (2009) Economic implications of Kras testing in metastatic colorectal cancer (mCRC). Presented at: the 2009 Gastrointestinal Cancers Symposium, San Fransisco, CA, USA.

167. Yabroff, K.R., Schrag, D. (2009) Challenges and opportunities for use of cost-effectiveness analysis. *J Natl Cancer Inst*, **101**, 1161–1163.

168. Kerr, D., Gray, R., Quirke, P. *et al.* (2009) A quantitative multigene RT-PCR assay for prediction of recurrence in stage II colon cancer: Selection of the genes in four large studies and results of the independent, prospectively designed QUASAR validation study. *J Clin Oncol*, **27**, 15s.

169. MedicalNewsToday (2009) Genomic Health's Oncotype DX(R) Colon Cancer Test Predicts Individualized Recurrence Risk For Stage II Colon Cancer Patients.

170. Oncotype DX® Colon Cancer Assay, Recurrent Risk. Recurrence Score® Result, Genomic Health, 2011. http://www.oncotypedx.com/enUS/Colon/HealthcareProfessionals/RecurrenceRisk/ScoreResult

171. Salazar, R., Roepman, P., Capella, G. *et al.* (2010) Gene expression signature to improve prognosis prediction of stage II and III colorectal cancer. *J Clin Oncol*, **29(1)**, 17–24.

172. Rosenberg, R. (2011) Independent validation of a prognostic genomic profile (ColoPrint) for stage II colon cancer (CC) patients. *J Clin Oncol*, **29(Suppl 4)**, abstract 358.

173. ColoPrint(R): A Gene Expression Profile that Identifies Patients at High Risk of Metastasis, Agendia.

174. Barbara, B. (2011) Expert point of view: genomic profile test again validated for colon cancer recurrence, THE ASCO POST.

175. Genomics, E. (2011) OncoDefender-CRC: Prognostic Test Questions and Answers for Physicians, Everist Genomics.

176. Bosset, J.F., Calais, G., Mineur, L., *et al.* (2005) Enhanced tumoricidal effect of chemotherapy with preoperative radiotherapy for rectal cancer: preliminary results–EORTC 22921. *J Clin Oncol*, **23**, 5620–5627.

177. Brown, G. (2007) Colorectal Cancer. 1st ed, Cambridge University Press.

178. Sinha, R. (2002) An epidemiologic approach to studying heterocyclic amines. *Mutat Res*, **506–507**, 197–204.

179. Bosset, J.F., Collette, L., Calais, G., *et al.* (2006) Chemotherapy with preoperative radiotherapy in rectal cancer. *N Engl J Med*, **355**, 1114–1123.

180. Onaitis, M.W., Noone, R.B., Hartwig, M., *et al.* (2001) Neoadjuvant chemoradiation for rectal cancer: analysis of clinical outcomes from a 13-year institutional experience. *Ann Surg*, **233**, 778–785.

181. Learn About Cancer, Colorectal Cancer, American Cancer Society, (2011). http://www.cancer.org/cancer/colonandrectumcancer/detailedguide/colorectal-cancer-treating-by-stage-colon

182. Gruenberger, B., Tamandl, D., Schueller, J., *et al.* (2008) Bevacizumab, capecitabine, and oxaliplatin as neoadjuvant therapy for patients with potentially curable metastatic colorectal cancer. *J Clin Oncol*, **26**, 1830–1835.

183. Bokemeyer, C., Bondarenko, I., Makhson, A., *et al.* (2009) Fluorouracil, leucovorin, and oxaliplatin with and without cetuximab in the first-line treatment of metastatic colorectal cancer. *J Clin Oncol*, **27**, 663–671.

184. Van Cutsem, E., Oliveira, J. (2009) Advanced colorectal cancer: ESMO clinical recommendations for diagnosis, treatment and follow-up. *Ann Oncol*, **20(Suppl 4)**, 61–63.

185. Dahabre, J., Vasilaki, M., Stathopoulos, G.P., *et al.* (2007) Surgical management in lung metastases from colorectal cancer. *Anticancer Res*, **27**, 4387–4390.

186. Venook, A., Curley, S.A. (2010) Management of potentially resectable colorectal cancer liver metastasis, UptoDate. UpToDate.com, UpToDate, pp. 1–39.

187. National Comprehensive Cancer Network (2010) *Colon Cancer Clinical Practice Guidelines in Oncology*—v.1.2007.

188. Kelly, H., Goldberg, R.M. (2005) Systemic therapy for metastatic colorectal cancer: current options, current evidence. *J Clin Oncol*, **23**, 4553–4560.

189. Mitry, E., Fields, A.L., Bleiberg, H., *et al.* (2008) Adjuvant chemotherapy after potentially curative resection of metastases from colorectal cancer: a pooled analysis of two randomized trials. *J Clin Oncol*, **26**, 4906–4911.

190. Alden, T.D., Gianino, J.W., Saclarides, T.J. (1996) Brain metastases from colorectal cancer. *Dis Colon Rectum*, **39**, 541–545.

191. Baek, J.Y., Kang, M.H., Hong, Y.S., *et al.* (2011) Characteristics and prognosis of patients with colorectal cancer-associated brain metastases in the era of modern systemic chemotherapy. *J Neurooncol*, **104(4)**, 745–753.

192. Power, D.G., Kemeny, N.E. (2010) Role of adjuvant therapy after resection of colorectal cancer liver metastases. *J Clin Oncol*, **28**, 2300–2309.

193. Young, A., Rea, D. (2000) ABC of colorectal cancer: treatment of advanced disease. *BMJ*, **321**, 1278–1281.

194. Wong, S.L., Mangu, P.B., Choti, M.A., *et al.* (2010) American Society of Clinical Oncology 2009 clinical evidence review on radiofrequency ablation of hepatic metastases from colorectal cancer. *J Clin Oncol*, **28**, 493–508.

195. Alberts, S.R., Roh, M.S., Mahoney, M.R., *et al.* (2010) Alternating systemic and hepatic artery infusion therapy for resected liver metastases from colorectal cancer: a North Central Cancer Treatment Group (NCCTG)/ National Surgical Adjuvant Breast and Bowel Project (NSABP) phase II intergroup trial, N9945/CI-66. *J Clin Oncol*, **28**, 853–858.

196. Kemeny, N., Huang, Y., Cohen, A.M., *et al.* (1999) Hepatic arterial infusion of chemotherapy after resection of hepatic metastases from colorectal cancer. *N Engl J Med*, **341**, 2039–2048.

197. Mocellin, S., Pilati, P., Lise, M., *et al.* (2007) Meta-analysis of hepatic arterial infusion for unresectable liver metastases from colorectal cancer: the end of an era? *J Clin Oncol*, **25**, 5649–5654.

198. Laohavinij, S., Maneechavakajorn, J., Techatanol, P. (2010) Prognostic factors for survival in colorectal cancer patients. *J Med Assoc Thai*, **93**, 1156–66.

199. Sorbye, H. (2008) Prognostic clinical factors in metastatic colorectal cancer, *Advances in Gastrointestinal Cancer*. findarticles.com.

200. Kohne, C.H., Cunningham, D., Di, C.F., *et al.* (2002) Clinical determinants of survival in patients with 5-fluorouracil-based treatment for metastatic

colorectal cancer: results of a multivariate analysis of 3825 patients. *Ann Oncol*, **13**, 308–317.

201. Locker, G.Y., Hamilton, S., Harris, J., *et al.* (2006) ASCO 2006 update of recommendations for the use of tumor markers in gastrointestinal cancer. *J Clin Oncol*, **24**, 5313–5327.

202. Moertel, C.G., Fleming, T.R., Macdonald, J.S., *et al.* (1993) An evaluation of the carcinoembryonic antigen (CEA) test for monitoring patients with resected colon cancer. *JAMA*, **270**, 943–947.

203. Soeth, E., Wirth, T., List, H.J., *et al.* (2001) Controlled ribozyme targeting demonstrates an antiapoptotic effect of carcinoembryonic antigen in HT29 colon cancer cells. *Clin Cancer Res*, **7**, 2022–30.

204. Popat, S., Hubner, R., Houlston R (2005) Systematic review of microsatellite instability and colorectal cancer prognosis. *J Clin Oncol*, **23(3)**, 609–618.

205. DeCosse, J.J., Cennerazzo, W.J. (1997) Quality-of-life management of patients with colorectal cancer. *CA Cancer J Clin*, **47**, 198–206.

206. Kim, J., Takeuchi, H., Lam, S.T., *et al.* (2005) Chemokine receptor CXCR4 expression in colorectal cancer patients increases the risk for recurrence and for poor survival. *J Clin Oncol*, **23**, 2744–2753.

207. Desch, C.E., Benson, A.B. III, Somerfield, M.R., *et al.* (2005) Colorectal cancer surveillance: 2005 update of an American Society of Clinical Oncology practice guideline. *J Clin Oncol*, **23**, 8512–8519.

208. Kornek, G.V., Scheithauer, W. (2003) Follow-up investigations in colorectal cancer. *Onkologie*, **26**, 303–307.

209. Imperiale, T.F., Glowinski, E.A., Lin-Cooper, C., *et al.* (2008) Five-year risk of colorectal neoplasia after negative screening colonoscopy. *N Engl J Med*, **359**, 1218–1224.

210. American Society of Clinical Oncology (2009) What to know: ASCO's Guideline on Tumor Markers for Gastrointestinal Cancers. www.cancer.net.

211. Miles, K., Burkill, G. (2007) Colorectal cancer: imaging surveillance following resection of primary tumour. *Cancer Imaging*, **7**(Spec No A), S143–S149.

212. Chau, I., Allen, M.J., Cunningham, D., *et al.* (2004) The value of routine serum carcino-embryonic antigen measurement and computed tomography in the surveillance of patients after adjuvant chemotherapy for colorectal cancer. *J Clin Oncol*, **22**, 1420–1429.

213. Roy, H.K., Bianchi, L.K. (2008) Colorectal cancer risk: black, white, or shades of gray? *JAMA*, **300**, 1459–1461.

214. Platz, E.A., Willett, W.C., Colditz, G.A., *et al.* (2000) Proportion of colon cancer risk that might be preventable in a cohort of middle-aged US men. *Cancer Causes Control*, **11**, 579–588.

215. Colditz, G.A., Atwood, K.A., Emmons, K., *et al.* (2000) Harvard report on cancer prevention volume 4: Harvard Cancer Risk Index. Risk Index Working Group, Harvard Center for Cancer Prevention. *Cancer Causes Control*, **11**, 477–488.

216. Takahashi, H. (2007) Metabolic syndrome and precancerous lesions of colon cancer. Presented at: the 2007 Gastrointestinal Cancers Symposium, Orlando, FL, USA.

217. Huxley, R.R., Ansary-Moghaddam, A., Clifton, P., *et al.* (2009) The impact of dietary and lifestyle risk factors on risk of colorectal cancer: a quantitative overview of the epidemiological evidence. *Int J Cancer*, **125**, 171–180.

218. Stein, C.J., Colditz GA (2004) Modifiable risk factors for cancer. *Br J Cancer*, **90**, 299–303.

219. Clevers, H. (2006) Colon cancer–understanding how NSAIDs work. *N Engl J Med*, **354**, 761–763.

220. Giovannucci, E., Rimm, E.B., Ascherio, A., *et al.* (1995) Alcohol, low-methionine–low-folate diets, and risk of colon cancer in men. *J Natl Cancer Inst*, **87**, 265–273.

221. Chan, J.A., Meyerhardt, J.A., Chan, A.T., *et al.* (2006) Hormone replacement therapy and survival after colorectal cancer diagnosis. *J Clin Oncol*, **24**, 5680–5686.

222. Santarelli, R.L., Pierre, F., Corpet, D.E. (2008) Processed meat and colorectal cancer: a review of epidemiologic and experimental evidence. *Nutr Cancer*, **60**, 131–144.

223. Kabat, G.C., Miller, A.B., Jain, M., *et al.* (2007) A cohort study of dietary iron and heme iron intake and risk of colorectal cancer in women. *Br J Cancer*, **97**, 118–122.

224. Friedenreich, C., Norat, T., Steindorf, K., *et al.* (2006) Physical activity and risk of colon and rectal cancers: the European prospective investigation into cancer and nutrition. *Cancer Epidemiol Biomarkers Prev*, **15**, 2398–2407.

225. Howard, R.A., Freedman, D.M., Park, Y., *et al.* (2008) Physical activity, sedentary behavior, and the risk of colon and rectal cancer in the NIH-AARP Diet and Health Study. *Cancer Causes Control*, **19**, 939–953.

226. Samad, A.K., Taylor, R.S., Marshall, T., *et al.* (2005) A meta-analysis of the association of physical activity with reduced risk of colorectal cancer. *Colorectal Dis*, **7**, 204–213.

227. Wolin, K.Y., Yan, Y., Colditz, G.A., *et al.* (2009) Physical activity and colon cancer prevention: a meta-analysis. *Br J Cancer*, **100**, 611–616.

228. Chan, A.T., Giovannucci, E.L. (2010) Primary prevention of colorectal cancer. *Gastroenterology*, **138**, 2029–2043 e10.

229. Larsson, S.C., Orsini, N., Wolk, A. (2005) Diabetes mellitus and risk of colorectal cancer: a meta-analysis. *J Natl Cancer Inst*, **97**, 1679–1687.

230. Bonovas, S., Filioussi, K., Flordellis, C.S., *et al.* (2007) Statins and the risk of colorectal cancer: a meta-analysis of 18 studies involving more than 1.5 million patients. *J Clin Oncol*, **25**, 3462–3468.

231. Rock, C.L. (2011) Milk and the risk and progression of cancer. *Nestle Nutr Workshop Ser Pediatr Program*, **67**, 173–185.

232. Weingarten, M.A., Zalmanovici, A., Yaphe J (2008) Dietary calcium supplementation for preventing colorectal cancer and adenomatous polyps. *Cochrane Database Syst Rev*, CD003548.

233. Bustin, S.A. (unknown) *Role of VDR-Signalling in Colorectal Tumourigenesis*, London.

234. Steinbach, G., Lynch, P.M., Phillips, R.K., *et al.* (2000) The effect of celecoxib, a cyclooxygenase-2 inhibitor, in familial adenomatous polyposis. *N Engl J Med*, **342**, 1946–1952.

235. Sinicrope, F.A., Half, E., Morris, J.S., *et al.* (2004) Cell proliferation and apoptotic indices predict adenoma regression in a placebo-controlled trial of celecoxib in familial adenomatous polyposis patients. *Cancer Epidemiol Biomarkers Prev*, **13**, 920–927.

236. Lin, J.H., Giovannucci, E. (2010) Sex hormones and colorectal cancer: what have we learned so far? *J Natl Cancer Inst*, **102**, 1746–1747.

237. Borgelt, L., Umland, E. (2000) Benefits and challenges of hormone replacement therapy. *J Am Pharm Assoc (Wash)*, **40**, S30–S31.

238. Sprangers, M.A., Taal, B.G., Aaronson, N.K., *et al.* (1995) Quality of life in colorectal cancer. Stoma vs. nonstoma patients. *Dis Colon Rectum*, **38**, 361–369.

239. Grumann, M.M., Noack, E.M., Hoffmann, I.A., *et al.* (2001) Comparison of quality of life in patients undergoing abdominoperineal extirpation or anterior resection for rectal cancer. *Ann Surg*, **233**, 149–156.
240. Engel, J., Kerr, J., Schlesinger-Raab, A., *et al.* (2003) Quality of life in rectal cancer patients: a four-year prospective study. *Ann Surg*, **238**, 203–213.
241. Ustun, C., Ceber, E. (2004) Ethical issues for cancer screenings. Five countries–four types of cancer. *Prev Med*, **39**, 223–229.
242. Bagai, A., Parsons, K., Malone, B., *et al.* (2007) Workplace colorectal cancer-screening awareness programs: an adjunct to primary care practice? *J Community Health*, **32**, 157–167.

6 Anal Cancer

Jeffrey J. Meyer,[1] Christopher G. Willett,[2] and Brian G. Czito[2]
[1]UT-Southwestern Medical Center, Dallas, TX, USA
[2]Duke University Medical Center, Durham, NC, USA

Key Points

- A variety of tumor types can arise in the anal canal and surrounding perianal skin; squamous cell tumors are the most common.
- Infection with human papillomavirus is strongly associated with development of squamous cell anal tumors.
- Treatment of anal canal cancer has evolved from abdominoperineal resection to sphincter-preserving, "definitive" concurrent radiation therapy and chemotherapy in most cases.
- A number of ongoing clinical studies will continue to refine the combined modality approach to squamous cell anal cancer in an effort to improve tumor outcomes while minimizing toxicity.

Key Web Links

http://www.nccn.org
US National Comprehensive Cancer Network—provides guidelines for diagnosis, staging, and management of various cancer

http://www.asco.org
American Society of Clinical Oncology—provides resources on cancer education and policies

Potential Pitfalls

- Different types of tumors can arise in the anal canal. Treatments are tailored to the histology, with concurrent radiation therapy and chemotherapy usually the treatment of choice in localized squamous cell tumors, with surgery reserved for local tumor persistence or recurrence. Surgery can play an important role in the treatment of anal canal adenocarcinomas.

Handbook of Gastrointestinal Cancer, First Edition. Edited by Janusz Jankowski and Ernest Hawk.
© 2013 John Wiley & Sons, Ltd. Published 2013 by John Wiley & Sons, Ltd.

- Concurrent radiation therapy and chemotherapy can provide long-term disease-free survival in the management of squamous cell anal cancer, and requires close monitoring of acute and late toxicities.

Epidemiology

Prior to reviewing the epidemiology of anal cancer, one must first understand the anatomical relations and histological features of the "anal canal." A variety of terms regarding anatomical classification and histology of the anal canal are present in the literature, which can lead to some confusion.

Histologically, the dentate, or pectinate, line marks the separation between the squamous mucosa of the distal anal canal and the transitional epithelium that "transitions" into the glandular mucosa of the distal rectum. As noted, definitions have varied in the literature, but the anal canal can be considered to extend from the anal verge, or orifice, where the perianal skin merges with the squamous cell mucosal lining of the distal anal canal, to the top of the anal sphincter mechanism, where the external anal sphincter muscle joins the puborectalis segment of the levator ani muscle at the anorectal ring. Although variable, the length of the canal typically measures about 4 cm. Some series define the anal canal as the canal between the anorectal ring and the dentate line.[1] As opposed to exact location within the canal proximal to the anal verge, histology is generally the more important feature of a tumor with regard to management options. The term "anal margin" is also variably used in the literature, but it is frequently defined as the perianal skin within 5 cm of the anal verge.[2] Figure 6.1 is a depiction of the anal canal.

A variety of malignancies can arise within the anal canal. To simplify matters, these can be divided into squamous cell and nonsquamous cell tumors. Squamous cell tumors are the most common presentation. Histological descriptions such as basaloid/cloacogenic (tumors arising in the transitional mucosa of the proximal canal) are not as relevant for practical management and are no longer commonly used in histopathologic descriptions.[3] Tumors arising in this area are considered squamous cell tumors and are managed accordingly. Nonsquamous cell tumors including adenocarcinomas, melanomas, lymphomas, and sarcomas have been described, but are less common. A suspected anal adenocarcinoma may in fact be an extension from a distal rectal adenocarcinoma in some scenarios. Ultimately, tumor location within the anal canal is not as important as histological subtype; true anal canal adenocarcinomas are treated as conventional rectal adenocarcinomas, as will be discussed later.

Tumors that lie near, but definitively outside of, the anal verge (perianal skin lesions) are typically squamous cell skin cancers that can be managed

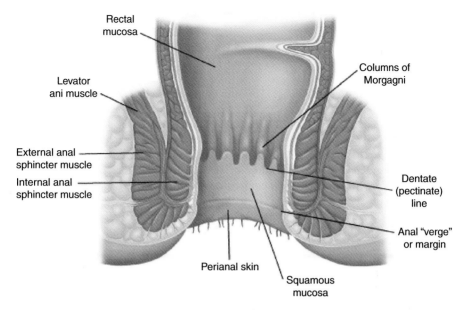

Rectal mucosa

Levator ani muscle

External anal sphincter muscle

Internal anal sphincter muscle

Columns of Morgagni

Dentate (pectinate) line

Anal "verge" or margin

Perianal skin

Squamous mucosa

Figure 6.1 Anatomy of the anal canal. Anatomical features of the anal verge, anal canal, and sphincter musculature. (Reproduced with permission from Ryan, D.P. & Willett, C.G. (2011) Classification and epidemiology of anal cancer. In: UpToDate, Basow, D.S. (ed), UpToDate, Waltham, MA. Copyright ©2011 UpToDate, Inc. For more information, visit www.uptodate.com.)

as such, although there is controversy regarding this point, which will be addressed later in this chapter. From a practical point of view, invasion locally up to or through the anal verge may impact treatment strategies for these tumors.

Squamous cell anal canal tumors are relatively uncommon, with about 5000 new presentations annually in the United States.[4] However, the incidence has climbed steadily in recent years. Epidemiological investigations have identified a number of risk factors associated with the development of squamous cell anal tumors. An increased number of sexual partners have been associated with an increased risk of developing anal cancer.[5] In one large case-control series, an increasing number of sexual partners were associated with the development of anal cancer in both men and women (odds ratio of 4.5 for women and 2.5 for men with ≥10 sexual partners).[5] This study also demonstrated that a history of anal warts was associated with a higher risk of developing anal cancer, as was receptive anal intercourse in women. Other reports have also shown a relationship between receptive anal intercourse in men who have sex with men and subsequent development of anal cancer.[6] Similarly, a prior history of cervical and genital malignancies has also been found to be associated with a higher risk of subsequent development of anal cancer.[7,8]

These results strongly suggest that a sexually transmitted factor is important in anal cancer carcinogenesis. Thus, it is not surprising that there is a clear association between viral infection with certain subtypes of human papillomavirus (HPV) and development of preinvasive and invasive squamous cell anal cancer, and the majority of squamous cell anal tumors harbor HPV DNA.[5,9,10] As with cervical cancer, there are certain subtypes of HPV, in particular HPV-16, commonly found in the cells of malignant lesions. The relationship between high-risk HPV subtype infection and subsequent malignant cellular transformation is well studied in squamous cell carcinomas of the uterine cervix, and as mentioned earlier, women with cervical cancer are also at significantly increased risk of developing squamous cell anal cancer compared with the general population.[7] Infection with HPV can lead to a procession from a preinvasive phase (anal intraepithelial neoplasia (AIN), similar to preinvasive cervical lesions) to frank invasive tumors.[11]

Other identified independent risk factors include non-HIV-related chronic immunosuppression and cigarette smoking.[12–14] In another series, patients receiving chronic steroid therapy for amelioration of autoimmunity were also found to be predisposed to HPV-associated anogenital tumor formation. Immunosuppression may prevent effective immune responses to HPV and also hinder antitumor immunity. Cigarette smoking is also associated with development of anal cancer, much as it is with cervical and other cancers.[15] The risk of anal cancer appears to be related to the pack-year history of smoking, with more extensive histories associated with a higher risk. The mechanism of the association of smoking with anal tumors is unclear, but there may be a cocarcinogen effect in the context of HPV infection.[16]

The association with HIV as an independent risk factor for the development of anal cancer is controversial. HIV may not be an independent risk factor for development of anal cancer but may facilitate development of anal cancer in HPV-positive patients[17,18] as a result of impaired immunity. In one series, patients who were simultaneously HPV and HIV positive appeared to have a higher risk of developing AIN and anal cancer as opposed to those who were HIV negative. In a separate analysis, patients with low CD4+ T-cell counts were at risk for more aggressive courses of HPV infection.

Diagnosis

Histological confirmation of malignancy by tissue biopsy is required prior to initiation of tumor-directed therapy. Staging, as with most tumors, involves determining local extent of the primary disease, whether or not nodal metastases are present, and whether or not there is evidence for distant spread of disease (outside of the pelvis). Computed tomography (CT) of the chest, abdomen, and pelvis is typically obtained, and digital and endoscopic examination of the anus and rectum, in addition to palpation of the inguinal region, is necessary to delineate the extent of gross tumor.

Positron emission tomography (PET) and PET–CT are also now routinely integrated into the staging algorithm for patients.[19–21] In one series, PET–CT appeared to have a higher sensitivity than conventional imaging (CT and/or MRI) for detecting regional lymph node metastases (89% vs. 62%), although for practical reasons, not all nodes could be biopsied for a true measure of sensitivity and specificity. PET was found to change planned radiation therapy fields in 13% of patients and thus worthy of inclusion in the staging process.[21] Of note, HIV-positive patients may have false-positive fluorodeoxyglucose (FDG)-avid lymph nodes. Biopsy may be necessary in these situations to determine whether or not there is true nodal metastatic disease versus a benign inflammatory process. Table 6.1 describes the current staging system.

Table 6.1 Anal cancer: Staging

Primary tumor (T)	
TX	Primary tumor cannot be assessed
T0	No evidence of primary tumor
Tis	Carcinoma in situ (Bowen's disease, high-grade squamous intraepithelial lesion (HSIL), anal intraepithelial neoplasia II-III (AIN II-III)
T1	Tumor 2 cm or less in greatest dimension
T2	Tumor more than 2 cm but not more than 5 cm in greatest dimension
T3	Tumore more than 5 cm in greatest dimension
T4	Tumor of any size invades adjacent organ(s), e.g., vagina, urethra, bladder*

*Note: Direct invasion of the rectal wall, perirectal skin, subcutaneous tissue, or the sphincter muscle(s) is not classified at T4.

Regional lymph nodes (N)	
NX	Regional lymph nodes cannot be assessed
N0	No regional lymph node metastasis
N1	Metastasis in perirectal lymph node(s)
N2	Metastasis in unilateral internal iliac and/or inguinal lymph node(s)
N3	Metastasis in perirectal and inguinal lymph nodes and/or bilateral internal iliac and/or inguinal lymph nodes

Distant metastasis (M)	
M0	No distant metastasis
M1	Distant metastasis

Anatomic stage/Prognostic groups			
0	Tis	N0	M0
I	T1	N0	M0
II	T2	N0	M0
	T3	N0	M0
IIIA	T1	N1	M0
	T2	N1	M0
	T3	N1	M0
	T4	N0	M0
IIIB	T4	N1	M0
	Any T	N2	M0
	Any T	N3	M0
IV	Any T	Any N	M0

Prevention

As mentioned earlier, AIN is thought to represent the precursor lesion to invasive anal cancer. AIN is broadly subdivided into low- and high-grade AIN. Given the success of cervical cancer screening in women, there has been a natural interest in the potential value of screening of patients at high risk for development of AIN and subsequent anal cancer. When performed, screening is usually in the form of analysis of anal cytology obtained by swabbing the anal canal ("anal Pap smear"). Sensitivity for detection of dysplasia appears higher (approximately 75%) in HIV-positive patients as opposed to HIV-negative patients (approximately 60%).[22,23] It is also higher in HIV-positive patients with lower CD4 counts.[22] In patients with abnormal cytology, anoscopy with administration of 3% acetic acid can then be performed to guide biopsies, much as is done with cervical colposcopy.

Treatment of high-grade AIN, thought to be the direct precursor to invasive anal cancer, can take many forms. Larger mucosal lesions can be ablated with anoscopic-directed electrocautery. Smaller lesions can be treated with topical trichloroacetic acid (TCA), topical 5-fluorouracil (5-FU), or imiquimod.[24-26] Topical applications yield lesion control in the range of 60–80%.

To date, however, there are no established guidelines for anal cancer screening in high-risk groups as there are for cervical cancer screening. The main debate regards the cost-effectiveness of screening programs. One important study showed annual screening in HIV-positive men who have sex with men to be of value.[27] The cost-effectiveness of screening was deemed comparable with the common practice of using prophylactic antibiotics in HIV-positive patients with very low CD4 counts.

Cancer management

Perianal skin tumors

Tumors that lie definitively distal to the anal verge (perianal skin) may be managed as skin tumors. Treatment options for squamous cell tumors of the perianal skin include local excision with or without adjuvant radiation, or radiation with or without chemotherapy. The treatment approach must take into account expected morbidity. Chapet et al.[2] reviewed their experience with 26 patients with tumors of the perianal skin (5 patients also had involvement of the anal canal). Twenty-one tumors were ≤5 cm in diameter. Fourteen patients were treated with definitive radiation (with or without chemotherapy), and 12 patients were treated with radiation after initial local excision. The initial crude local control rate was 61.4% (16/26). After salvage surgical treatment, this increased to 80.8%. Five-year cause-specific survival was 88.3%. Khanfir et al.[28] reported similar results in their series of 45 patients. Twenty-nine patients underwent local excision preceding radiation. Treatment fields were variable as a function of patient and tumor features. Five-year local–regional control was 78% and 5-year disease-free survival was 86%.

Balamucki *et al.*[29] recently updated the University of Florida experience with definitive radiotherapy and chemoradiotherapy for squamous cell tumors of the anal margin. Twenty-six patients were treated. Two patients developed local recurrence of disease and two patients had regional lymph node recurrence. Ten-year cause-specific survival was 92%. Of note, two patients with clinically node-negative disease who did not receive prophylactic inguinal nodal irradiation developed groin recurrences.

Anal canal adenocarcinoma

Adenocarcinomas of the anal canal are uncommon and in some cases will represent growth of distal rectal adenocarcinomas into the canal. A study of 82 patients from the Rare Cancer Network registry with a diagnosis of anal adenocarcinoma analyzed outcomes based on treatment approach—radiotherapy plus surgery, chemoradiotherapy, and abdominoperineal resection (APR).[30] Tumor and patient features were evenly distributed across the three groups. Local–regional control at 5 years was highest in the APR-treated patients (80% vs. 64% with chemoradiotherapy and 63% with radiation plus surgery), although the differences were not statistically significant. Moreover, 5-year survival was improved in the chemoradiotherapy group (58%) as opposed to the radiotherapy plus surgery (29%) and APR (21%) groups. In multivariate analysis, chemoradiotherapy was found to be a positive independent factor for disease-free and overall survival. A review of 165 patients with anal adenocarcinoma from the Surveillance, Epidemiology and End Results (SEER) database yielded differing conclusions.[31] Five-year survival for patients treated with APR was 58%, compared with 50% for APR plus radiation and 30% for radiation alone. These differences were statistically significant. Finally, a report from MD Anderson Cancer Center analyzed 16 patients with anal adenocarcinoma and compared outcomes with chemoradiotherapy treatment with similarly treated patients with squamous cell tumors.[32] Five-year rate of local failure was 54% for the adenocarcinoma group and 18% for the squamous cell group, with corresponding 5-year disease-free survival worse for the adenocarcinoma group (19% vs. 77%), as was overall survival (64% vs. 85%).

As a result, patients with anal adenocarcinoma are generally treated as if they had similarly staged rectal adenocarcinoma, with surgery the cornerstone of therapy and (neo) adjuvant chemoradiotherapy reserved for high-risk features (T3 or T4 disease and/or nodal involvement).

Anal canal melanomas

Melanomas of the anorectum are rare, representing about 1% of all anal canal tumors. Prognosis tends to be very poor, with 5-year overall survival rates as low as 6%, usually associated with development of distant metastases.

Appropriate local therapy remains a controversial area, although it appears that obtaining a negative surgical margin may be more important than the actual extent of the surgery. Nilsson reviewed 251 presentations from the Swedish National Cancer Registry, and on multivariate analysis, the two most important prognostic factors with respect to survival were surgical margin status and tumor stage.[33] Patients with an R0 surgery had a 5-year survival rate of 19% as opposed to 6% for those with positive margins. Iddings *et al.*[34] reviewed data regarding anorectal melanoma from the SEER database from 1973 to 2003. One hundred forty-three patients were recorded as having localized disease: 51 underwent APR and 92 underwent local excision. Patients between the two groups had "similar" pathologic features, and there were similar outcomes between the two treatments: median survival was 16 and 18 months in the APR and local excision groups, respectively, and 5-year survival was 16.8% and 19.3% for APR and local excision, respectively.

Investigators from MD Anderson Cancer Center reported on 23 patients with anorectal melanomas treated to the primary site with local excision, with or without nodal dissection based on clinical presentation.[35] Nine patients received some form of systemic therapy. A dose of 30 Gy was delivered in five fractions to the primary tumor site (to the level of the bottom of the sacroiliac joints) and inguinal nodes. Four patients received an additional 6-Gy boost dose to the primary site. Local and regional nodal control rates at 5 years were 74% and 84%, respectively. Five-year overall survival was 31%, and no patients with regional lymph node involvement at presentation were alive at 5 years.

Anal canal squamous cell cancer

Surgery
Prior to the use of curative-intent chemoradiotherapy, surgery was the mainstay of treatment for squamous cell anal canal tumors. Surgical options include local excision for small and minimally invasive tumors or more radical extirpation such as APR with formation of a permanent colostomy.

Boman *et al.*[36] reviewed the Mayo Clinic experience with 188 patients with anal canal carcinoma. One hundred seventy-two patients had squamous cell or nonkeratinizing basaloid carcinomas (tumors of the proximal anal canal in the transitional zone). Nineteen patients with small tumors confined to the "anal epithelium and subepithelial connective tissue" were treated with local excision only. Only one of these patients had disease failure and was salvaged with APR. Of 118 patients undergoing APR, disease failure was seen in 46 patients. Of these patients, patterns of failure were known in 38. Thirty-two of the 38 patients had a component of local–regional failure. In a separate series of results for anal cancer treatment from Roswell Park, the crude regional recurrence rate following local excision and APR for a variety of stages was 60%.[37]

As will be discussed in more detail in the following section, concurrent radiation therapy and chemotherapy emerged as a sphincter-sparing alternative to resection. Although there are no randomized trials comparing APR with chemoradiotherapy, local–regional tumor control rates and overall survival with chemoradiotherapy at least rival (if they are not superior to) those obtained with surgery with the added advantage of sphincter preservation. In an overview of the University of Minnesota's treatment experience with anal cancer, 21 patients with squamous cell anal cancer were treated with surgery, whereas 122 were treated with chemoradiotherapy.[38] Nearly half of the chemoradiotherapy-treated patients had T3 or T4 tumors, whereas only 14% of the surgery group had T3 tumors. Despite the more advanced tumors in the chemoradiotherapy cohort, overall 5-year survival was similar between the two groups—60% in those undergoing surgery and 55% in those treated with chemoradiotherapy. Tumor recurrence was found in 23% of the surgical group and 34% of the chemoradiotherapy group.

Concurrent chemotherapy and radiotherapy

Given the relatively poor local–regional control results obtained with surgery alone for locally advanced anal tumors, Nigro *et al.*[39] at Wayne State University instituted a protocol incorporating concurrent pelvic radiation therapy and chemotherapy (5-FU and mitomycin-C (MMC)) as induction therapy prior to surgery for anal canal cancers (defined in their series as tumors at and just proximal to the dentate line). The total radiation dose in the original report ranged from 30 to 35 Gy, and in subsequent series, it was 30 Gy, delivered at 2 Gy per fraction.[39,40] When pathologic complete responses were obtained in their original cohort, it became clear that chemoradiotherapy could provide definitive therapy, allowing preservation of the anal sphincter musculature, and APR could be reserved for locally persistent or recurrent disease. Other series using similar chemoradiotherapy treatment protocols also showed high rates of disease response, including pathologic complete response.[41,42] Radiation (typically to higher doses in the original Nigro series, at least 45 Gy) and concurrent 5-FU and MMC remain the "standard of care" treatment for most patients with squamous cell anal canal tumors.

Three randomized phase III clinical trials helped to establish this standard.[43–46] Two of the studies, the United Kingdom Coordinating Committee on Cancer Research (UKCCCR) Anal Cancer Trial (ACT I) and the European Organization for Research and Treatment of Cancer (EORTC), had similar designs. In the ACT I study, 568 eligible patients with anal canal or anal margin cancer were analyzed.[43,44] Randomization was to radiation (45 Gy in 20 or 25 fractions, followed by an additional dose to "good responders" of 15 or 25 Gy after a 6-week break) alone or radiation with infusional 5-FU (1000 mg/m^2 for 5 days or 750 mg/m^2 for 5 days, given during the first and last weeks of radiation) and MMC (12 mg/m^2 delivered on day 1 of treatment). Local–regional failure rates were significantly higher in the patients treated with radiation alone (25.3% absolute difference at 12 years), and relapse-free survival was similarly higher in the chemoradiotherapy group (12% absolute difference at 12 years). Cause-specific, but not overall, survival was higher in the chemoradiation group. There was no significant difference between the two groups with respect to late morbidity.

In the EORTC study, 103 eligible patients with T3-4N0-3 or T1-2N1-3 anal cancer were treated with radiation therapy (45 Gy, with a boost dose of 15 or 20 Gy following a 6-week break based on disease response) with or without concurrent chemotherapy (infusional 5-FU at a dose of 750 mg/m^2 daily for days 1–5 and 29–33, with MMC also given on day 1 at 15 mg/m^2).[45] Patients treated with chemotherapy had a higher complete response rate than those treated with radiation alone: 80% versus 54%. Local–regional control, colostomy-free survival, and event-free survival were all higher in the chemoradiotherapy group at 5 years. Rates of high-grade toxicity were similar between the two groups, although rates of late anal ulceration were higher in the combined modality group. Overall survival was superior in the chemoradiotherapy treatment arm, but this did not reach statistical significance.

A third study, conducted by the Radiation Therapy Oncology Group (RTOG) and the Eastern Cooperative Oncology Group (ECOG), attempted to de-intensify therapy by omitting MMC, hoping to maintain oncologic efficacy while eliminating the toxicities associated with MMC.[46] Patients with anal canal cancer of any T- or N-stage were randomized to radiation therapy and 5-FU plus MMC versus radiation and 5-FU alone. The radiation dose was 45–50.4 Gy depending on treatment response, with an additional 9 Gy delivered to patients with biopsy-proven persistent disease 4–6 weeks following completion of initial treatment, and an additional 9 Gy delivered to residual palpable inguinal lymph nodes. Infusional 5-FU was delivered at 1000 mg/m^2/day on days 1–4 and 29–32. MMC was delivered at 10 mg/m^2 on days 1 and 29 in patients randomized to receive it. In patients with an initial positive biopsy after the first 4–6-week break, a second biopsy was later obtained. If this was positive for residual tumor, patients proceeded to APR. Two hundred ninety-one patients could be assessed in the study analysis. At 4 years, colostomy-free survival was higher in the MMC-treated patients (71% vs. 59%), as was disease-free survival (73% vs. 51%). Overall survival at 4 years was also higher in the MMC group (76% vs. 67%), although this did not reach statistical significance. The rate of all grades 4 and 5 toxicities was considerably higher in the MMC group (23% vs. 7%). An important point relative to this trial design relating to general patient management is that there are very long regression periods in some patients after chemoradiotherapy (beyond 4 months). Therefore, one general recommendation is for patients to undergo biopsy of remaining lesions only in the presence of overt disease progression, assuming close follow-up.[47]

As oncologic efficacy was diminished with the omission of MMC, yet toxicity rates remained high, investigators next attempted to replace MMC with cisplatin in combined modality therapy. Cisplatin has established activity against squamous cell tumors of the head and neck, esophagus and cervix, and is also established as a radiosensitizing agent for tumors in these areas.[48] Moreover, its toxicity profile differs from that of MMC. Thus, it is logical to consider replacing MMC with cisplatin, maintaining the backbone of infusional 5-FU. Institutional and phase II clinical trial reports were supportive of further investigation in the phase III setting.[49–51] RTOG 98-11 was a phase III randomized trial that enrolled patients with

T2-4N0-3 anal cancers.[52] Six hundred twenty-four patients were included in the trial analysis. Randomization was to one of two arms. In the first arm, patients were treated with radiation (T3, T4, and node-positive tumors were treated to a total dose of 55–59 Gy, as were patients with T2 tumors with residual disease after 45 Gy was reached) concurrently with infusional 5-FU (1000 mg/m^2 days 1–4 and 29–32) and MMC (10 mg/m^2 delivered days 1 and 29). In the second arm, patients received induction chemotherapy with cisplatin (75 mg/m^2 delivered on days 1 and 29) and infusional 5-FU (1000 mg/m^2 on days 1–4 and 29–32) alone, followed by concurrent therapy (radiation delivered as above along with cisplatin repeated on days 57 and 85 and 5-FU delivered on days 57–60 and 85–88). Thus, in the second group, there was an 8-week break from initiation of induction chemotherapy and the start of radiation. The primary end point of the study was disease-free survival. Rates of high-grade hematologic toxicity were higher in the MMC-treated patients. Five-year disease-free survival (60% vs. 54%) and OS (75% vs. 70%) were higher in the MMC-treated patients, but these differences were not statistically significant. Local–regional control rates were lower at 5 years in the cisplatin group (67% vs. 75%, $p = 0.07$), and 5-year rates of colostomy requirement were higher in the cisplatin-treated patients (19% vs. 10%) ($p = 0.02$). This study has been criticized for the use of an induction chemotherapy component in the group of patients receiving cisplatin, as this prolonged overall treatment duration and may have allowed for accelerated repopulation of tumor cells prior to the initiation of radiation treatments.

Table 6.2 summarizes the most significant findings from these randomized trials.

The ACT II study was similar in concept to RTOG 98-11, but eliminated the component of induction chemotherapy, thus providing a more direct comparison of cisplatin as a direct replacement for MMC.[53] Patients with anal cancer were randomized to treatment with infusional 5-FU (delivered weeks 1 and 5) and pelvic radiation therapy 50.4 Gy plus MMC (delivered week 1) or cisplatin (delivered weeks 1 and 5). There was a second randomization following the completion of the combined treatment course, to no further therapy or two additional cycles of cisplatin and 5-FU. Preliminary results were recently reported. Hematologic toxicity was more common in the MMC-treated group, while nonhematologic toxicity rates were similar for the MMC- and cisplatin-treated patients. At a median follow-up of 3 years, there were no differences between the two arms with respect to complete response rates. Longer follow-up and comparison of survival outcomes are awaited.

The French Federation Nationale des Centres de Lutte Contre le Cancer ACCORD 03 study tested the value of induction therapy as well as dose escalation. Patients with T2 (>4 cm), T3-4, and/or node-positive anal cancer were randomized to one of four treatment arms.[54] The first arm consisted of induction therapy with 5-FU and cisplatin followed by combined therapy (radiation dose: 45 Gy). Patients then underwent a scheduled break and were subsequently treated with a 15-Gy boost. The second treatment arm was identical to the first, but the boost dose was

Table 6.2 Summary of major randomized phase III clinical trials of chemoradiotherapy for anal cancer.

Study (Reference)	Treatment Arms[a]	Local–Regional Failure[b]	Relapse-Free Survival[b]	Colostomy-Free Survival[b]	Overall Survival	Acute Toxicity
UKCCCR/ ACT I (44,45)	(1) Radiation versus (2) Radiation + 5-FU + MMC	(1) 59.1% (2) 33.8% (at 12 years)	(1) 17.7% (2) 29.7% (at 12 years)	(1) 20.1% (2) 29.6% (at 12 years)	(1) 27.5% (2) 33.1% (at 12 years) P = NS	(1) "Severe" skin toxicity = 39% "Severe" GI toxicity = 5% (2) "Severe" skin toxicity = 50% "Severe" GI toxicity = 14%
EORTC (46)	(1) Radiation versus (2) Radiation + 5-FU + MMC	18% improvement in arm 2 at 5 years	N/A	32% improvement in arm 2 (colostomy-free)		(1) Grades 3–4 diarrhea = 8% Grades 3–4 dermatologic = 50% (2) Grades 3–4 diarrhea = 20% Grades 3–4 dermatologic = 57%
RTOG/ECOG (47)	(1) Radiation + 5-FUversus (2) Radiation + 5-FU + MMC	(1) 34% (2) 16%	(1) 51% (2) 73% (disease-free survival at 4 years)	(1) 59% (2) 73% (at 4 years)	(1) 67% (2) 76% (at 4 years) P = NS	(1) Grades 4–5 heme = 3% grades 4–5 nonheme = 4% (2) Grades 4–5 heme = 18% Grades 4–5 nonheme = 7%
RTOG 98-11 (53)	(1) Radiation + 5-FU + MMC versus (2) Cisplatin > radiation + 5-FU + cisplatin	(1) 25% (2) 33%	(1) 60% (2) 54% (disease-free survival at 5 years) P = NS	(1) 10% (2) 19% (cumulative incidence of colostomy)	(1) 75% (2) 70% (at 5 years) P = NS	(1) Grades 3–4 heme = 61% Grades 3–4 nonheme = 74% (2) Grades 3–4 heme = 42% Grades 3–4 nonheme = 74%

[a]Details of treatment arms noted in the text.
[b]p values significant for comparisons unless otherwise noted.

20–25 Gy. Arms 3 and 4 were the same as arms 1 and 2, respectively, but without the component of induction therapy. At a median follow-up of 43 months, preliminary results showed that there were no differences in 3-year colostomy-free survival rates (ranging from 80% to 86%). Cause-specific and overall survival rates were also similar.

Results of the EORTC study 22011-40014, a randomized phase II trial evaluating the omission of 5-FU, were recently reported in a preliminary form.[55] Patients with anal tumors >4 cm and/or node-positive were treated with radiation to 36 Gy, followed by a 2-week break and subsequent delivery of an additional 23.4 Gy. MMC was delivered on the first day of each sequence, to all patients. Patients were randomized to either 5-FU or cisplatin. High-grade hematologic toxicity was more pronounced in the MMC plus cisplatin group, and patients receiving these therapies were less likely to complete all intended treatments. However, at 8 weeks following therapy completion, patients receiving MMC and cisplatin had higher overall response rates. Further follow-up is needed to determine if this finding will translate into improved survival.

New and investigational drug agents in combined modality therapy

With the constant goal of improving on tumor control while minimizing toxicity, a variety of new and investigational drug agents are under study as new components of combined modality therapy regimens for the treatment of squamous cell anal canal cancer. In this section, we will focus on two cytotoxic chemotherapeutic agents, capecitabine and oxaliplatin, and one "molecular-targeted" agent, cetuximab, an antibody directed against the epidermal growth factor receptor (EGFR).

Capecitabine is an orally delivered prodrug formulation of 5-FU.[56] A series of enzymatic modifications converts capecitabine to 5-FU. The last enzyme involved in this series is thymidine phosphorylase, which is often preferentially expressed in tumors as opposed to normal tissues.[57] Thus, in addition to the convenience of oral dosing, there is an important theoretical backing to study capecitabine as an alternative to infusional 5-FU. Capecitabine as a replacement for infusional 5-FU in anal cancer treatment was studied in the multi-institutional phase II EXTRA trial.[58] Thirty-one patients with anal cancer were treated with concurrent capecitabine (given on days of radiation treatment), MMC (given on day 1 of the treatment course), and radiation (total dose: 50.4 Gy). One patient had high-grade acute diarrhea and three patients developed grade 3 neutropenia. At 4 weeks following treatment completion, 77% of patients had a clinical complete response; at a median follow-up of 14 months, three patients had developed local–regional tumor failure.

Oxaliplatin is a third-generation platinum agent that appears to have radiosensitizing properties, although there is some controversy regarding its true role as a sensitizer, especially in the context of concurrent therapy with 5-FU.[59] In a study of HIV-negative patients with stage II or III anal cancer, investigators from MD Anderson Cancer Center tested a combination of oxaliplatin, capecitabine, and radiation.[60] Preliminary results were recently reported. Radiation dose was prescribed based on the T-stage of the tumor. Initially, capecitabine was given twice daily on weekdays and oxaliplatin delivered once weekly; when high rates of high-grade acute gastrointestinal toxicity were seen, the protocol was modified to hold chemotherapy during the third and sixth weeks. Rates of high-grade acute gastrointestinal toxicity were reduced in subsequently enrolled patients. At a median follow-up of 19 months, there were no local recurrences; one patient developed distant disease failure.

Cetuximab is a humanized antibody targeted against the EGFR. EGFR is implicated in tumorigenesis in a number of malignancies. A variety of EGFR antagonists, including small molecule inhibitors (gefitinib, erlotinib) and antibodies (cetuximab, panitumumab) are available and under study in cancer treatment. In addition, there is a rationale for employing anti-EGFR therapy specifically in conjunction with radiation, as the EGFR signaling pathway is implicated in radioresistance.[61] In preclinical study, radiation has been shown to activate EGFR signaling with subsequent pleiotropic pro-survival effects on tumor cells, and use of cetuximab counters these effects.[61,62] Radiation combined with cetuximab for the treatment of squamous cell head and neck cancer yielded an overall survival advantage when compared with radiation alone in a randomized phase III clinical trial.[63] Activating mutations in downstream components of EGFR signaling, including k-ras and B-raf mutations, have been implicated as negative predictive factors for response to anti-EGFR therapies, at least in the treatment of colorectal cancer.[64,65] K-ras mutations appear to be uncommon in squamous cell anal cancers, increasing interest in use of this therapy.[66] Of note, special consideration of treatment sequencing needs to be considered with chemotherapy is used in conjunction with cetuximab, as there may be potential antagonistic effects rooted in cell cycle disruption induced by cetuximab.[67]

Personalized medicine in anal cancer treatment
To date, the major randomized clinical trials that have shaped the contemporary treatment of squamous cell anal cancer have enrolled patients without specific regard to biological features of their tumor (outside of histology). There is a strong need for more tailored treatments to match treatment intensity with a given patient's tumor sensitivity, particularly given the potential morbidities associated with therapy. Molecular profiling of tumors to predict tumor growth and metastasis behavior as well as sensitivity to drug and radiation treatments is an intense area of investigation for many tumor sites. Such efforts in anal cancer management are generally lacking to date, although attempts to define mutations in proteins involved in important signaling pathways are now emerging.[66]

Improvements in imaging may also allow more accurate staging, in particular detection of nodal metastases. As described previously, PET imaging has resulted in improved detection of nodal involvement as compared with conventional CT. As further example, lymphotropic particles with superparamagnetic properties have been used to detect nodal micrometastatic disease in patients with prostatic adenocarcinomas.[68] Extension of this or similar technologies would potentially have significant implications for design of clinical target volumes (CTVs) in the radiation treatment planning process.

Radiation therapy planning

Radiation treatment plans require careful identification of target volumes. The gross target volume (GTV) is defined as any site of grossly identifiable cancer as revealed by physical examination, endoscopy, and imaging studies. The CTV consists of the GTV as well as regions thought to be at high risk for harboring occult micrometastatic disease. The planning target volume (PTV) is the CTV expanded by variable margins to account for uncertainties in patient positioning and organ location. CTV-to-PTV margins can be reduced by reproducible positioning of patients with immobilization devices and in some cases by use of image-guidance technology to ascertain patient alignment immediately prior to treatment.

Based on patterns of regional disease spread, the "full" lymph node component of the CTV for anal cancer treatments has included the mesorectal and presacral space nodal regions, as well as the internal and external iliac regions, along with the latter extending into the femoral–inguinal region. Lymph nodes along the obturator branch of the internal iliac vessels are also at risk. In traditional 2-dimensional (2D) treatment planning, vascular (and thus lymph node) location was inferred based on appearance of bony anatomy, and traditional treatment "portals" were employed to treat the pelvic–inguinal–anal CTV. With the advent of CT-based treatment simulation, the GTV and CTV can be defined in three dimensions specific to a patient's anatomy. In 2D- and 3D-conformal treatment planning, there are multiple CTVs (and PTVs) that are progressively smaller in volume while receiving progressively higher radiation doses as a function of their higher likelihood of harboring disease.

Traditional radiation treatment portals encompass a large volume of tissue, and although they cover gross disease and at-risk nodal volumes easily, they are also relatively unforgiving with respect to irradiation of normal tissues, thus accounting for much of the treatment-related toxicity (dermatologic, gastrointestinal, urinary, sexual, and hematopoietic) discussed previously. Intensity-modulated radiation therapy (IMRT) is an advanced form of 3D-conformal radiation treatment that makes use of multiple beams with nonuniform dose delivery. In dynamic IMRT, collimating leaves sweep across the beam path during x-ray delivery at a given gantry angle. High-quality IMRT plans conform high doses of radiation to irregularly shaped target volumes, providing a relative sparing of nearby normal tissues. IMRT is commonly used in radiotherapy of head and neck cancers to spare salivary glands from receiving high doses and in prostate cancer to limit dose to rectum and bladder.[69,70] IMRT may be of particular benefit to patients who are HIV positive with anal cancer, as the normal tissue injury can be accentuated.[71] IMRT also allows for "simultaneous integrated boosting," in which different target subvolumes can be treated to different doses during the same treatment.[72] For example, an area of gross disease can be treated to a higher dose in the same treatment fraction relative to an area being treated prophylactically for possible micrometastatic disease. This style of treatment is also sometimes referred to as "dose painting."

IMRT is under active investigation for its role in reducing treatment-related toxicity during radiation therapy for anal cancer.[73–77] RTOG 0529 is a phase II study that evaluated the role of IMRT in reducing chemoradiotherapy-associated toxicity.[76,77] Patients with T2-4N0-3 anal cancer were treated with concurrent MMC, 5-FU, and IMRT. Dose painting was employed with subvolume doses selected as a function of tumor stage. The initial report compared acute toxicity outcomes with results from RTOG 9811, where IMRT was not implemented. Grade 3 or higher dermatologic toxicity rates were lower in the IMRT study (20% vs. 47%), as were rates of grade 3 or higher gastrointestinal and genitourinary toxicity (22% vs. 36%). Importantly, rates of local failure, colostomy-free survival, and disease-free and overall survival were similar between the two studies, indicating no loss of oncologic efficacy and thus a possibly improved therapeutic ratio with the employment of IMRT.

Figure 6.2 is a demonstration of an IMRT treatment plan.

Radiation dose–time factors

As previously noted, the original reports from Nigro *et al.* employed radiation doses of about 30 Gy. The major randomized trials have employed at least 45 Gy, and doses in the range of 45–59.4 Gy are used in clinical practice. Dose escalation through conventional external beam approaches or brachytherapy may improve on tumor control rates but can also increase treatment morbidity.

Retrospective studies have indicated that higher doses of radiation (≥54 Gy as opposed to less) were associated with improved local tumor control

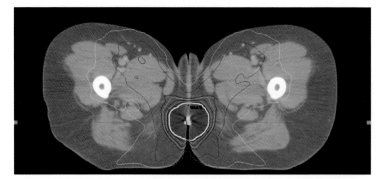

Figure 6.2 Axial CT slice showing sparing of the genitalia in a female patient with anal cancer, treated with intensity-modulated radiation therapy. The target volume (anus) is shaded in light brown and relative dose lines are displayed on the figure. The "bowing-in" of the dose lines is a typical feature of IMRT treatment plans and allows for relative sparing on normal, critical tissues. (Figure courtesy of Rodney Hood, CMD.)

as well as superior overall survival.[78] Two clinical trials have examined the role of dose escalation. RTOG 92-08 was a phase II study that treated 47 patients with at least T2 anal tumors.[79,80] In RTOG 92-08, the total radiation dose was 59.4 Gy delivered at 1.8 Gy per fraction, but there was a mandated 2-week treatment break following 36 Gy.[79] Patients also received concurrent 5-FU and MMC. The 2-year rate of colostomy requirement was 30%, considerably higher than expected based on previous experience. One possible explanation for this finding was the use of split-course therapy, which allows for tumor cell repopulation. A similar study conducted by the ECOG showed high rates of tumor response but also high rates of hematologic toxicity.[80] Increased radiation dose has also been associated with increased rates of late toxicity, including need for APR for management of treatment-related morbidity.[81]

Radiation alone for early-stage tumors?

Although patients with T1-2N0 tumors were eligible for treatment on the ACT I study, there are no randomized phase III data specifically supporting a need for chemotherapy in this group of early-stage tumors. Various retrospective series have shown good control rates with radiation alone, especially for T1 tumors.[82,83] In one series from Vancouver, patients with anal cancer were treated with radiation alone (usually 50 Gy in 20 fractions). Local control was 89% (8 out of 9 patients) for those presenting with T1 disease and 79% (34 out of 43 patients) for those with T2 tumors.

Concurrent chemotherapy and radiation therapy remain the standard treatment for patients with anal cancer. However, radiation alone can be considered for definitive therapy in patients deemed as poor candidates for combined therapy, especially if they have early-stage (T1) tumors.

Treatment of metastatic disease

The liver is the most common distant organ involved by metastatic anal cancer. Cisplatin and 5-FU is a commonly employed first-line regimen for patients who develop metastatic disease.[84–86] Other chemotherapy agents including irinotecan, mitomycin, carboplatin, and doxorubicin have also been employed, as has cetuximab, in small series.[87–90]

Aggressive surgical resection of liver metastases (or thermal ablation) can be considered in selected patients. In one of the reports of the experience across eight centers, 52 patients with squamous cell tumors (27 with anal cancer primary tumors) with limited metastatic liver involvement (median number of live metastases: 1) underwent resection, resection plus radiofrequency ablation (RFA), or RFA alone.[91] The median disease-free survival for the patients with metastatic squamous cell anal cancer was 9.6 months, and the actuarial 5-year overall survival was 22.9%. Patients presenting with synchronous metastases, hepatic lesions >5 cm, and those with positive resection margins had worse survival outcomes. These results indicate that in selected presentations of liver-limited metastatic disease, liver-directed treatments have the potential to play an important role in improving survival outcomes.

Case Study

A 48-year-old man with history of HIV-positive status presented with a slowly growing mass at the anal verge. The mass grew over a period of about 10 years. On examination, a 10 × 15 cm mass was seen protruding from the anal verge. On anoscopic examination, the mass stretched proximally a few millimeters into the anal canal. The mass was thought to represent a large condylomatous lesion and had the clinical features of a Buschke–Löwenstein tumor. The mass was resected and there was a component of poorly differentiated invasive squamous cell carcinoma arising within an anal condyloma. The carcinoma portion measured 4.5 cm. A second, re-excision of perianal skin showed no evidence for tumor. A follow-up PET–CT scan showed FDG avidity within the perianal region, reflecting postsurgical inflammation versus recurrent tumor, as well as two lymph nodes within the left inguinal region that were also FDG avid. The largest of these nodes measured 1.2 cm and a fine-needle aspiration biopsy revealed metastatic squamous cell tumor.

On physical examination, the anal tumor had been completely grossly excised, although there was concern for possible microscopic residual disease. After consultation with the radiation oncology and medical oncology teams, a plan for concurrent chemotherapy and radiation therapy was devised. The chemotherapy consisted of 5-FU and MMC, both delivered during weeks 1 and 5 of treatment. The site of the excised primary tumor, the bilateral inguinal nodal regions, external and internal iliac nodal regions, and mesorectum and presacral nodal regions were treated to a total dose of 36 Gy at 1.8 Gy per fraction, with an intensity-modulated radiation treatment plan. A boost dose of 9 Gy (at 1.8 Gy per fraction) was delivered to the primary tumor and bilateral inguinal regions, as well as the external and internal iliac nodes below the level of the bottom of the sacroiliac joints. Following this, a boost dose of 9 Gy (at 1.8 Gy per fraction) was delivered with electron irradiation to the two lymph nodes in the left inguinal region.

The patient tolerated the treatment well, developing moist desquamation in the perianal skin as well as the inguinal region treated to high dose (the involved side). Six weeks following completion of treatment, there was no evidence for local tumor recurrence in the anal canal on physical examination, and no palpable inguinal lymphadenopathy. This was confirmed on subsequent follow-up, and at most recent follow-up, 1 year after treatment, there was no evidence for disease recurrence. CT scan obtained 6 months following treatment completion showed resolution of the inguinal lymphadenopathy and no new lesions. The patient continues on a course of posttreatment surveillance.

References

1. Greenall, M.J., Quan, S.H.Q., Stearns, M.W. et al. (1985) Epidermoid cancer of the anal margin. Pathologic features, treatment, and clinical results. *Am J Surg*, **149**, 95–101.
2. Chapet, O., Gerard, J-P., Mornex, F. et al. (2007) Prognostic factors of squamous cell carcinoma of the anal margin treated by radiotherapy: the Lyon experience. *Int J Colorectal Dis*, **22**, 191–199.

3. Robb, B.W., Mutch, M.G. (2006) Epidermoid carcinoma of the anal canal.*Clin Colon Rect Surg*, **19**, 54–60.

4. Jemal, A., Siegel, R., Xu, J. *et al.* (2010) Cancer statistics, 2010. *CA Cancer J Clin*, **60**, 277–300.

5. Frisch, M., Glimelius, B., van den Brule, A.J. *et al.* (1997) Sexually transmitted infection as a cause of anal cancer. *New Engl J Med*, **337**, 1350–1358.

6. Daling, J.R., Weiss, N.S., Hislop, T.G. *et al.* (1987) Sexual practice, sexually transmitted diseases, and the incidence of anal cancer. *New Engl J Med*, **317**, 973–977.

7. Melbye, M., Sprøgel, P. (1991) Aetiological parallel between anal cancer and cervical cancer. *Lancet,* **338**, 657–659.

8. Rabkin, C.S., Biggar, R.J., Melbye, M. *et al.* (1992) Second primary cancers following anal and cervical carcinoma: evidence of shared etiologic factors. *Am J Epidemiol*, **136**, 54–58.

9. Bjorge, T., Engeland, A., Luostarinen, T. *et al.* (2002) Human papillomavirus infection as a risk factor for anal and perianal skin cancer in a prospective study. *Br J Cancer*, **87**, 61–64.

10. Daling, J.R., Madeleine, M.M., Johnson, L.G. *et al.* (2004) Human papillomavirus, smoking, and sexual practices in the etiology of anal cancer. *Cancer,* **101**, 270–280.

11. Palefsky, J.M., Holly, E.A., Hogeboom, C.J. *et al.* (1998) Virologic, immunologic, and clinical parameters in the incidence and progression of anal squamous intraepithelial lesions in HIV-positive and HIV-negative homosexual men. *J Acquir Immune Defic Syndr Hum Retrovirol*, **17**, 314–319.

12. Penn, I. (1986) Cancers of the anogenital region in renal transplant recipients. Analysis of 65 cases. *Cancer,* **58**, 611–616.

13. Arends, M.J., Benton, E.C., McLaren, K.M. *et al.* (1997) Renal allograft recipients with high susceptibility to cutaneous malignancy have an increased prevalence of human papillomavirus DNA in skin tumors and a greater risk of anogenital malignancy. *Br J Cancer*, **72**, 722–728.

14. Sillman, F., Sedlis, A. (1991) Anogenital papillomavirus infection and neoplasia in immunodeficient women: an update. *Dermatol Clin,* **9**, 353–369.

15. Holley, E.A., Whittemore, A.S., Aston, D.A. *et al.* (1989) Anal cancer incidence: genital warts, anal fissure or fistula, hemorrhoids, and smoking. *J Natl Cancer Inst*, **81**, 1726–1731.

16. Sook, A.K. (1991) Cigarette smoking and cervical cancer: meta-analysis and critical review of recent studies. *Am J Prev Med,* **7**, 208–213.

17. Palefsky, J.M., Holly, E.A., Ralston, M.L. *et al.* (1998) Prevalence and risk factors for human papillomavirus infection of the anal canal in human immunodeficiency virus (HIV)-positive and HIV-negative homosexual men. *J Infect Dis*, **177**, 361–367.

18. Sobhani, I., Vuagnat, A., Walker, F. *et al.* (2001) Prevalence of high-grade dysplasia and cancer in the anal canal in human papillomavirus-infected individuals. *Gastroenterology,* **120**, 857–866.

19. Trautmann, T.G., Zuger, J.H. (2005) Positron emission tomography for pretreatment staging and posttreatment evaluation in cancer of the anal canal. *Mol Imaging Biol,* **7**, 309.

20. Cotter, S.E., Grigsby, P.W., Siegel, B.A. *et al.* (2006) FDG-PET/CT in the evaluation of anal carcinoma. *Int J Radiat Oncol Biol Phys,* **65**, 720.

21. Winton, E., Heriot, A.G., Ng, M. *et al.* (2009) The impact of 18-fluorodeoxyglucose positron emission tomography on the staging, management and outcome of anal cancer. *Br J Cancer*, **100**, 693.

22. Nathan, M., Singh, N., Garrett, N. *et al.* (2010) Performance of anal cytology in a clinical setting when measured against histology and high-resolution anoscopy findings. *AIDS,* **24**, 373–379.

23. Palefsky, J.M., Holly, E.A., Hogeboom, C.J., Berry, J.M., Jay, N., Darragh, T.M. (1997) Anal cytology as a screening tool for anal squamous intraepithelial lesions. *J Acquir Immune Defic Syndr Hum Retrovirol,* **14(5)**, 415–422.

24. Singh, J.C., Kuohong, V., Palefsky, J.M. (2009) Efficacy of trichloroacetic acid in the treatment of anal intraepithelial neoplasia in HIV-positive and HIV-negative men who have sex with men. *J Acquir Immune Defic Syndr,* **52**, 474–479.

25. Richel, O., Wieland, U., de Vries, H.J. *et al.* (2010) Topical 5-fluorouracil treatment of anal intraepithelial neoplasia in HIV-positive men. *Br J Dermatol,* **163**, 1301–1307.

26. Fox, P.A., Nathan, M., Francis, N. *et al.* (2010) A double-blind, randomized controlled trial of the use of imiquimod cream for the treatment of anal canal high-grade anal intraepithelial neoplasia in HIV-positive MSM on HAART, with long-term follow-up data including use of open-label imiquimod. *AIDS,* **24**, 2331–2335.

27. Goldie, S.J., Kuntz, K.M., Weinstein, M.C. *et al.* (1999) The clinical effectiveness and cost-effectiveness of screening for anal squamous intraepithelial lesions in homosexual and bisexual HIV-positive men. *JAMA,* **281**, 1822–1829.

28. Khanfir, K., Ozsahin, M., Bieri, S. *et al.* (2008) Patterns of failure and outcome in patients with carcinoma of the anal margin. *Ann Surg Oncol,* **15**, 1092–1098.

29. Balamucki, C.J., Zlotecki, R.A., Rout, W.R. *et al.* (2010) Squamous cell carcinoma of the anal margin: the university of Florida experience. *Am J Clin Oncol,* **34(4)**, 406–410.

30. Belkacemi, Y., Berger, C., Poortmans, P. *et al.* (2003) Management of primary anal canal adenocarcinoma: a large retrospective study form the rare cancer network. *Int J Radiat Oncol Biol Phys,* **56**, 1274–1283.

31. Kounalakis, N., Artinyan, A., Smith, D. *et al.* (2009) Abdominal perineal resection improves survival for nonmetastatic adenocarcinoma of the anal canal. *Ann Surg Oncol,* **16**, 1310–1315.

32. Papagikos, M., Crane, C.H., Skibber, J. *et al.* (2003) Chemoradiation for adenocarcinoma of the anus. *Int J Radiat Oncol Biol Phys,* **55**, 669–678.

33. Nilsson, P.J., Ragnarsson-Olding, B.K. (2010) Importance of clear resection margins in anorectal malignant melanoma. *Br J Surg,* **97**, 98–103.

34. Iddings, D.M., Fleisig, A.J., Chen, S.L. *et al.* (2010) Practice patterns and outcomes for anorectal melanoma in the USA, reviewing three decades of treatment: is more extensive surgical resection beneficial in all patients? *Ann Surg Oncol,* **17**, 40–44.

35. Ballo, M.T., Gershenwald, J.E., Zagars, G.K. *et al.* (2002) Sphincter-sparing local excision and adjuvant radiation for anal-rectal melanoma. *J Clin Oncol,* **20**, 4555–4558.

36. Boman, B.M., Moertel, C.G., O'Connell, M.J. *et al.* (1984) Carcinoma of the anal canal. A clinical and pathologic study of 188 cases. *Cancer,* **54**, 114–125.

37. Singh, R., Nime, F., Mittelman, A. (1981) Malignant epithelial tumors of the anal canal. *Cancer,* **48**, 411–415.

38. Klas, J.V., Rothenberger, D.A., Wong, W.D. *et al.* (1999) Malignant tumors of the anal canal. The spectrum of disease, treatment, and outcomes. *Cancer,* **85**, 1686–1693.

39. Nigro, N.D., Vaitkevicius, V.K., Considine Jr, B. (1974) Combined therapy for cancer of the anal canal. A preliminary report. *Dis Colon Rec*, **17**, 354–356.
40. Nigro, N.D., Seydel, H.G., Considine, B. *et al.* (1983) Combined preoperative radiation and chemotherapy for squamous cell carcinoma of the anal canal. *Cancer*, **51**, 1826–1829.
41. Meeker Jr, W.R., Sickle-Santanello, B.J., Philpott, G. *et al.* (1986) Combined chemotherapy, radiation, and surgery for epithelial cancer of the anal canal. *Cancer*, **57**, 525–529.
42. Michaelson, R.A., Magill, ZGB, Quan, SHQ, *et al.* (1983) Preoperative chemotherapy and radiation therapy in the management of anal epidermoid carcinoma. *Cnacer*, **51**, 390–395.
43. Northover, J., Glynne-Jones, R., Sebag-Montefiore, D. *et al.* (2010) Chemoradiation for the treatment of epidermoid anal cancer: 13-year follow-up of the first randomised UKCCCR Anal Cancer Trial (ACT I). *Br J Cancer*, **103**, 1123–1128.
44. UKCCCR Anal Cancer Trial Working Party. UK Co-ordinating Committee on Cancer Research. (1996). Epidermoid anal cancer: results from the UKCCCR randomised trial of radiotherapy alone versus radiotherapy, 5-fluorouracil, and mitomycin. *Lancet*, **348**, 1049–1054.
45. Bartelink, H., Roelofsen, F., Eschwege, F. *et al.* (1997) Concomitant radiotherapy and chemotherapy is superior to radiotherapy alone in the treatment of locally advanced anal cancer: results of a phase III randomized trial of the European organization for research and treatment of cancer radiotherapy and gastrointestinal cooperative groups. *J Clin Oncol*, **15**, 2040–2049.
46. Flam, M., John, M., Pajak, T.F. *et al.* (1996) Role of mitomycin in combination with fluorouracil and radiotherapy, and of salvage chemoradiation in the definitive nonsurgical treatment of epidermoid carcinoma of the anal canal: results of a phase III randomized intergroup study. *J Clin Oncol*, **14**, 2527–2539.
47. Cummings, B.J., Keane, T.J., O'Sullivan, B. *et al.* (1991) Epidermoid anal cancer: treatment by radiation alone or by radiation and 5-fluorouracil with and without mitomycin c. *Int J Radiat Oncol Biol Phys*, **21**, 1115–1125.
48. Vokes, E.E., Weichselbaum, R.R. (1990) Concomitant chemoradiotherapy: rationale and clinical experience in patients with solid tumors. *J Clin Oncol*, **8**, 911–934.
49. Rich, T.A., Ajani, J.A., Morrison, W.H. *et al.* (1993) Chemoradiation therapy for anal cancer: radiation plus continuous infusion fluorouracil with or without cisplatin. *Radiother Oncol*, **27**, 209–215.
50. Gerard, J.P., Ayzac, L., Hun, D. *et al.* (1998) Treatment of anal carcinoma with high-dose radiation and concomitant fluorouracil-cisplatin: long-term results in 95 patients. *Radiother Oncol*, **46**, 249–256.
51. Peiffert, D., Giovannini, M., Ducreux, M. *et al.* (2001) High-dose radiation therapy and neoadjuvant plus concomitant chemotherapy with 5-fluorouracil and cisplatin in patients with locally advanced squamous-cell anal carcinoma: final results of a phase II study. *Ann Oncol*, **12**, 397–404.
52. Ajani, J.A., Winter, K.A., Gunderson, L.L. *et al.* (2008) Fluorouracil, mitomycin, and radiotherapy vs fluorouracil, cisplatin, and radiotherapy for carcinoma of the anal canal: a randomized clinical trial. *JAMA*, **299**, 1914–1921.
53. James, R., Wan, S., Glynne-Jones, R. *et al.* (2009) A randomized trial of chemoradiation using mitomycin or cisplatin, with or without maintenance

cisplatin/5FU in squamous cell carcinoma of the anus (ACT II) [Suppl; abstract LBA4009]. *J Clin Oncol,* **27**, 18s.

54. Conroy, T., Ducreux, M., Lemanski, C. *et al.* (2009) Treatment intensification by induction chemotherapy (ICT) and radiation dose escalation in locally advanced squamous cell anal carcinoma (LAAC): definitive analysis of the intergroup ACCORD 03 trial. *J Clin Oncol,* **27(Suppl 1)**, abstract 4033.

55. Matzinger, O., Roelofsen, F., Mineur, L. *et al.* (2009) Mitomycin C with continuous fluorouracil or with cisplatin in combination with radiotherapy for locally advanced anal cancer (European organization for research and treatment of cancer phase II study 22011-40014). *Eur J Cancer,* **45**, 2782–2791.

56. Aprile, G., Mazzer, M., Moroso, S. *et al.* (2009) Pharmacology and therapeutic efficacy of capecitabine: focus on breast and colorectal cancer. *Anticancer Drugs,* **20**, 217–229.

57. Miwa, M., Ura, M., Nishida, M. *et al.* (1998) Design of a novel oral fluoropyrimidine carbamate, capecitabine, which generated 5-fluorouracil selectively in tumors by enzymes concentrated in human liver and cancer tissue. *Eur J Cancer,* **34**, 1274–1281.

58. Glynne-Jones, R., Meadows, H., Wan, S. *et al.* (2008) EXTRA—a multicenter phase II study of chemoradiation using a 5 day per week oral regimen of capecitabine and intravenous mitomycin C in anal cancer. *Int J Radiat Oncol Biol Phys,* **72**, 119–126.

59. Folkvord, S., Flatmark, K., Seierstad, T. *et al.* (2008) Inhibitory effects of oxaliplatin in experimental radiation treatment of colorectal carcinoma: does oxaliplatin improve 5-fluorouracil-dependent radiosensitivity? *Radiother Oncol,* **86**, 428–434.

60. Eng, C., Chang, G.J., Das, P. *et al.* (2009) Phase II study of capecitabine and oxaliplatin with concurrent radiation therapy (XELOX-RT) for squamous cell carcinoma of the anal canal [abstract 4116]. *J Clin Oncol,* **27(Suppl)**, 15s.

61. Chen, D.J., Nirodi, C.S. (2007) The epidermal growth factor: a role in repair of radiation-induced DNA damage. *Clin Cancer Res,* **12**, 6555–6560.

62. Milas, L., Mason, K., Hunter, N. *et al.* (2000) In vivo enhancement of tumor radioresponse by C225 antiepidermal growth factor receptor antibody. *Clin Cancer Res,* **6**, 701–707.

63. Bonner, J.A., Harari, P.M., Giralt, J. *et al.* (2010) Radiotherapy plus cetuximab for locoregionally advanced head and neck cancer: 5-year survival data from a phase 3 randomised trial, and relation between cetuximab-induced rash and survival. *Lancet Oncol,* **11**, 21–28.

64. Karapetis, C.S., Khambata-Ford, S., Jonker, D.J. *et al.* (2008) K-ras mutations and benefit from cetuximab in advanced colorectal cancer. *New Engl J Med,* **359**, 1757–1765.

65. De Roock, W., Claes, B., Bernasconi, D. *et al.* (2010) Effects of KRAS, BRAF, NRAS, and PIK3CA mutations on the efficacy of cetuximab plus chemotherapy in chemotherapy-refractory metastatic colorectal cancer: a retrospective consortium analysis. *Lancet Oncol,* **11**, 753–762.

66. Zampino, M.G., Magni, E., Sonzogni, A. *et al.* (2009) K-ras status in squamous cell canal carcinoma (SCC): it's time for targeted-oriented treatment? *Cancer Chemother Pharmacol,* **65**, 197–199.

67. Glynne-Jones, R., Mawdsley, S., Harrison M. (2010) Cetuximab and chemoradiation for rectal cancer—is the water getting muddy? *Acta Oncol,* **49**, 278–286.

68. John, S.S., Zietman, A.L., Shipley, W.U. *et al.* (2008) Newer imaging modalities to assist with target localization in the radiation treatment of

prostate cancer and possible lymph node metastases. *Int J Radiat Oncol Biol Phys,* **71** (1 Suppl), S43–S47.

69. Nutting, C.M., Morden, J.P., Harrington, K.L. *et al.* (2011) Parotid-sparing intensity modulated versus conventional radiotherapy in head and neck cancer (PARSPORT): a phase 3 multicentre randomised controlled trial. *Lancet Oncol,* **12**, 127–136.

70. Lee, C.T., Dong, L., Ahamad, A.W. *et al.* (2005) Comparison of treatment volumes and techniques in prostate cancer radiation therapy. *Am J Clin Oncol,* **28**, 618–625.

71. Hoffman, R., Welton, M.L., Klencke, B. *et al.* (1999) The significance of pretreatment CD4 count on the outcome and treatment tolerance of HIV-positive patients with anal cancer. *Int J Radiat Oncol Biol Phys,* **44**, 127–131.

72. Orlandi, E., Palazzi, M., Pignoli, E. *et al.* (2010) Radiobiological basis and clinical results of the simultaneous integrated boost (SIB) in intensity modulated radiotherapy (IMRT) for head and neck cancer: A review. *Crit Rev Oncol Hematol,* **72**, 111–125.

73. Salama, J.K., Mell, L., Schomas, D.A. *et al.* (2007) Concurrent chemotherapy and intensity-modulated radiation therapy for anal canal cancer patients: a multicenter experience. *J Clin Oncol,* **25**, 4581–4586.

74. Pepek, J.M., Willett, C.G., Clough, R.W. *et al.* (2010) Intensity modulated radiation therapy (IMRT) for anal cancer: the duke university experience. *Int J Radiat Oncol Biol Phys,* **78**, 1413–1419.

75. Kachnic, L.A., Tsai, H.K., Coen, J.J. *et al.* (2010) Dose-painted intensity-modulated radiation therapy for anal cancer: a multi-institutional report of acute toxicity and response to therapy. *Int J Radiat Oncol Biol Phys,* **82** (1), 153–158.

76. Kachnic, L.A., Winter, K.A., Myerson, RJ. *et al.* (2011) Two-year outcomes of RTOG 0529: a phase II evaluation of dose-painted IMRT in combination with 5-fluorouracil and mitomycin-C for the reduction of acute morbidity in carcinoma of the anal canal. *J Clin Oncol,* **29(Suppl 4)**, abstract 368.

77. Kachnic, L., Winter, K., Myerson, R. *et al.* (2009) RTOG 0529: a phase II evaluation of dose-painted IMRT in combination with 5-fluorouracil and mitomycin-C for reduction of acute morbidity in carcinoma of the anal canal. *Int J Radiat Oncol Biol Phys,* **75(Suppl)**, S5.

78. Constantinou, E.C., Daly, W., Fung, C.Y. *et al.* (1997) Time-dose considerations in the treatment of anal cancer. *Int J Radiat Oncol Biol Phys,* **39**, 651–657.

79. John, M., Pajak, T., Flam, M. *et al.* (1996) Dose escalation in chemoradiation for anal cancer: preliminary results of RTOG 92-08. *Cancer J Sci Am,* **2**, 205–211.

80. Martenson, J.A., Lipsitz, S.R., Wagner Jr, H. *et al.* (1996) Initial results of a phase II trial of high dose radiation therapy, 5-fluorouracil, and cisplatin for patients with anal cancer (E4292): an eastern cooperative oncology group study. *Int J Radiat Oncol Biol Phys,* **35**, 745–749.

81. Allal, A.S., Memillod, B., Roth, A.D. *et al.* (1997) Impact of clinical and therapeutic factors on major late complications after radiotherapy with or without concomitant chemotherapy for anal carcinoma. *Int J Radiat Oncol Biol Phys,* **39**, 1099–1105.

82. Newman, G., Calvery, D.C., Acker, B.D. *et al.* (1992) The management of carcinoma of the anal canal by external beam radiotherapy, experience in Vancouver 1971-1988. *Radiother Oncol,* **25**, 196–202.

83. Deniaud-Alexandre, E., Touboul, E., Tiret, E. *et al.* (2003) Results of definitive irradiation in a series of 305 epidermoid carcinomas of the anal canal. *Int J Radiat Oncol Biol Phys*, **5**, 1259–1273.

84. Faivre, C., Rougier, P., Ducreux, M. *et al.* (1999) 5-fluorouracil and cisplatinum combination chemotherapy for metastatic squamous-cell anal cancer. *Bull Cancer*, **86**, 861–865.

85. Jaiyesimi, I.A., Parzdur, R. (1993) Cisplatin and 5-fluorouracil as salvage therapy for recurrent metastatic squamous cell carcinoma of the anal canal. *Am J Clin Oncol*, **16**, 536–540.

86. Tanum, G. (1993) Treatment of relapsing anal carcinoma. *Acta Oncol*, **32**, 33–35.

87. Fisher, W.B., Herbst, K.D., Sims, J.E. *et al.* (1978) Metastatic cloacogenic carcinoma of the anus: sequential responses to adriamycin and cis-diclorodiammineplatinum (II). *Cancer Treat Rep*, **62**, 91–97.

88. Grifaichi, F., Padovani, A., Romeo, F. *et al.* (2001) Response of metastatic epidermoid anal cancer to single agent irinotecan: a case report. *Tumori*, **87**, 58–59.

89. Phan, L.K., Hoff, P.M. (2007) Evidence of clinical activity for cetuximab combined with irinotecan in a patient with refractor anal canal squamous-cell carcinoma: report of a case. *Dis Colon Rectum*, **50**, 395–398.

90. Lukan, N., Strobel, P., Willer, A. *et al.* (2009) Cetuximab-based treatment of metastatic anal cancer: correlation of response with KRAS mutational status. *Oncology*, **77**, 293–299.

91. Pawlik, T.M., Gleisner, A.L., Bauer, T.W. *et al.* (2007) Liver-directed surgery for metastatic squamous cell carcinoma to the liver: results of a multi-center analysis. *Ann Surg Oncol*, **14**, 2807–2816.

7 Primary Hepatic Cancer

Anan H. Said,[1] Kirti Shetty,[2] Ying Li,[3] Boris Blechacz,[3] Ernest Hawk,[3] and Lopa Mishra[3]

[1]University of Maryland Medical Center, Baltimore, MD, USA
[2]MedStar Georgetown University Hospital, Washington, DC, USA
[3]The University of Texas MD Anderson Cancer Center, Houston, TX, USA

Key Points

- Primary hepatic or hepatocellular cancer (HCC) is among the most common tumors worldwide, and its incidence is rising in many countries, including the United States.
- In the majority of cases, HCC occurs against a background of chronic liver disease or cirrhosis, providing a well-defined "at-risk" population for whom surveillance strategies may be employed. Diagnosis of HCC depends primarily on imaging studies. However, biopsy and serum biomarkers are also utilized.
- Although outcome is poor for patients with advanced HCC, those diagnosed at an early stage can be managed effectively with a variety of curative options. Treatment is dependent on a range of factors, particularly on the size and stage of the tumor, as well as hepatic function.
- Novel biomarkers and molecular therapy aimed at earlier diagnosis and more effective treatment therapy carries significant potential for more effective management of HCC.

Key Web Links

http://www.aasld.org/practiceguidelines/Pages/SortablePractice GuidelinesAlpha.aspxAASLD Practice Guidelines

http://www.nccn.org/professionals/physician_gls/f_guidelines.asp NCCN Clinical Practice Guidelines in Oncology

http://depts.washington.edu/uwhep/calculations/childspugh.htm Child-Pugh Score Calculator

Handbook of Gastrointestinal Cancer, First Edition. Edited by Janusz Jankowski and Ernest Hawk.
© 2013 John Wiley & Sons, Ltd. Published 2013 by John Wiley & Sons, Ltd.

Potential Pitfalls

- Only 15% of hepatocellular carcinoma (HCC) patients are potentially amenable to curative therapies at the time of presentation. Hence, screening at-risk populations for the development of HCC is essential.
- Alpha-fetoprotein as a serum marker for HCC lacks adequate sensitivity and specificity for effective surveillance and diagnosis of HCC. Therefore, screening needs to be based on imaging studies such as abdominal ultrasound at 6-month intervals.
- A single dynamic imaging technique (i.e., four-phase multidetector computed tomography or dynamic contrast-enhanced MRI) is sufficient for diagnosing HCC of more than 1 cm in size if arterial enhancement is observed followed by "washout" in the venous-delayed phase.
- These characteristic, radiologic patterns can be missing in the following situations and should prompt consideration of a targeted liver biopsy:
  - HCC of less than 2 cm can be hypovascular and present hypointense on the arterial as well as portal venous phase. In this situation, a liver biopsy will aid in distinguishing between HCC and a dysplastic nodule.
  - Cholangiocarcinomas can present as false positive for HCC. Therefore, a targeted liver biopsy of such lesions is required in cases of discrepancies between imaging studies.
- 5-year survival rates after orthotopic liver transplantation for HCC are 70%. In contrast, 5-year survival rates for intrahepatic cholangiocarcinomas outside of carefully conducted treatment protocols are less than 20%. Therefore, certainty of the diagnosis of HCC is highly important.

Epidemiology

Primary hepatic cancer is the fifth most common cancer worldwide and the third leading cause of cancer mortality in the United States, after lung and stomach cancer.[1] An estimated 24,120 new cases from liver and intrahepatic bile duct cancer in the United States are expected to occur during 2010, resulting in approximately 18,910 deaths. The incidence of hepatocellular carcinoma (HCC) has been steadily increasing since the early 1980s, with approximately 80% of cases due to an underlying chronic hepatitis B virus (HBV) and hepatitis C virus (HCV) infection.[2] HCC is second only to thyroid cancer with regard to the increase in rates of incidence from 1994 to 2003.[3]

The incidence of HCC varies widely according to geographic location with differences in distribution likely due to variations in exposure to the hepatitis viruses. High incidence regions of HCC (>20/100,000) occur in sub-Saharan Africa and eastern Asia, with China alone accounting for more than 50% of new cases.[1] North and South America, most of

Europe, Oceania, and parts of the Middle East are areas of low incidence (<5/100,000).

HCC is the fastest growing cause of cancer-related death in men in the United States.[4] Both incidence and mortality rates are twice as high in men as in women (incidence rates of 5.0 and 1.3 per 100,000 population, respectively).[4] HCV is the leading contributor to HCC in the United States and other Western nations.[5,6] Of the estimated 2.7–3.9 million people in the United States who are chronic carriers of hepatitis C, approximately 20% will develop cirrhosis and 5% will ultimately die from HCC.[5] High infection rates with hepatitis C between 1960 and 1990 and the lag time of 20–30 years between virus acquisition and development of cirrhosis and carcinoma have been largely responsible for the tripling of HCC incidence in the United States between 1975 and 2005.[7] HCC disproportionately affects minorities—the age-adjusted incidence rates are higher in those of Asian descent (8/100,000 population), Hispanics (6/100,000 population), and African Americans (5/100,000 population) as compared with Caucasians (2.5/100,000 population).[8]

Recently, the combination of insulin resistance, hypertension, dyslipidemia, and obesity, termed "metabolic syndrome," has been recognized as a cause of nonalcoholic fatty liver disease (NAFLD). There is increasing evidence that the risk of developing HCC in NAFLD cirrhosis is between 18% and 27%, which is greater than the risk of developing HCC in HCV-related cirrhosis.[9] Hemochromatosis is also a significant risk factor for HCC, with an increased relative risk 200 times that of the normal population.

Diagnosis

There are a number of tests utilized in the diagnosis of HCC including radiological studies, histopathology, and analysis of serum biomarkers.[10] The American Association for the Study of Liver Diseases (AASLD) guidelines on the management of HCC provide a framework for the approach to diagnosis.[11]

Clinical features

HCC is typically asymptomatic and most signs and symptoms of the disease relate to the patient's chronic liver disease. The most commonly reported symptoms are nonspecific and include phrenic irritation causing vague upper abdominal pain or right shoulder discomfort. Patients may also report fatigue, weight loss, jaundice, early satiety, anorexia, and fever, although these symptoms are more often found in advanced lesions. On physical examination, patients with HCC may have hepatomegaly, ascites, splenomegaly, jaundice, a palpable upper abdominal mass, hepatic bruit, or fever.[12] A paraneoplastic syndrome may also develop in patients with HCC, and such patients may present with hypercalcemia, hypoglycemia, diarrhea, erythrocytosis, hypercholesterolemia, gynecomastia, and virilization.[13]

Imaging studies

HCC is a highly vascular tumor, receiving the majority of its blood supply from branches of the hepatic artery, as opposed to the liver parenchyma that receives 70% of its supply from the portal vein.[14] This "arterialization" of the vascular supply to the tumor accounts for its classic imaging hallmark: enhancement in the arterial phase and washout of contrast media in the portal venous phase.[15] Imaging modalities used in diagnosis include ultrasound, computed tomography (CT), magnetic resonance imaging (MRI), and angiography.[16] Contrast-enhanced studies allow for the diagnosis of HCC without necessitating biopsy; four-phase helical CT and multiphase dynamic contrast-enhanced MRI are the most reliable imaging tests for HCC.[17]

Ultrasound is the preferred test in screening for HCC. However, imaging quality is dependent both on the operator and patient body habitus. Neoplastic lesions less than 3 cm in size are typically hypoechoic, well circumscribed, and homogenous. As tumor size exceeds 3 cm, the appearance on ultrasound is more heterogenous, isoechoic, or hyperechoic, and central hypoechoic regions representing fibrous septae may be observed.[18] Ultrasound can also reveal vascular patency or intrahepatic thrombosis, and color Doppler ultrasound can provide an estimate of mean velocity blood flow of the hepatic vessels. Contrast-enhanced ultrasonography is not widely utilized in the United States, but has been shown in several studies to have superior accuracy to standard ultrasound.

Four-phase helical CT consists of unenhanced, hepatic arterial, portal venous, and delayed phases, and it is often carried out after detection of an abnormality on ultrasound. The typical CT findings of HCC during the arterial phase 25 seconds after contrast injection are increased enhancement of the tumor as compared with nontumorous liver parenchyma. Seventy seconds after contrast injection, during the portal venous phase, the lesion is either isodense or hypodense; 300 seconds later, during the delayed phase, HCC is typically hypodense due to the early "washout" of contrast.[18]

MRI has been shown to be more accurate than CT in the detection of neoplastic lesions. Gadolinium-enhanced MRI demonstrates a hyperintense image of the tumor in the arterial phase, isointensity in the portal phase, and hypointensity in the delayed phase. T2-weighted images typically demonstrate hyperintensity; T1-weighted images reveal variable intensity. Sensitivity of MRI and CT in detecting HCC has been noted to be 81% and 68%, respectively, and specificity of MRI and CT is 85% and 93%, respectively. MRI can more reliably differentiate HCC from regenerating or dysplastic nodules as compared with CT.[19,20]

Biopsy

Percutaneous biopsy confirmation of HCC should only be performed if radiologic studies demonstrate uncertainty in the diagnosis, as there are several risks associated with biopsy such as needle track seeding and bleeding.[21] Needle core biopsy is preferred over fine needle aspiration biopsy (FNAB), since it provides a more reliable specimen.[22] FNAB has been reported to have high false-negative rates and is highly dependent on the expertise of the cytopathologist.[23] However, FNAB has the advantages of being a less invasive test lowering the complication rates of this procedure, as well as providing for an instant assessment of whether sufficient tissue samples were obtained.[24]

The risk of malignant needle track seeding is a recognized complication of biopsy, and is clinically significant in patients who are under consideration for liver transplantation (LT) or resection. A recent review reported 14 series with 66 cases of seeding following biopsy. The risk of seeding ranged from 0% to 11%, with a median value of 2.29%.[25] Numerous factors have been related to the risk of neoplastic dissemination: larger diameter needles, more passes, superficial location of the tumor in the liver, intrinsic metastatic property of the tumor related to either or both tumor size/aggressiveness, and patients' immunodepression resulting in reduced tumor surveillance.

Serology

Although the use of alpha-fetoprotein (AFP) has been used for both surveillance and diagnosis in the past, recent studies have discounted its utility. The Hepatitis C Antiviral Long-Term Treatment Against Cirrhosis (HALT-C) trial analyzed the accuracy of both AFP and descarboxyprothrombin (DCP) in diagnosing HCC among 1031 randomized patients with hepatitis C-related cirrhosis. Among this group, 39 patients developed HCC over the course of the study; however, neither biomarker alone was sufficiently sensitive or specific for the detection of HCC, warranting the continued need for radiological or histological diagnosis.[26] Serum AFP levels have been shown to be normal in patients with fibrolamellar HCC, which generally occurs in young adults without underlying cirrhosis.[27] Furthermore, elevations in serum AFP are noted in a number of other diseases such as intrahepatic cholangiocarcinoma or other nonmalignant conditions, and the serum level rarely correlates with size, stage, or prognosis.

Surveillance

HCC is unique among cancers in that it is usually preceded by chronic liver disease and cirrhosis, thus providing a well-defined target population for whom surveillance strategies may be devised. Unfortunately, many questions remain about the feasibility and efficacy of surveillance for HCC. In order to make informed decisions about which patients should be entered into a surveillance program for HCC, we need to address some important issues:

1. What is the objective of HCC surveillance?

    The ideal objective would be to decrease mortality from the disease. There is a single randomized controlled study of surveillance versus no surveillance that has shown a survival benefit. This study that was conducted in China and recruited 18,816 at-risk patients demonstrated a 37% reduction in HCC-related mortality. Due to adherence rates of only 60%, this result probably represents the minimum benefit that may be expected from surveillance, and ideally should be replicated in other study populations. However, ethical issues probably preclude such a study being performed in the future.[28]

2. What is the population that should be entered into a surveillance program?

    The decision to enter a patient into a surveillance program is determined by the level of risk for HCC. There is no population-based data estimating such a risk, and therefore current guidelines are based on decision analysis studies. In general, surveillance for HCC in cirrhosis of various etiologies was found to be cost-effective if the risk of HCC was 1.5%/year or greater. The only exceptions to this are patients with chronic HBV infection who develop HCC even in the absence of cirrhosis. Analysis of this population suggests that surveillance was cost-effective when the incidence of HCC exceeds 0.2%/year,[11] see Table 7.1.

    An additional group of patients who should undergo surveillance for HCC are patients on the liver transplant waiting list, as current United Network of Organ Sharing (UNOS) criteria gives priority for transplantation to patients who develop HCC. Conversely, identification of a neoplastic lesion that exceeds guidelines during the waiting period would result in the elimination of that patient from transplant candidacy.[11]

Table 7.1 Recommended surveillance populations and the associated annual incidence of hepatocellular carcinoma.

Population group for which surveillance is recommended	HCC incidence/year
HBV carrier	
• Asian male ≥age 40	0.4–0.6%
• Asian female ≥age 50	0.3–0.6%
• Family history of HCC	Unclear but higher than those without family history
• African/North American Black	Occurs at younger age
Cirrhosis due to	
• HBV	3–8%
• HCV	3–5%
• PBC	3–5%
• Genetic hemochromatosis	Unknown but >1.5%/year
• Alpha-1 antitrypsin deficiency	Unknown but >1.5%/year

Source: Reproduced with permission from the American Association for the Study of Liver Diseases. Bruix, J., Sherman, M. (2010) *Management of Hepatocellular Carcinoma: An Update*. American Association for the Study of Liver Diseases, Alexandria, VA. This updates a previous version: Bruix J, Sherman M. Management of Hepatocellular Carcinoma. Hepatology 2005 **42(5)**, 1208–1236.

Proposed Work-up of Suspicious Hepatic Nodules:

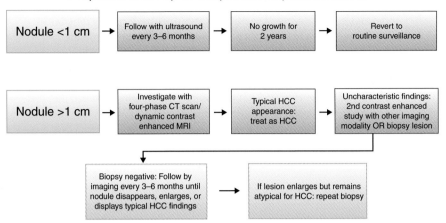

Figure 7.1 Biopsies of small lesions should be evaluated by expert pathologists. Tissue that is not clearly HCC should be stained with all the available markers including CD34, CK7, glypican 3, HCP-70, and glutamine synthetase to improve diagnostic accuracy. (Adapted from AASLD Practice Guidelines.[11])

3. What are ideal surveillance modalities?

Screening or surveillance tests for HCC fall into two categories—serological and radiological. Of the serological tests, the performance characteristics of AFP have been best studied. Despite its widespread use for HCC surveillance, AFP has suboptimal accuracy, with sensitivity of 66% and specificity of 82%. As such, its continued utility as a tumor marker for HCC has been questioned. Other serological tests are DCP, glypican 3, and heat-shock protein 70, as well as the ratio of glycosylated AFP (L3 fraction) to total AFP. None of these can be recommended as a screening test at the current time.

The radiological test most commonly used for surveillance is ultrasonography. Ultrasound is reported to have a sensitivity of 65–80% and specificity of more than 90% when used for screening. Its performance characteristics are negatively impacted by the presence of cirrhotic nodules, subject obesity, and operator inexperience. However, its easy availability and relative cost-efficacy make it the test of choice for surveillance. Surveillance intervals should be between 6 and 12 months based on reported tumor doubling times.

The latest update to the AASLD practice guidelines for management of patients with HCC based on surveillance screening is summarized in Figure 7.1.

Prognosis and staging

Cancer staging systems are vital prognostic tools, and guide treatment decisions while stratifying different key factors into a common algorithm. Many different staging systems exist for HCC and there is no uniform consensus for the use of any single system. Most of these staging systems take into account the following parameters: aggressiveness and growth rate of the tumor, the presence of vascular invasion, hepatic synthetic function, and performance status. The most commonly used staging systems are the Barcelona Clinic Liver Cancer (BCLC) staging classification, the American Joint Committee on Cancer Tumor Node Metastasis (AJCC-TNM) system, the Okuda system, and the Cancer of the Liver Italian Program (CLIP) system.[29–32] AASLD Practice Guidelines recommend the use of the BCLC staging system for patients with HCC (Figure 7.2).[11] The BCLC system is unique in that it incorporates tumor stage, liver function as defined by Child–Turcotte–Pugh (CTP) class, and performance status, linking these to individualized treatment modalities. This staging system's ability to stratify patients into different prognostic categories has been well documented in a meta-analysis of untreated patients with HCC in randomized clinical trials, as well as other major trials of HCC therapy.[33–36]

Based on the BCLC staging classification, patients are classified into the following five stages:

1. *Very early stage (0)*: These patients have a solitary lesion under 2 cm in size, usually detected incidentally. Their 5-year survival rate is near 100% with resection or radiofrequency ablation.
2. *Early stage (A)*: Defined by those with preserved liver function (CTP class A and B), and up to three nodules each being ≤3 cm in size, or one solitary lesion between 2 and 5 cm. This is effectively treated by resection, transplantation, or percutaneous ablation. The 5-year survival rate ranges from 50% to 75%.

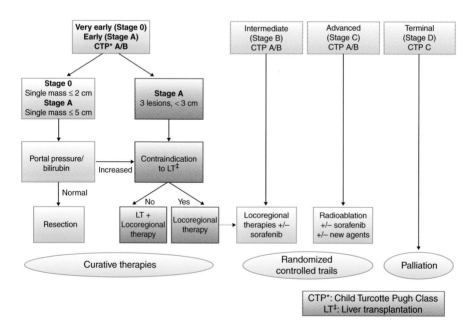

Figure 7.2 Multidisciplinary Approach to Hepatocellular Carcinoma. (Adapted from the BCLC staging classification and treatment schedule.[34])

3. *Intermediate stage (B)*: It includes patients with compensated cirrhosis but without cancer-related symptoms, extrahepatic spread, or macrovascular invasion. These patients have a 3-year survival rate of approximately 50% without therapy and are usually suitable candidates for transarterial chemoembolization (TACE) therapy.
4. *Advanced stage (C)*: These patients present with mild cancer-related symptoms and/or portal invasion or extrahepatic spread and have a survival rate of approximately 50% at 1 year. These patients are candidates for sorafenib or other chemotherapeutic agents.
5. *Terminal disease (D)*: These patients present with extensive impairment in their liver function (CTP class C), vascular involvement, cancer-related symptoms, extrahepatic spread, and physical impairment (WHO performance status >2). They have an approximate survival time of less than 3 months and should receive symptomatic treatment to avoid unnecessary suffering.

Although the BCLC staging classification has been proven to be a more accurate prognostic model than other staging systems, it has been faulted for its algorithmic rather than multidisciplinary approach.[37,38] There are limitations to other classification systems as well. The AJCC TNM staging system identifies the size and number of tumors, as well as the presence of vascular invasion. Even though this system is most predictive of long-term outcome, its applicability is limited by the fact that it is usually based on analysis of a surgical specimen and cannot be utilized in treatment decisions.[36,39]

The Okuda system incorporates parameters of hepatic synthetic function (ascites, albumin, and bilirubin) and tumor characteristics.[29] This system does not include macrovascular invasion or extrahepatic spread, and it seems most suited to those with advanced disease.

The CLIP system is a mathematical score incorporating subscores in CTP, tumor morphology, AFP levels, and the presence of vascular invasion. Although the CLIP system is particularly useful in assessing prognosis of patients who undergo transarterial embolization (TAE) or those patients treated in palliative settings, it is limited in its ability to adequately assess patients undergoing therapies such as resection or transplantation.[40]

Cancer management

Surgery

Surgical resection is the mainstay of therapy for HCC in noncirrhotic patients, especially in populations with limited access to orthotopic liver transplantation (OLT).[41] However, this modality is restricted to solitary tumors without vascular invasion in suitable anatomical locations. Other important presurgical selection criteria include adequate hepatic synthetic function and the absence of portal hypertension. If both these criteria are met, the 5-year survival is approximately 70%.[42] Patients with portal hypertension, defined as hepatic vein pressure gradient measuring

>10 mm Hg, are at risk of postoperative decompensation, with 5-year survival under 50%. Those with both elevated bilirubin levels and portal hypertension have 5-year survival rates under 30%. Tumor size per se is not a limitation for surgery, although increasing tumor size does increase the risk of vascular invasion and dissemination.[43]

The risk of recurrence is affected by a number of factors, with the presence of vascular invasion and the number of tumors beyond the primary lesion being the most predictive. One large study showed that patients with three or more nodules have a 26% 5-year survival compared with a 57% rate of patients with solitary tumors.[44] No effective adjuvant therapy has been demonstrated to reduce the rate of postsurgical recurrence.[45]

Liver transplantation

LT for HCC is an attractive option, as it simultaneously removes cancerous lesions and replaces the cirrhotic premalignant liver. The role of LT in the management of HCC has evolved significantly over the past two decades. The initial experience with LT was limited to those with extensive tumors and was marked by uniformly dismal outcomes.[46,47]

The first suggestion that favorable tumor characteristics may be associated with decreased recurrence came from the University of Pittsburgh experience wherein a series of unexpected or "incidental" tumors were found to have surprisingly good survival rates.[48] This led to the recognition that early cancer detection and meticulous pretransplant staging were key to successful outcomes. An important study in 1996 by Mazzaferro and his colleagues from Milan confirmed this view. By carefully selecting patients who satisfied specific tumor criteria, the Milan group was able to achieve excellent recurrence-free survivals of 92% at 3 years and a 4-year overall survival rate of 85%.[49]

Against this encouraging backdrop, HCC once again became an important indication for transplantation. Recognizing that these patients were disadvantaged by an organ allocation system based solely on decompensated cirrhosis, the UNOS decided to prioritize allocation of organs to those HCC patients who met the tumor criteria recognized in the Milan experience to have the best outcomes. The Milan criteria are based on tumor burden and limit prioritization for LT to those who have either a single tumor less than 5 cm or those with three or less tumors each less than 3 cm, without evidence of metastatic disease or vascular invasion. Patients satisfying Milan criteria are afforded additional priority on the transplant waiting list. Despite this prioritization, the scarcity of available organs translates into prolonged waiting times, which causes approximately 30% of patients to suffer tumor progression, and "drop-out" of the waiting list.[50]

Adult-to-adult living donor liver transplantation (LDLT) has been utilized to shorten the waiting time and potentially decrease waiting list mortality in HCC. A large multicenter study conducted by the Adult-to-Adult Living Donor Liver Transplantation Cohort Study (A2ALL) group found that HCC patients who underwent LDLT had a significantly higher HCC recurrence rate than deceased donor liver transplant (DDLT) recipients. It is hypothesized that putting patients with HCC on a "fast track" to LT may not provide adequate time to assess the tumor's biological behavior. Inclusion of patients with more aggressive tumors in the LDLT group may account for the higher recurrence rate compared with DDLT recipients who had a significantly longer waiting time (median 95 vs. 373 days from listing to transplant).[11,51,52]

Percutaneous ablation

Ablation therapy using radiofrequency ablation (RFA) or percutaneous ethanol injection (PEI) under ultrasound guidance is a very good option for patients who are not surgical candidates or as a "bridge" to definitive therapy such as LT. RFA utilizes radiofrequency thermal energy, which is applied through high frequency alternating currents into the tissue surrounding a lesion. This results in a wide region of cell death and tissue necrosis. PEI is administered over a number of days and involves direct injection of ethanol into the tumor, which also induces tissue necrosis. This method is used sparingly in the West. Both methods have relatively low complication rates, and the efficacy of therapy can be monitored by dynamic CT/MRI after treatment sessions: necrotic areas indicate successful tumor ablation, whereas persistent contrast enhancement indicates tumor viability.[53]

Both RFA and PEI are equally effective in tumors <2 cm, with necrosis rates of between 90% and 100%.[54] For tumors >2 cm, RFA results in more extensive tumor necrosis rates than PEI, and has the added advantage of requiring fewer treatment sessions.[55] Survival rates at 1 and 2 years were 100% and 98%, respectively, in patients treated with RFA as compared with 96% and 88%, respectively, in patients undergoing PEI. Furthermore, 1 and 2 years recurrence rates were 86% and 64%, respectively, with RFA therapy as compared with 77% and 43%, respectively, in patients undergoing PEI, showing that among all tumor sizes, RFA has a more predictable necrotic effect and increased efficacy as compared with PEI.[55]

Transarterial embolization

Utilizing the principle of "arterialization" of HCC, TAE selectively occludes a branch of the hepatic artery that supplies the tumor, inducing ischemic tumor necrosis with relative sparing of nonmalignant liver parenchyma. Transarterial Chemoembolization (TACE) is the injection of chemotherapy prior to arterial obstruction. Although little data exists to guide choice of chemotherapy in TACE, agents that have been used commonly include cisplatin, adriamycin, doxorubicin, and mitomycin coupled with lipiodol, an oily contrast agent that prolongs exposure of the chemotherapy to tumor cells.[56] Extensive tumor necrosis is observed in upward of 50% of patients who undergo TACE. However, less than 2% of patients have a durable response, since the tumor revascularizes weeks to months after therapy.[56] A randomized controlled trial done in 2002 has clearly demonstrated the benefits of TACE.[57] Patients with unresectable HCC were assigned to TAE, TACE, or conservative therapy. TACE was demonstrated to have a survival benefit compared with conservative treatment (hazard ratio of death 0.47 (95% CI 0.25–0.91), $p = 0.025$). Survival probabilities at 1 and 2 years were 75% and 50%, respectively, for TAE; 82% and 63%, respectively, for TACE, and 63% and 27%, respectively, for control (TACE vs. control $p = 0.009$). TACE-induced objective responses were sustained for at least 6 months in 35% of cases, and TACE was associated with a significantly lower rate of portal vein invasion than conservative treatment.

Locoregional therapies are used in those with multiple tumors without extrahepatic spread or vascular invasion. They are also utilized to "bridge" patients to LT, so as to prevent tumor progression and "drop-out" of the transplant waiting list.[58] The main contraindications to TACE are extensive portal vein thrombosis (PVT) and advanced liver disease. Those with CTP class C liver function have been demonstrated to have poor outcomes with locoregional therapies.[59] A relative contraindication to TACE therapy as stated by the National Comprehensive Cancer Network (NCCN) Practice Guidelines is a bilirubin level >3 mg/mL because of the increased risk of hepatic necrosis and hepatic decompensation in patients with limited synthetic reserve.[60]

A newer method of HCC ablation involves the injection of yttrium-90 (Y90) tagged glass or resin microspheres directly through the hepatic artery, delivering a high dose of internal radiation when the particles become trapped in the tumor-associated capillary bed. This method of internal radiation delivery results in tumor necrosis due to beta radiation and allows for sparing of nontumorous tissue.[61] In a recently reported cohort study of 291 patients with HCC who were treated with Y90, response rates were 42% and 57% based on WHO and EASL (European Association for the Study of the Liver) guidelines, respectively. Patients with CTP A disease, with or without PVT, benefited from most treatment. A retrospective comparison between HCC patients treated by chemoembolization or Yttrium-90 radioembolization demonstrated similar survival times. However, radioembolization resulted in delayed time to progression and less toxicity than chemoembolization.[62]

Molecular therapy

For patients with intermediate or advanced stage HCC and preserved liver function, sorafenib has been shown to prolong life. This drug is an oral multikinase inhibitor of the vascular endothelial growth factor (VEGF) receptor, the platelet-derived growth factor receptor, and Raf that inhibit tumor cell angiogenesis and proliferation.[63] A large randomized, placebo-controlled phase III trial of patients with advanced HCC (Sorafenib HCC Assessment Randomized Protocol or SHARP trial) was recently concluded. It showed a 31% decrease in the risk of death, with a median survival of 10.7 versus 7.9 months, and time to progression of 5.5 versus 2.8 months in the sorafenib and placebo groups, respectively.[64] The majority of patients (83%) in this trial had evidence of portal vein invasion, and 20% had extrahepatic spread of disease. Sorafenib is currently the only agent approved by the Food and Drug Administration for the treatment of advanced HCC. Even though its survival benefit appears modest, sorafenib has highlighted the role for molecular therapy in HCC. Ongoing studies have focused on growth factors involved in the angiogenesis of HCC.[65] One such promising drug targeting VEGF is bevacizumab, a recombinant, humanized IgG1 anti-VEGF monoclonal antibody. Phase II studies using bevacizumab monotherapy have revealed a partial response in 8–13% of patients and stable disease in 54–72% of patients.[66,67] Other promising anti-VEGF/VEGF receptor therapies in phase II development include vatalanib, cediranib, and linifanib.

Endothelial growth factor (EGF) has also been shown to be involved in the development of HCC through binding to the EGF receptor and activation of the RAF/MEK/ERK and PI3K/AKT/mTOR pathways. Erlotinib is an oral tyrosine kinase inhibitor of EGF receptor in phase II development that has shown antitumor activity in a study of 38 patients with unresectable or metastatic HCC.[68] In this study, a partial response was observed in 9% of patients with a disease control rate of 59%. Twelve of the thirty eight patients taking daily erlotinib were progression free at 6 months and median overall survival was noted to be 13 months. Currently, a phase III placebo-controlled, double-blind study is in progress, and it is aimed at analyzing the effect of combination therapy with erlotinib and either bevacizumab or sorafenib in advanced HCC.

Other novel approaches toward targeting the intracellular signaling pathways involved in the generation of HCC are currently under investigation. The transforming growth factor-β (TGF-β) signaling pathway is involved in tumor suppression, and the adaptor protein β-2SP is emerging as a potent regulator of tumorigenesis through its ability to affect TGF-β tumor suppressor function. It has been demonstrated that mice with downregulated β-2SP develop HCC at a higher rate, and β-2SP expression is lost in human HCC. This indicates a possible role for β-2SP in suppression of early HCC. E3 ligases, KEAP1, and PRAJA are dramatically increased in human and mouse HCC when TGF-β signaling is inactivated and are strong potential therapeutic targets.[69,70] In light of these observations, small molecule inhibitors and other drugs that specifically inhibit PRAJA and KEAP1 in addition to other signaling pathways have been proposed and tested in studies to test the utility of these molecules in HCC therapy as well as other neoplasms (Table 7.2).

Prevention

The prevention of HCC is through avoidance of risk factors, as approximately 90–95% of cases are a result of chronic infection with either HBV or HCV. Chronic viral hepatitis leads to liver injury and regeneration, with subsequent fibrosis and cirrhosis. The pathogenesis of HBV-associated HCC may be related to the hepatitis B x (HBx) gene product, which is a transcriptional activator of genes involved in cell growth.[71] In the United States, universal infant vaccination against HBV has been utilized since 1991 and vaccination is also aimed at other at-risk populations, with the aim to eliminate transmission of the virus. Taiwan is

Table 7.2 List of representative drugs targeting different signaling pathways.

Targeting Wnt signaling			
Agent name	Type	Target	Indications
Sulindac and derivatives	NSAID	β-Catenin	Hereditary forms of colon cancer
Retinoids	Vitamin A	β-Catenin	Colon cancer
1α, 25-dihydroxyvitamin D3 and synthetic derivatives	Vitamin D	β-Catenin	Colon, breast, and prostate cancers
Specific antibodies	Monoclonal antibodies	Wnt and FZD receptors	Preclinical
PKF115-584, PKF-222-815	Small molecule inhibitors	β-Catenin-Tcf	Preclinical
H101	Virus	Promoter containing Tcf-responsive elements	Phase I trial

Targeting CDKs			
Agent name	Type	Target	Indications
AG-024322	Small molecule inhibitors	CDK1, CDK2, CDK4	Phase I, advanced cancer
AT-7519	Small molecule inhibitors	CDK1, CDK2, CDK4, CDK5, GSK3β	Phase I/II, advanced or metastatic tumors
P276-00	Small molecule inhibitors	CDK1, CDK4, CDK9	Phase I/II, advanced refractory neoplasms
P1446A-05	Small molecule inhibitors	CDK4	Phase I, advanced refractory malignancies
PD-0332991	Small molecule inhibitors	CDK4, CDK6	Phase I, advanced cancer
R547 (also known as Ro-4584820)	Small molecule inhibitors	CDK1, CDK2, CDK4, CDK7	Phase I, advanced solid tumors
Roscovitine (also known as seliciclib and CYC202)	Small molecule inhibitors	CDK2, CDK7, CDK8, CDK9	Phase II, non-small cell lung cancer, nasopharyngeal cancer, hematological tumors
SNS-032 (also known as BMS-387032)	Small molecule inhibitors	CDK1, CDK2, CDK4 CDK7, CDK9, GSK3β	Phase I, B-lymphoid malignancies Phase I, solid tumors

Targeting telomerase			
Agent name	Type	Target	Indications
GRN163L	Small molecule inhibitors	Telomerase	Phase I/II for chronic lymphocytic leukemia patients; Phase I/II for multiple myeloma; Phase I for solid tumors; Phase I/II for breast cancer; and Phase I/II for NSCLC lung cancer
GV1001	Peptide vaccine	*TERT* epitopes	Phase III trial for advanced pancreatic patients

Table 7.2 *Continued*

Targeting telomerase			
Agent name	Type	Target	Indications
Telomelysin®	Adenovirus	Containing the *hTERT* promoter	Phase I solid tumor clinical trials

Targeting stat3 signaling			
Agent name	Type	Target	Indications
PY*LKTK Y*LPQTV	Peptide	STAT3 SH2	Preclinical
ISS 610 S3I-M2001 STA-21	Small molecule inhibitors	STAT3 SH2	Preclinical
IS3-295 CPA-1, CPA-7 Galiellalactone	Small molecule inhibitors	STAT3 DBD	Preclinical
Peptide aptamers	Peptide	STAT3 DBD	Preclinical

Targeting TGF-β signaling			
Agent name	Type	Target	Indications
Lerdelimumab	Monoclonal antibody	TGF-β2 and TGF-β3	Postoperative scarring in glaucoma patients
Metelimumab	Monoclonal antibody	TGF-β1	Renal fibrosis
Belagenpumatucel-L	Anti-TGF-β2 vaccine	TGF-β2	Non-small-cell lung cancer
AP 12009	Antisense oligonucleotide	TGF-β2	Glioma, pancreatic carcinoma, melanoma
LY550410	Small molecule	TβRI kinase domain	Preclinical
SB-505124	Small molecule	TβRI kinase domain	Preclinical

the first country in the world that has been able to demonstrate a decline in HCC incidence directly related to universal HBV immunization.[72] Reducing viral load through the use of antiviral therapy may reduce HCC risk, as cancer risk is greatest in patients with the highest serum levels of HBV DNA.[73] Although research into therapeutic and prophylactic vaccines against HCV has been ongoing, there is no currently approved vaccine.

Prevention of cirrhosis from other etiologies such as alcohol, NAFLD, or hemochromatosis would involve lifestyle changes, effective management of obesity, diabetes and dyslipidemia, and regular phlebotomies for hemochromatosis. Identification of patients with cirrhosis and enrollment of an "at-risk" population into a surveillance program for HCC would facilitate diagnosis of this lethal cancer at an early and treatable stage. New hypotheses aimed at suppressing the fibrotic and inflammatory processes that eventually lead to HCC are also being tested. Agents such as P38 inhibitors, vitamin D, Cox-2 inhibitors, and pentoxifylline are in preclinical studies to examine if these agents suppress the growth or induce death of malignant or premalignant hepatocytes with the aim of preventing the development and progression of HCC in at-risk patients.

Case Study

During staging evaluation for a recurrent, metastatic tonsillar carcinoma, a 63-year-old gentleman was incidentally found to have an intrahepatic mass lesion on magnetic resonance imaging (MRI). His past medical history is significant for chronic hepatitis C virus (HCV) infection and chronic alcohol consumption. He was found to have cirrhosis based upon his hepatic synthetic function markers and the radiologic morphology. His Child–Pugh score was 5 consistent with grade A cirrhosis. The intrahepatic mass was located in segment IV of the liver and 4.3 × 2.6 cm in size; there was no evidence for metastases, vascular invasion, or PVT (Figure 7.3). The mass showed an enhancing pattern on the arterial phase of the MRI and "washout" on the portal venous phase. The patients' alpha-fetoprotein serum concentration was within the normal range with 4.3 ng/mL. Due to his coexisting tonsillar carcinoma, an ultrasound-guided liver biopsy of the mass was obtained to rule out metastatic disease; the biopsy confirmed the diagnosis of hepatocellular carcinoma (HCC). Although the patient was within Milan criteria in regard to the characteristics of his HCC, orthotopic liver transplantation (OLT) was not an option due to coexisting metastatic tonsillar carcinoma. Given the limited prognosis due to his recurrent, metastatic tonsillar carcinoma, it was recommended to proceed with transarterial chemoembolization (TACE). However, the patient decided against any further treatment for either of his two malignancies.

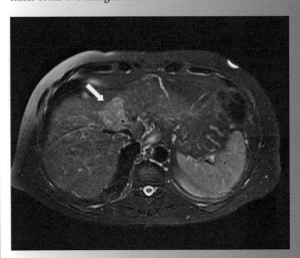

Figure 7.3 Hepatocellular carcinoma.

Shown is a T2-weighted axial MRI of the liver. In segment IV of the liver, a hyperintense mass lesion during the arterial phase is noticeable (*white arrow*). This lesion became hypointense during the portal venous phase of the MRI study; this phenomenon is known as "washout" and specific for hepatocellular carcinoma (HCC). The diagnosis was later confirmed by a targeted liver biopsy.

References

1. El-Serag, H.B., Marrero, J.A., Rudolph, L., Reddy, K.R. (2008) *Diagnosis and treatment of hepatocellular carcinoma. Gastroenterology*, **134(6)**, 1752–1763.
2. Cancer Facts and Figures 2010. American Cancer Society. Available at: http://www.cancer.org/acs/groups/content/@nho/documents/document/acspc-024113.pdf
3. Surveillance Epidemiology & End Results. National Cancer Institute. Available at: http://seer.cancer.gov/statistics/
4. El-Serag, H.B. (2004) Hepatocellular carcinoma: recent trends in the United States. *Gastroenterology*, **127(5, Suppl 1)**, S27–S34.
5. Centers for Disease Control and Prevention. (1998) Recommendations for prevention and control of hepatitis C virus (HCV) infection and HCV-related chronic disease. Centers for Disease Control and Prevention. *MMWR*, **47(No. RR-19)**, 1–39
6. Thomas, M.B., Jaffe, D., Choti, M.M. *et al.* (2010) Hepatocellular carcinoma: consensus recommendations of the national cancer institute clinical trials planning meeting. *J Clin Oncol*, **28(25)**, 3994–4005.
7. El-Serag, H.B., Mason, A.C. (1999) Rising incidence of hepatocellular carcinoma in the United States. *N Engl J Med*, **340(10)**, 745–750.
8. El-Serag, H.B., Davila, J.A., Petersen, N.J., McGlynn, K.A. (2003) The continuing increase in the incidence of hepatocellular carcinoma in the United States: an update. *Ann Intern Med*, **139(10)**, 817–823.
9. Siegel, A.B., Zhu, A.X. (2009) Metabolic syndrome and hepatocellular carcinoma: two growing epidemics with a potential link. *Cancer*, **115**, 5651–5661.
10. Llovet, J.M., Burroughs, A., Bruix, J. (2003) Hepatocellular carcinoma. *Lancet*, **362(9399)**, 1907–1917.
11. Bruix, J., Sherman, M. (2010) Management of hepatocellular carcinoma: an update; Practice Guidelines Committee, American Association for the Study of Liver Diseases. *Hepatology*, 1–35.
12. Takamatsu, S., Noguchi, N., Kudoh, A. *et al.* (2008) Influence of risk factors for metabolic syndrome and non-alcoholic fatty liver disease on the progression and prognosis of hepatocellular carcinoma. *Hepatogastroenterology*, **55(82–83)**, 609–614.
13. Eastman, R.C., Carson, R.E., Orloff, D.G. *et al.* (1992) Glucose utilization in a patient with hepatoma and hypoglycemia. Assessment by a positron emission tomography. *J Clin Invest*, **89(6)**, 1958–1963.
14. Budhu, A., Forgues, M., Ye, Q.H. *et al.* (2006) Prediction of venous metastases, recurrence, and prognosis in hepatocellular carcinoma based on a unique immune response signature of the liver microenvironment. *Cancer Cell*, **10(2)**, 99–111.
15. Torzilli, G., Minagawa, M., Takayama, T. *et al.* (1999) Accurate preoperative evaluation of liver mass lesions without fine-needle biopsy. *Hepatology*, **30(4)**, 889–893.
16. Shinmura, R., Matsui, O., Kadoya, M. *et al.* (2008) Detection of hypervascular malignant foci in borderline lesions of hepatocellular carcinoma: comparison of dynamic multi-detector row CT, dynamic MR imaging and superparamagnetic iron oxide-enhanced MR imaging. *Eur Radiol*, **18(9)**, 1918–1924.
17. Kim, M.J., Choi, J.Y., Chung, Y.E., Choi, S.Y. (2008) Magnetic resonance imaging of hepatocellular carcinoma using contrast media. *Oncology*, **75(Suppl 1)**, 72–82.

18. Gomaa, A.I., Khan, S.A., Leen, ELS., Waked, I., Taylor-Robinson, S.D. (2009) Diagnosis of hepatocellular carcinoma. *World J Gastroenterol*, **15(11)**, 1301–1331.

19. Colli, A., Fraquelli, M., Casazza, G. *et al.* (2006) Accuracy of ultrasonography, spiral CT, magnetic resonance, and alpha fetoprotein in diagnosing hepatocellular carcinoma: a systemic review. *Am J Gastroenterol*, **101**, 513.

20. Yu, S.C., Yeung, D.T., So, N.M. (2004) Imaging features of hepatocellular carcinoma. *Clin Radiol*, **59(2)**, 145–156.

21. Bialecki, E.S., Ezenekwe, A.M., Brunt, E.M. *et al.* (2006) Comparison of liver biopsy and noninvasive methods for diagnosis of hepatocellular carcinoma. *Clin Gastroenterol Hepatol*, **4(3)**, 361–368.

22. The International Consensus Group for Hepatocellular Neoplasia (2009) Pathologic diagnosis of early hepatocellular carcinoma: a report of the international consensus group for hepatocellular neoplasia. *Hepatology*, **49(2)**, 658–664.

23. Forner, A., Vilana, R., Ayuso, C. *et al.* (2008) Diagnosis of hepatic nodules 20 mm or smaller in cirrhosis: Prospective validation of the noninvasive diagnostic criteria for hepatocellular carcinoma. *Hepatology*, **47(1)**, 97–104.

24. Stewart, C.J., Coldewey, J., Stewart, I.S. (2002) Comparison of fine needle aspiration cytology and needle core biopsy in the diagnosis of radiologically detected abdominal lesions. *J Clin Pathol*, **55(2)**, 93–97.

25. Stigliano, R., Marelli, L., Yu, D., Davies, N., Patch, D., Burroughs, A.K. (2007) Seeding following percutaneous diagnostic and therapeutic approaches for hepatocellular carcinoma. What is the risk and the outcome? Seeding risk for percutaneous approach of HCC. *Cancer Treat Rev*, **33(5)**, 437–447.

26. Lok, A.S., Sterling, R.K., Everhart, J.E. *et al.* (2010) Des-gamma-carboxy prothrombin and alpha-fetoprotein as biomarkers for the early detection of hepatocellular carcinoma. *Gastroenterology*, **138(2)**, 493–502.

27. Stipa, F., Yoon, S.S., Liau, K.H. *et al.* (2006) Outcome of patients with fibrolamellar hepatocellular carcinoma. *Cancer*, **106(6)**, 1331–1338.

28. Zhang, B.H., Yang, B.H., Tang, Z.Y. (2004) Randomized controlled trial of screening for hepatocellular carcinoma. *J Cancer Res Clin Oncol*, **130**, 140417–140422.

29. Okuda, K., Ohtsuki, T., Obata, H. *et al.* (1985) Natural history of hepatocellular carcinoma and prognosis in relation to treatment. Study of 850 patients. *Cancer*, **56(4)**, 918–928.

30. Cancer of the Liver Italian Program (CLIP). (1998) Investigators A new prognostic system for hepatocellular carcinoma: a retrospective study of 435 patients. *Hepatology*, **28(3)**, 751–755.

31. Edge, S.B., Compton, C.C. (2010) The American Joint Committee on Cancer: the 7th edition of the AJCC cancer staging manual and the future of TNM. *Ann Surg Oncol*, **17(6)**, 1471–1474.

32. Forner, A., Reig, M.E., de Lope, C.R., Bruix, J. (2010) Current strategy for staging and treatment: the BCLC update and future prospects. *Semin Liver Dis*, **30(1)**, 61–74.

33. Cabibbo, G., Enea, M., Attanasio, M., Bruix, J., Craxì, A., Cammà, C. (2010) A meta-analysis of survival rates of untreated patients in randomized clinical trials of hepatocellular carcinoma. *Hepatology*, **51(4)**, 1274–1283.

34. Llovet, J.M., Brú C., Bruix, J. (1999) Prognosis of hepatocellular carcinoma: the BCLC staging classification. *Semin Liver Dis*, **19(3)**, 329–338.

35. Kamath, P.S., Wiesner, R.H., Malinchoc, M. *et al.* (2001) A model to predict survival in patients with end-stage liver disease. *Hepatology*, **33(2)**, 464–470.

36. Vauthey, J.N., Lauwers, G.Y., Esnaola, N.F. *et al.* (2002) Simplified staging for hepatocellular carcinoma. *J Clin Oncol*, **20(6)**, 1527–1536.

37. Cillo, U., Vitale, A., Grigoletto, F. *et al.* (2006) Prospective validation of the Barcelona Clinic Liver Cancer staging system. *J Hepatol*, **44(4)**, 723–731.

38. Marrero, J.A., Fontana, R.J., Barrat, A. *et al.* (2005) Prognosis of hepatocellular carcinoma: comparison of 7 staging systems in an American cohort. *Hepatology*, **41(4)**, 707–716.

39. Vauthey, J.N., Ribero, D., Abdalla, E.K. *et al.* (2007) Outcomes of liver transplantation in 490 patients with hepatocellular carcinoma: validation of a uniform staging after surgical treatment. *J Am Coll Surg*, **204(5)**, 1016–1027.

40. Cho, Y.K., Chung, J.W., Kim, J.K. *et al.* (2008) Comparison of 7 staging systems for patients with hepatocellular carcinoma undergoing transarterial chemoembolization. *Cancer*, **112(2)**, 352–361.

41. Chok, K.S., Ng, K.K., Poon, R.T., Lo, C.M., Fan, S.T. (2009) Impact of postoperative complications on long-term outcome of curative resection for hepatocellular carcinoma. *Br J Surg*, **96(1)**, 81–87.

42. Bruix, J., Castells, A., Bosch, J. *et al.* (1996) Surgical resection of hepatocellular carcinoma in cirrhotic patients: prognostic value of preoperative portal pressure. *Gastroenterology*, **111(4)**, 1018–1022.

43. Pawlik, T.M., Poon, R.T., Abdalla, E.K. *et al.* (2005) Critical appraisal of the clinical and pathologic predictors of survival after resection of large hepatocellular carcinoma. *Arch Surg*, **140(5)**, 450–457

44. Ikai, I., Arii, S., Kojiro, M. *et al.* (2004) Reevaluation of prognostic factors for survival after liver resection in patients with hepatocellular carcinoma in a Japanese nationwide survey. *Cancer*, **101(4)**, 796–802.

45. Schwartz, J.D., Schwartz, M., Mandeli, J., Sung, M. (2002) Neoadjuvant and adjuvant therapy for resectable hepatocellular carcinoma: review of the randomised clinical trials. *Lancet Oncol*, **3(10)**, 593–603.

46. Ringe, B., Pichlmayr, R., Wittekind, C., Tusch, G. (1991) Surgical treatment of hepatocellular carcinoma: experience with liver resection and transplantation in 198 patients. *World J Surg*, **15**, 270–285.

47. Penn, I. (1991) Hepatic transplantation for primary and metastatic cancers of the liver. *Surgery*, **110**, 726–735.

48. Iwatsuki, S., Gordon, R.D., Shaw, B.W. Jr., Starzl, T.E. (1985) Role of liver transplantation in cancer therapy. *Ann Surg*, **202(4)**, 401–407.

49. Mazzaferro, V., Regalia, E., Doci, R. *et al.* (1996) Liver transplantation for the treatment of small hepatocellular carcinomas in patients with cirrhosis. *N Engl J Med*, **334(11)**, 693–699.

50. Freeman, R.B. Jr. (2002) Diagnosing hepatocellular carcinoma: a virtual reality. *Liver Transpl*, **8(9)**, 762–764.

51. Strong, R.W., Lynch, S.V., Ong, T.H., Matsunami, H., Koido, Y., Balderson, G.A. (1990) Successful liver transplantation from a living donor to her son. *N Engl J Med*, **322(21)**, 1505–1507.

52. Fisher, R.A., Kulik, L.M., Freise, C.E. *et al.* (2007) Hepatocellular carcinoma recurrence and death following living and deceased donor liver transplantation. *Am J Transplant*, **7(6)**, 1601–1608.

53. Bruix, J., Sherman, M., Llovet, J.M. *et al.* (2001) Clinical management of hepatocellular carcinoma. Conclusions of the Barcelona-2000 EASL conference. European Association for the Study of the Liver. *J Hepatol*, **35(3)**, 421–430.

54. Okada, S. (1999) Local ablation therapy for hepatocellular carcinoma. *Semin Liver Dis*, **19**, 323–328.

55. Lencioni, R.A., Allgaier, H.P., Cioni, D. *et al.* (2003) Small hepatocellular carcinoma in cirrhosis: randomized comparison of radio-frequency thermal ablation versus percutaneous ethanol injection. *Radiology*, **228(1)**, 235–240.

56. Bruix, J., Sala, M., Llovet, J.M. (2004) Chemoembolization for hepatocellular carcinoma. *Gastroenterology*, **127(5, Suppl 1)**, S179–S188.

57. Llovet, J.M., Real, M.I., Montaña X. *et al.* (2002) Arterial embolisation or chemoembolisation versus symptomatic treatment in patients with unresectable hepatocellular carcinoma: a randomised controlled trial. *Lancet*, **359(9319)**, 1734–1739.

58. Heckman, J.T., deVera, MB., Marsh, JW. *et al.* (2008) Bridging locoregional therapy for hepatocellular carcinoma prior to liver transplantation. *Ann Surg Oncol*, **15**, 3169–3177.

59. Lladó L, Virgili, J., Figueras, J. *et al.* (2000) A prognostic index of the survival of patients with unresectable hepatocellular carcinoma after transcatheter arterial chemoembolization. *Cancer*, **88(1)**, 50–57.

60. NCCN Clinical Practice Guidelines in Oncology 2010, Hepatobiliary Cancers. Available at: http://www.nccn.org/professionals/physiciangls/fguidelines.asp

61. Kulik, L.M., Carr, B.I., Mulcahy, MF. *et al.* (2008) Safety and efficacy of 90Y radiotherapy for hepatocellular carcinoma with and without portal vein thrombosis. *Hepatology*, **47**, 71–81.

62. Salem, R., Lewandowski, R.J., Kulik, L. *et al.* (2010) Radioembolization Results in Longer Time to Progression and Reduced Toxicity Compared With Chemoembolization in Patients With Hepatocellular Carcinoma. *Gastroenterology*, **140(2)**, 497–507.

63. Wilhelm, S.M., Adnane, L., Newell, P., Villanueva, A., Llovet, J.M., Lynch, M. (2008) Preclinical overview of sorafenib, a multikinase inhibitor that targets both Raf and VEGF and PDGF receptor tyrosine kinase signaling. *Mol Cancer Ther*, **7(10)**, 3129–3140.

64. Llovet, J.M., Ricci, S., Mazzaferro, V. *et al.* (2008) Sorafenib in advanced hepatocellular carcinoma. *N Engl J Med*, **359(4)**, 378–390.

65. Whittaker, S., Marais, R., Zhu, A.X. (2010) The role of signaling pathways in the development and treatment of hepatocellular carcinoma. *Oncogene*, **29(36)**, 4989–5005.

66. Siegel, A.B., Cohen, E.I., Ocean, A. *et al.* (2008) Phase II trial evaluating the clinical and biologic effects of bevacizumab in unresectable hepatocellular carcinoma. *J Clin Oncol*, **26(18)**, 2992–2998.

67. Zhu, A.X., Stuart, K., Blaszkowsky, L.S. *et al.* (2007) Phase 2 study of cetuximab in patients with advanced hepatocellular carcinoma. *Cancer*, **110(3)**, 581–589.

68. Philip, P.A., Mahoney, M.R., Allmer, C. *et al.* (2005) Phase II study of Erlotinib (OSI-774) in patients with advanced hepatocellular cancer. *J Clin Oncol*, **23(27)**, 6657–6663.

69. Baek, H.J., Lim, S.C., Kitisin, K. *et al.* (2008) Hepatocellular cancer arises from loss of transforming growth factor beta signaling adaptor protein embryonic liver fodrin through abnormal angiogenesis. *Hepatology*, **48(4)**, 1128–1137.

70. Thenappan, A., Li, Y., Kitisin, K. *et al.* (2010) Role of transforming growth factor beta signaling and expansion of progenitor cells in regenerating liver. *Hepatology*, **51(4)**, 1373–1382.

71. Muroyama, R., Kato, N., Yoshida, H. *et al.* (2006) Nucleotide change of codon 38 in the X gene of hepatitis B virus genotype C is associated with an increased risk of hepatocellular carcinoma. *J Hepatol*, **45(6)**, 805–812.

72. Chang, M.H., Chen, C.J., Lai, M.S. *et al.* (1997) Universal hepatitis B vaccination in Taiwan and the incidence of hepatocellular carcinoma in children. Taiwan Childhood Hepatoma Study Group. *N Engl J Med*, **336(26)**, 1855–1859.

73. Chen, C.-J., Yang, H.-I., Iloeje, U.H.; REVEAL-HBV Study Group. (2009) Hepatitis B virus DNA levels and outcomes in chronic hepatitis B. *Hepatology*, **49**, S72–S84.

8 Pancreatic and Biliary Cancer

Neil Bhardwaj and David M. Lloyd
University Hospitals of Leicester, Leicester, UK

Key Points/Potential Pitfalls for Pancreatic Cancer

- Surgery is the only treatment that offers a long-term cure.
- All inoperable diseases have a dismal prognosis.
- The majority of patients are inoperable at presentation.
- Smoking is a major risk factor for developing pancreatic cancer.
- Postoperative adjuvant therapy improves survival but more randomized controlled trials are required.

Key Web Links

http://www.esmo.org
European cancer network

http://www.macmillan.org.uk
UK based support and palliative care information

http://www.cancerresearchuk.org/
Latest incidence, prevalence, and research in pancreatic and biliary cancer in United Kingdom

http://www.cancerstaging.org/
American Joint Committee on Cancer (AJCC) latest TNM staging of HPB cancer

Pancreatic cancer

Epidemiology

Pancreatic cancer is the fourth commonest cause of cancer-related death in the Western world. More than 43,000 new cases in the United States and more than 7500 cases in the United Kingdom are diagnosed yearly with a slightly increased incidence in males.[1,2] More than 75%

Handbook of Gastrointestinal Cancer, First Edition. Edited by Janusz Jankowski and Ernest Hawk.
© 2013 John Wiley & Sons, Ltd. Published 2013 by John Wiley & Sons, Ltd.

of pancreatic cancer occurs in patients older than 65 years and peak incidence occurs in the seventh and eighth decades of life.[2] The majority of pancreatic cancers are incurable at presentation and these patients have a median survival of 5–8 months.[3,4] Only 20% of patients present with localized disease that is potentially resectable, yet only 20% of these survive 5 years.[5,6]

Histology of pancreatic tumors

Exocrine carcinomas represent more than 95% of all pancreatic carcinomas and the majority (>90%) of these are adenocarcinomas with more than 75% occurring in the head of the gland. Other types include cystic tumors of the pancreas and endocrine tumors.

Molecular biology of pancreatic carcinomas

Pancreatic ductal carcinoma results from the accumulation of acquired mutations. The multigenic nature of most pancreatic ductal cancer is reflected in the abnormalities of three broad classifications of genes: oncogenes such as *K-ras*; tumor-suppressor genes such as *p16*, *p53*, and *SMAD4*; and genomic maintenance genes such as *hMLH1* and *MSH2*.[6] The *K-ras* oncogene, which mediates signal transduction in the growth factor receptors, undergoes a point mutation and is present in almost 75–100% of pancreatic tumors.[7,8] The *P16* tumor-suppressor gene is inactivated in around 95% of pancreatic cancers and typically occurs later in pancreatic carcinogenesis.[9,10] Similarly, *p53*, another tumor-suppressor gene, is also inactivated late in the progression of pancreatic carcinoma, prior to metastatic spread, and is present in 50–75% cases.[11,12]

It is suggested that the mutations occur in a predictable time course, leading to the development of a progression model, which describes the changes that occur as normal pancreatic epithelium transforms into intraepithelial neoplasia and finally to invasive cancer. The concept was first suggested when atypical ductal papillary hyperplasia was noticed adjacent to resected adenocarcinomas.[13] Subsequently, a unified nomenclature to classify intraductal precursor lesions of the pancreas, known as pancreatic intraepithelial neoplasia (PanINs), has been proposed.[14] *PanIN-1A* lesions are flat, tall columnar cells with basally located nuclei. *PanIN-1B* lesions exhibit papillary architecture. *PanIN-2* lesions are characterized by nuclear abnormalities such as loss of polarity or nuclear crowding and *PanIN-3* have marked nuclear and cytological abnormalities and were previously referred to as carcinoma *in situ*. Invasion through the basement membrane marks the transition from *PanIN-3* to invasive carcinoma.[15] Genetic aberrations are apparent at different stages through the PanIN sequence; for example, *K-ras* mutations are observed as early as the *PanIN-1* stage[16] and *P16* inactivation usually occurs by the *PanIN-2* stage.[17] In addition, loss of *BRCA2* function,[18] *DPC4 and p53* tumor-suppressor genes, occurs in advanced PanIN lesions.[17,19]

Adenocarcinoma of the pancreas

Risk factors and prevention

Smoking
Smoking is the only preventable risk factor. It increases the risk of pancreatic cancer up to 2.5-fold compared with that of nonsmokers and is estimated to be responsible for 20% of pancreatic cancers. The risk increases with greater tobacco use and longer exposure, although does drop off significantly after cessation of smoking.[3,20,21] The pathophysiology behind nicotine-induced pancreatic carcinoma is unclear, but it is believed that N-nitroso compounds in tobacco are carried to the pancreas in the blood.[22]

Diabetes mellitus
A systematic review and meta-analysis concluded that type I diabetes mellitus increases the risk of pancreatic carcinoma by twofold.[23] Similarly, a meta-analysis of 36 studies concluded that type II diabetics have a 1.8-fold increased risk of developing pancreatic cancer. The study also concluded that risk was 50% higher if diabetes was diagnosed within the preceding 5 years.[24]

Chronic pancreatitis
Chronic pancreatitis is defined as a progressive inflammatory disease of the pancreas, associated with irreversible histological changes and subsequent loss of function. Chronic pancreatitis increases the risk of pancreatic cancer, which increases over time.[25,26]

Familial pancreatic cancer
Familial pancreatic cancer is defined as ductal adenocarcinoma of the pancreas affecting at least two first-degree relatives who do not fulfil the criteria for another inherited tumor syndrome.[3] Inherited mutations account for 2–10% of all pancreatic cancers.[15] Individuals with one, two, or three first-degree relatives with a history of pancreatic cancer demonstrate a 6-, 18- and 57-fold increase risk, respectively, compared with the normal population.[27]

Hereditary syndromes/conditions associated with pancreatic cancer
Five hereditary tumor predisposition syndromes/conditions have been identified that increase the risk of pancreatic cancer.

Peutz–Jeghers syndrome
Peutz–Jeghers syndrome (PJS) is a rare autosomal-dominant condition with an incidence of 1:25,000 births. It is characterized by mucocutaneous pigmentation and hamartomatous gastrointestinal polyps. These patients

have a 132-fold increase in developing pancreatic cancer and a lifetime risk of greater than 30%.[28]

Hereditary nonpolyposis colorectal cancer

Hereditary nonpolyposis colorectal cancer (HNPCC) is an autosomal-dominant disorder and has an incidence of 1:174 births. It is responsible for 20% of all colorectal carcinomas.[29] In addition to a 1–5% increased risk of developing pancreatic cancer, patients have an increased risk of developing extracolonic cancers such as endometrial (60%), stomach (10%), ovarian (12%), genitourinary (4%), biliary (2%), nervous system (4%), and small bowel cancer (1–4%).[15,30,31]

Familial atypical multiple mole melanoma

Familial atypical multiple mole melanoma (FAMMM) is an autosomal-dominant condition characterized by multiple nevi, melanomas, and extracutaneous tumors. It accounts for 12% of all familial pancreatic cancers and affected individuals have a 20-fold increased risk of developing pancreatic cancer and a lifetime risk of 15%.[31,32]

Hereditary breast and ovarian cancer carriers

Familial breast and ovarian cancer syndromes are due to mutations in the *BRCA1* or *BRCA2* genes. Patients with the *BRCA1* mutation have a twofold risk increase of pancreatic cancer and those with *BRCA2* mutation (responsible for 17% of all familial pancreatic carcinomas) have between 4- and 13-fold risk increase. The risk is highest in Ashkenazi Jews as 1% of the population have the *BRCA2* mutation.[15,33,34]

Hereditary pancreatitis

Sufferers of hereditary pancreatitis, an autosomal-dominant disease causing 1% of all cases of pancreatitis, have a 50-fold increase risk of developing pancreatic cancer and their lifetime risk approaches 40%.[35]

Presentation and diagnosis

In order to understand the presentation of pancreatic lesions, it is imperative to appreciate pancreatic anatomy. The pancreas is a retroperitoneal structure, divided into the head, neck, body, and tail. It lies in a C-shaped groove formed by the first three parts of the duodenum and is intimately attached to it. It is formed by the fusion of dorsal and ventral buds, by the ventral bud rotating posteriorly to fuse with the dorsal bud. The ventral duct, which becomes the main pancreatic duct (of Wirsung), fuses with the dorsal duct, also referred to as the minor pancreatic duct (of Santorini), which drains the body and tail of the pancreas. The ventral duct usually joins the common bile duct in the head of the pancreas and continues forward as a "common channel" before entering the midpoint of the second part of the duodenum as the ampulla of Vater.

The majority of exocrine pancreatic tumors occur in the head of the gland and often the patient may present with painless jaundice due to compression of the common bile duct.[36] This is in keeping with Courvoisier's law which states that "a palpable gallbladder in the setting of painless jaundice is rarely due to stone disease." However, the patient may present with a myriad of vague symptoms including anorexia, weight loss, and abdominal pain. In addition, compression of structures intimately related to this part of the gland such as the duodenum and coeliac nerves may present as gastric outlet obstruction and severe epigastric and back pain, respectively. Rarely, the tumor may cause obstruction of the pancreatic duct causing the patient to present with acute pancreatitis.

The purpose of any investigations in a patient suspected of pancreatic cancer is to confirm the diagnosis, the stage of the disease, assess resectability, and, if unresectable, plan palliative interventions. Investigations include basic blood tests including full blood count, which may demonstrate anemia due to occult loss from tumor invasion of the duodenum. Liver function tests may demonstrate an obstructive picture with high conjugated bilirubin and raised alkaline phosphatase. A raised amylase may demonstrate pancreatitis, and in addition, a low albumin may reflect the patient's low nutritional state. Carbohydrate antigen 19.9 (CA19.9) is the only tumor marker that is sensitive and specific for pancreatic tumors. Preoperatively, it has been demonstrated as a useful predictor of resectability, and postoperatively, it is a useful predicator of recurrence, disease-free, and median survival.[37–40] However, it must be used with caution as it has been demonstrated to be elevated in benign causes of obstructive jaundice,[41] although levels should return to normal post relief of jaundice. It is also reported to be absent in patients with blood Lewis antigen a or b deficiency despite advanced malignancy.[42] As always, the clinical picture in addition to thorough radiological or histological investigations must be taken into account when interpreting abnormal levels of any tumor markers.

Cross-sectional imaging of the thorax, abdomen, and pelvis by thin cut intravenous contrast-enhanced multidetector computerized tomography (CT) scan is the radiological investigation of choice.[43] Other investigations such as magnetic resonance cholangiopancreatography (MRCP) is usually reserved for patients where the diagnosis of pancreatic carcinoma is in doubt and an intraductal or periampullary lesion has to be excluded prior to endoscopic retrograde cholangiography (ERCP). Tissue diagnosis, either in the form of ultrasound or CT-guided biopsy or endoscopic ultrasound-guided fine needle aspiration, is essential. Patients with liver metastases may undergo biopsy of the liver lesions on the background of strong radiological suspicion of pancreatic carcinoma.

Cancer management

Surgical resection provides the only possible cure. All patients should be discussed by a multidisciplinary team involving surgeons, anesthetists, oncologists, radiologists, hepatobiliary nurse specialists, and nutritionists.

According to the TNM staging for pancreatic exocrine tumors (Table 8.1), T1, 2, and 3 are potentially resectable; however, any evidence of locally advanced carcinoma, particularly major vascular involvement, such as superior mesenteric artery or coeliac axis involvement, precludes curative resection. Patients with local invasion of portal vein with no evidence of thrombosis should be treated on their merit, as vein excision with reconstruction can be successful in experienced hands.[44] All patients suitable for resection should be considered for a staging laparoscopy and intraoperative ultrasound scan. This not only provides a real-life simulation of a general anesthetic but it has also been shown to detect occult peritoneal or locally invasive tumor, thus altering the prognosis in up to 20% of patients.[45] Preoperative drainage of biliary obstruction has been shown to increase postoperative sepsis, pancreatic fistula, and wound infections[46,47], and most centers now follow a policy of early resection. However, if there is an envisaged delay in treatment, then often patients undergo preoperative relief of obstruction either via a percutaneous route or an ERCP.

The operation depends on the location of the tumor. A head or neck of pancreas tumor requires a pancreaticoduodenectomy (the Whipple procedure) and tumors involving the tail should undergo a distal pancreatectomy.

Allen Oldfather Whipple first described the procedure synonymous with his name in 1935.[48] Initially a two-stage procedure, it was later developed as a one-stage procedure. Considerable advances in

Table 8.1 TNM staging of pancreatic cancer.[131]

Tumor (T)	Node (N)	Metastases (M)
Tx: Primary tumor cannot be assessed	N0: No nodes	M0: No metastases
T0: No evidence of tumor	N1: Positive nodes	M1: Spread to distant organs or nonregional nodes
Tis: Carcinoma in situ (includes PanIN-III classification.		
T1: <2 cm within the pancreas		
T2: >2 cm within the pancreas		
T3: adjacent extrapancreatic spread (duodenum, bile duct)		
T4: nonadjacent spread (stomach, colon, large vasculature)		
Stage 0: Tis, N0, M0		
Stage IA T1, N0, M0		
Stage IB: T2, 2, N0, M0		
Stage IIA: T3, N0, M0		
Stage IIB: T1, 2, 3, N1, M0		
Stage III: T4, any N, M0		
Stage IV: any T, any N, M1		

preoperative patient selection restricting surgery to high volume centers with expert surgical knowledge and skill along with improved intra- and postoperative anesthetic expertise has remarkably reduced the morbidity and mortality associated with this procedure.[49] Numerous variations of the surgical technique, dissection, and anastomotic reconstruction have been described, but the end result involves resection of the head and neck of pancreas, together with the attached duodenum (some surgeons prefer to resect the pylorus to aid gastric emptying while others preserve it in the belief that it prevents biliary reflux) and reconstruct drainage of the bile duct, stomach, and the pancreas using the jejunum as conduits. Most high volume centers (>18 procedures/year) report a mortality of less than 5% and this has decreased considerably over the last two decades. In addition, the 5-year survival is 20% in experienced centers and is influenced by tumor size of less than 3 cm, negative margins, negative nodal involvement, low-grade tumor, diploid tumor DNA content, and low postoperative CA19.9 levels.[5,49–51]

Distal pancreatectomy with en-bloc splenectomy is performed for resectable tumors of the body and tail.[52] As these patients are often rendered immunocompromised, all patients should be immunized against *Streptococcus pneumoniae, Neisseria meningitides*, and *Haemophilus influenzae* (type b) preoperatively and are required to take prophylactic antibiotics, usually in the form of penicillin V for life.

Patients with unresectable disease require symptom control. Jaundice is usually relieved by stenting the common bile duct via ERCP. Often a combination of external biliary drainage and radiologically guided internal biliary drainage is required if ERCP is unable to stent the common bile duct due to distortion of anatomy by local invasion of the pancreatic tumor. If unresectable disease is encountered at laparotomy, a biliary bypass should be performed and a gastrojejunostomy should be considered as 20% of patients with inoperable pancreatic cancer may develop duodenal obstruction during the course of their disease.[53] Pain and nausea control usually requires the input of palliative care nurses.

Neoadjuvant and adjuvant treatment of pancreatic cancer

The aim of surgery is to resect the tumor with normal pancreas at the margin and no evidence of residual tumor, commonly referred to as R0 resection. Preoperative chemoradiotherapy can be beneficial as it theoretically increase the likelihood of R0 resection margins by reducing tumor load. However, in patients with resectable disease, it may deem them unresectable while undergoing treatment and the toxicity of the treatment itself may delay them undergoing potentially curative surgery. Neoadjuvant chemoradiotherapy therefore is reserved for patient with nonmetastatic unresectable carcinoma with a view to shrinking the tumor and deeming patients resectable. All trials involve the use of external beam radiotherapy and usually multimodal chemotherapy agents with the greatest success achieved by gemcitabine-based regimens.[54,55] It is reported that up to a third of patients initially deemed unresectable may become resectable post-neoadjuvant therapy with similar median survival to those who initially underwent resection.[4] Local policies and a wide variation in treatment protocols make conducting large multicenter trials difficult.

Controversies exist regarding the optimal adjuvant treatment of patients postpancreatic resection. Unsurprisingly, patients with R0 resection have significantly prolonged survival compared with those with a R1 resection margin. The Gastrointestinal Tumour Study Group was one of the first of its kind to demonstrate improved survival and establish the role of 5-FU-based adjuvant chemoradiotherapy in patients undergoing pancreatic cancer surgery.[56] This study, however, was criticized for its poor accrual, low statistical power, suboptimal radiotherapy schedule, and low chemotherapy compliance.[57] Following this, the European Study Group for Pancreatic Cancer (ESPAC) conducted a large phase III trial and demonstrated improved survival with adjuvant 5-FU-based chemotherapy compared with chemoradiotherapy and concluded that chemoradiotherapy should be abandoned as it can lead to delay in starting chemotherapy.[58] However, this trial again generated significant controversy as it was criticized for its use of suboptimal radiotherapy schedule and nonstandardized randomization criteria.[57] Several studies have reanalyzed the data from the original ESPAC trial and have all concluded that adjuvant chemotherapy has significant benefit compared with chemoradiotherapy.[59] The Radiation Therapy Oncology Group trial 97-04 (RTOG 97-04) established the superior nature of gemcitabine-based chemoradiotherapy regimens for patients with resected head of pancreas tumors and other trials including the latest results from the ESPAC-3 trial tend to support the use of gemcitabine-based adjuvant chemotherapy compared with 5-FU due to its superior safety profile.[60,61] The need for good quality, randomized, multicentre trials still remain, particularly those comparing chemotherapy and chemoradiotherapy and in patients with R1 resections.

Patients with unresectable pancreatic carcinoma have an extremely dismal prognosis. Traditionally, 5-FU-based chemotherapy regimens in association with radiotherapy demonstrated a survival benefit of up to 44 weeks.[62] In addition, there was evidence that radiotherapy palliated the pain,[63] a common side effect of locally advanced carcinoma. Newer gemcitabine-based chemotherapy regimens seem to offer an increased survival benefit compared with 5-FU and radiotherapy with comparatively lower toxicity.[64] Unfortunately all patients relapse regardless of strategy used and succumb to the debilitating effects of metastatic pancreatic cancer. Patients require specialist palliative care input particularly for the intractable pain, nausea, and cachexia.

Cystic tumors of the pancreas

Intraductal papillary mucinous neoplasms

Intraductal papillary mucinous neoplasm (IPMN) was first described in 1982[65] and have since been defined as mucin-producing epithelial tumors, often with papillary architecture, of either the main pancreatic duct (main-duct IPMN) or one of its branches (branch-duct IPMN).[66] They are estimated to account for 1–3% of all exocrine pancreatic tumors and recognized as a premalignant condition with more than 30–72% of tumors presenting with either invasive carcinoma or carcinoma in situ.[67,68] Branch-duct IPMNs are less likely to be associated with malignancy.[69,70] IPMN mostly occurs in the sixth to seventh decade and usually presents with abdominal discomfort and weight loss, often mimicking chronic or relapsing pancreatitis, possibly due to intermittent obstruction of the main pancreatic duct by mucus plugs.[71] Patients may also present with weight loss, jaundice, vomiting, and diabetes, although these symptoms are highly suggestive of invasive malignancy.[72] A thorough history, particularly preceding episodes of alcohol-induced pancreatitis, and targeted investigations help distinguish IPMN from other malignant cystic lesions such as mucinous cystic neoplasm and benign conditions such as chronic pancreatitis and pancreatic pseudocysts. The majority of IPMNs involve the head of the pancreas, and CT and MRCP show a grossly dilated pancreatic duct in main-duct IPMN and "grape-like" dilatations associated with branch-duct IPMN.[53] An elevated serum CA19.9 suggests a neoplastic lesion and a patulous ampulla extruding mucus associated with main pancreatic duct filling defects at ERCP is associated with main-duct IPMN. The International Association of Pancreatology recommends that all patients with main-duct IPMN should undergo resection due to their malignant potential and branch-duct should be intensively followed up with a rise in CA19.9, increase in tumor size, or the presence of mural nodules or thick wall cysts either at presentation or on follow-up, an indication for resection.[53,73] There is significant morbidity associated with a total pancreatectomy and no added advantage compared with segmental tumor resection with negative margins.[74] Postresection, the presence of invasive disease is the main determinant of survival with 5-year survival— up to 100% with noninvasive disease compared with 13–60% in those with incomplete resection.[75,76] In addition, jaundice at presentation, tubular tumor type, vascular invasion, and positive lymph node status all relate to poor 5-year survival.[53,77]

Mucinous cystic neoplasms

Mucinous cystic neoplasms are the commonest cystic neoplasm of the pancreas.[78] Eighty percent occur in females, with a median age of 50 and unlike IPMNs almost never communicate with the duct. Histologically, they are formed by mucin-producing epithelial cells supported by an ovarian-type stroma.[79] They almost always arise *de novo* and are often located in the body tail of the pancreas.[79,80] They often present with vague symptoms of abdominal pain, weight loss, nausea, and vomiting. The presence of calcifications and multiseptae distinguish this from other cysts.[78] The imaging triad of calcifications, thick walls, and mural vegetation on CT scanning is predictive of malignant degeneration in up to 95% of cases.[81] A combination of cross-sectional imaging, endoscopic ultrasound assessment, and fine needle aspiration of cyst fluid confirms the diagnosis in the majority of cases.[71,78] The prognosis depends on the extent of local tumor invasion, tumor size, location, and type. All tumors resected with oncological techniques have a good prognosis with greater than 50% survival.[78,79]

Endocrine carcinomas of the pancreas

These tumors are also known as islet cell tumors or neuroendocrine tumors (NET) are part of the diffuse endocrine system (DES) and the gastroenteropancreatic axis (GEP) and are now collectively known as GEP–NETs. They make up around 5% of all pancreatic tumors and can be benign or malignant, functional or nonfunctional, and can often be part of a multiple endocrine neoplasia (MEN) syndrome. They usually take their name from the hormone produced by these cells such as insulinomas, gastrinomas, glucagonomas, VIPomas, somatostatinomas, and carcinoids. The majority are nonfunctional, and insulinomas followed by gastrinomas are the commonest functional tumors.[82] It is estimated from postmortem studies that pancreatic NETs are identifiable in up to 10% of individuals.[83]

Presentation

Nonfunctioning tumors usually present with either mass effect secondary to local invasion or due to secondary spread. Functioning tumors present with symptoms secondary to the hormones they produce, for example, Insulinomas present with confusion, sweating, weakness, and unconsciousness relieved by eating or dextrose administration. Gastrinomas (Zollinger–Ellison syndrome) may present with severe peptic ulceration and diarrhea. Glucagonomas present with vague symptoms of necrolytic migratory erythema, weight loss, diabetes mellitus, stomatitis, and diarrhea. VIPomas (Werner-Morrison syndrome) present with profuse watery diarrhea associated with marked hypokalemia and somatostatinomas also present with similar symptoms of diarrhea, steatorrhea, and diabetes mellitus.[84,85]

Investigations

They can be difficult to investigate due to the site, which can be anywhere in the gastrointestinal tract or the pancreas, lung thyroid, pituitary, and other sites. They are frequently small and can present with unusual symptoms. Usually, the investigations are easier to focus when a functioning tumor is suspected. Biochemical investigations include measuring serum glucose, insulin, C-peptide, chromogranin A, and 24-hour urinary 5-hydroxyindoleacetic acid (5-HIAA). A suggestion of MEN-1 (susceptible to parathyroid, pituitary, and pancreas neoplasms) should prompt calcium, parathyroid hormone, calcitonin, and thyroid function tests to be measured. Radiological localization of nonfunctioning tumors is done by high quality CT scanning. Somatostatinomas, VIPomas, and glucagonomas tend to be large and easily identified on imaging, whereas insulinomas and gastrinomas are more difficult to localize. Extrapancreatic sites such as gastric and colonic tumors may require endoscopic evaluation. An "octreoscan" may be useful, particularly when assessing secondaries or following up patients who have had a primary resection. These are usually done in specialized nuclear medicine departments.

Treatment

Patients should be referred to specialist hepatobiliary centers. Surgical treatment offers the best cure, and the extent of disease and completeness of resection are major predictors of survival.[82] Insulinomas, which have the lowest chance of malignant potential of all GEP–NETs can occur in extrapancreatic sites and can be difficult to localize. Single, solid, nonfunctioning tumors in MEN syndromes can be excised for cure or surgery can be employed to debulk tumors for the sake of symptom control. Essentially, all patients after undergoing extensive radiological and histological diagnoses, followed by search for metastases, should be offered resection.

Biliary cancer

Epidemiology

Cholangiocarcinoma is the malignant transformation of cholangiocytes, which line the intra- and extrahepatic bile ducts, and gallbladder carcinoma is the commonest biliary tract tumor. Bile duct tumors account for 2% of all reported cancers and 3% of all gastrointestinal cancers. The peak incidence is in the eight decade and is 1.5 times commoner in males than in females.[86,87] Southeast Asia has one of the highest rates of cholangiocarcinoma and may be due to the endemic infestation of the liver fluke parasite. Anatomically, cholangiocarcinomas are divided into intra- and extrahepatic tumors. Extrahepatic cholangiocarcinomas are further subdivided into proximal, mid-, and distal carcinomas depending on their location in the bile duct. Due to the unique risk factors, clinical presentation and management of gallbladder cancer compared with other extrahepatic carcinomas, it will be dealt with separately in this chapter. Although intrahepatic cholangiocarcinoma is a relatively rare tumor in the general population, it is the second most common primary liver tumor[88] and recent epidemiological studies suggest an increase in incidence in the western world.[88,89] Hilar or proximal tumors, also eponymously known as Klatskin tumors, were first described in 1965[90] and after gallbladder carcinoma are the second commonest site of bile duct tumors.[91]

Histology of bile duct tumors

Traditionally, extrahepatic cholangiocarcinomas are divided into three main histological subtypes: nodular, sclerosing, and papillary.[92] The liver cancer study group of Japan have subdivided intrahepatic carcinomas into mass-forming, periductal-infiltrating, and intraductal growth types, which corresponds to the extrahepatic subtypes of nodular, sclerosing, and papillary, respectively.[93] The majority of extrahepatic tumors are firm sclerotic tumors with few cellular components on a background of fibrous tissue. This may account for the poor preoperative biopsy yield associated with these tumors.[91,92] Papillary tumors represent around 10% of all tumors types and are often fleshy with a stalk and have a very good prognosis if resected early and completely.[94]

Risk factors and prevention

Several risk factors have been recognized that lead to the development of cholangiocarcinomas, such as autoimmune diseases, congenital anatomic anomalies, abnormal tumor suppress genes, infections, and iatrogenic causes.

Autoimmune diseases

Chronic inflammation may initiate molecular change, which leads to the development of cholangiocarcinoma. Primary sclerosing cholangitis (PSC) is an autoimmune chronic inflammatory disease of the bile ducts and increases the lifetime risk of developing cholangiocarcinoma by 10–15%.[95,96] The risk of cholangiocarcinoma is not related to the duration or severity of PSC,[97] and it is estimated that up to 40% of patients with PSC have evidence of cholangiocarcinoma at autopsy or liver explantation.[87] However, more than 50% of patients diagnosed with PSC present with cholangiocarcinoma within the first year[98]; therefore, all patients should be screened for the disease on initial diagnosis of PSC. The majority of patients with PSC (80%) have associated ulcerative colitis; thus, this is also associated with an increase risk of developing cholangiocarcinoma. Potential screening strategies for patients with PSC include regular Ca 19.9 measurements and yearly abdominal ultrasound scanning (USS).[99] However, several reports suggest that Ca 19.9 is not sensitive enough and is only elevated in patients with advanced malignancy.[100] In addition, as discussed later in this chapter, biomarkers can often be misleading and USS is not the gold standard imaging modality recommended for detection of cholangiocarcinoma.

Congenital and anatomical disorders

Caroli disease, a rare congenital disorder characterized by dilatation of intrahepatic bile ducts and choledochal cysts (abnormal extrahepatic bile duct dilatations), predisposes to cholangiocarcinoma.[101–103] Other risk factors that predispose to the development of cholangiocarcinoma on the background of chronic inflammation and cholangitis include an anomalous choledochopancreatic junction, particularly a long common channel that leads to reflux of pancreatic secretions up the biliary tree[104,105] and hepatolithiasis.[106]

Abnormal tumor-suppressor genes

Chronic inflammation is thought to promote carcinogenesis by causing damage to DNA mismatch repair genes, proto-oncogenes, and tumor-suppressor genes. The overexpression of the *p53* tumor-suppressor gene in patients with PSC and cholangiocarcinoma[107] and mutations in the K-ras and c-erbB-2 proto-oncogenes have been identified in cholangiocarcinoma patients.[108–110]

Infections

Infestation with liver flukes, particularly *Clonorchis sinensis* and *Opisthorchis viverrini*, is endemic in parts of Thailand and Far East Asia. These cause local and chronic inflammation, leading to malignant transformation and hence significantly increase the risk of cholangiocarcinoma in this region.[111,112] In addition, hepatitis C or B infections have been implicated in the development of intrahepatic cholangiocarcinoma.[88,113,114]

Iatrogenic causes

Thorotrast, a contrast medium used in radiological investigations between 1920 and 1950, increases the risk of developing cholangiocarcinoma by up to 300-fold compared with the general population with peak incidence 20–30 years after exposure.[115,116]

Presentation and diagnosis

More than 90% of extrahepatic cholangiocarcinomas present with painless jaundice, pruritus, pale stools, dark urine and the hematological hallmarks of obstructive jaundice, a high alkaline phosphatase, high bilirubin, and mildly elevated or normal transaminases. Intrahepatic cholangiocarcinomas are often detected incidentally while investigating nonspecific symptoms of lethargy, malaise, weight loss, and upper abdominal pain/fullness.[91,117] Carbohydrate antigen 19.9 is the most widely used serum marker for cholangiocarcinoma; however, it may also be raised in pancreatic cancer (as mentioned earlier in this chapter), gastric cancer, and primary biliary cirrhosis. At a cutoff value of 129 U/mL, it has a sensitivity and specificity for detecting cholangiocarcinoma of 79% and 98%, respectively. However, most studies report that a high CA19.9 indicates advanced stages of malignancy, when radical treatment is not indicated.[100,118] Therefore, although a good marker for malignancy, it lacks the sensitivity or specificity to be used as a reliable screening tool.

Histological confirmation of malignancy, particularly of extrahepatic lesions, is extremely difficult. Brush biopsies performed at ERCP for cytological analyses are often inadequate and unhelpful. Thus, a combination of clinical history and examination with radiological investigations is usually employed in order to stage the disease and subsequently plan curative or palliative procedures. Extrahepatic cholangiocarcinoma classically spreads along bile ducts, invades perineural and vascular tissues, and it may infiltrate adjacent structures including lymph nodes or metastasize to distant organs.[119,120] Ultrasound can be as successful as a CT scan in expert centers in establishing the etiology of the site of obstruction.[121] However, most centers use CT scanning as it often demonstrates intrahepatic bile duct dilatation up to the site of obstruction, assesses vessel encasement and associated liver atrophy, and detects lymphadenopathy. The accuracy with which MRCP determines the extent of bile duct tumors ranges from 71% to 96%.[122,123] The soft tissue contrast allows easier identification of the tumor and the evaluation of infiltrating tumors of the duct wall. It also assesses the extent of peripheral ductal involvement, which is essential for surgical planning and is superior to ERCP as ducts proximal to an obstructing cholangiocarcinoma may not adequately fill during ERCP.[124,125]

In addition, both ERCP and percutaneous transhepatic cholangiography are invasive, operator dependent, and associated with procedural risks, including duodenal perforation, biliary leakage, cholangitis, bleeding, and pancreatitis.[126,127]

Intrahepatic cholangiocarcinoma must be suspected in patients with a solitary solid-looking lesion on imaging in a noncirrhotic liver with a normal α-fetoprotein. MRI of the liver demonstrates a hypointense lesion relative to normal liver on T1-weighted images, and T2-weighted images show predominant isointensity or slight hyperintensity relative to the liver parenchyma. The lesions demonstrate initial rim enhancement; however, intravenous administration of gadolinium-based contrast material results in concentric contrast enhancement. There is usually associated capsular retraction.[128] A needle biopsy with specific immunocytochemical staining in addition to suspicious imaging is usually diagnostic.[129] However, this must be balanced against the theoretical risk of tumor seeding and most centers would only biopsy if the tumor is unresectable and a tissue biopsy was needed prior to palliative oncological therapy.

Cancer management

Surgical resection provides the only possible cure. Traditionally, intrahepatic cholangiocarcinomas are staged in a similar fashion to hepatocellular carcinomas, which unfortunately has no bearing on survival. Hilar cholangiocarcinomas are staged according to the Bismuth-Corlette classification, which describes tumor location and spread along the biliary tree (Table 8.2).[130] Similarly, extrahepatic mid and distal cholangiocarcinomas can be staged by the TNM classification as per the guidelines (Table 8.3).[131] However, neither of these systems predicts resectability. Four main factors have been demonstrated to predict resectability and consequently influence survival: the extent of tumor within the biliary tree, vascular invasion with subsequent associated lobar atrophy, and metastatic disease. Ipsilateral lobar atrophy implies portal vein involvement and commits the surgeon to performing a hepatectomy; however, contralateral lobar atrophy suggests extensive inflow involvement and precludes surgical resection.[91,132]

Table 8.2 The Bismuth-Corlette classification of perihilar tumors.[130]

Type I	Tumor involves the common hepatic duct
Type II	Tumor involves the bifurcation of the common hepatic duct
Type IIIa	Tumor involves the right hepatic duct
Type IIIb	Tumor involves the left hepatic duct
Type IV	Tumor involves both the right and left hepatic duct

Table 8.3 TNM staging extrahepatic cholangiocarcinoma.[131]

Tumor (T)	Node (N)	Metastases (M)
TX: Primary tumor cannot be assessed	NX: Regional lymph nodes cannot be assessed	MX: Presence of metastases cannot be assessed
T0: No evidence of primary tumor	N0: No metastases in regional lymph nodes	M0: No distant metastases
TIS: Carcinoma in situ	N1: Regional lymph node metastasis	M1: Distant metastases
T1: Tumor confined to bile duct		
T2: Tumor invades beyond the wall of the bile duct		
T3: Tumor invades liver, gallbladder, duodenum stomach, pancreas, or colon.		
T4: Tumor involves the coeliac axis or the superior mesenteric artery		
Stage 0: TIS, N0, M0		
Stage IA: T1, N0, M0		
Stage IB: T2, N0, M0		
Stage IIA: T1, 2, 3 N1, M0		
Stage III: T4, any N, M0		
Stage IV: any T, any N, M1		

The 5-year survival for completely resected intrahepatic cholangiocarcinoma, which usually involves a formal lobectomy, is 22–44%.[133–135] Similarly, hilar cholangiocarcinomas if treated with early radical R0 resection, including an ipsilateral hepatectomy, is associated with a 1-year survival of 80% and a 5-year survival of 39%.[86,136,137] Distal bile duct cholangiocarcinomas usually require a pancreatico-duodenectomy (Whipple's operation described earlier) and complete (R0) resections is associated with 5-year survival up to 40%.[138,139] Preoperative laparoscopy has been shown to detect occult metastases in up to 42% of all patients and is an essential part of the preoperative assessment, as it may prevent patients from undergoing an unnecessary laparotomy.[140]

The majority of patients present with advanced unresectable disease and they require palliation of their symptoms. In the case of obstructive jaundice, this usually requires biliary drainage. This can be done by the radiologist via a percutaneous route or via an ERCP. Often a combination of approaches is required. Unresectable extrahepatic cholangiocarcinomas discovered at laparotomy may be amenable to undergoing biliary-enteric bypass. However, this is usually at the discretion of the surgeon.

Neoadjuvant and adjuvant treatment of cholangiocarcinomas

No meaningful randomized trials exist, which advocate the use of adjuvant or neoadjuvant radio- or chemotherapy in completely resected R0 tumors. Locally advanced tumors without widespread disease may be treated with external beam radiotherapy or photodynamic therapy.[141–143] However, the actual benefit is debatable and little robust data exists to recommend these therapies routinely to patients with unresectable cholangiocarcinomas.

Gallbladder carcinoma

Epidemiology
Gallbladder carcinoma, although a rare gastrointestinal malignancy with only 600–700 cases diagnosed in the United Kingdom each year, is the commonest cancer of the biliary tract. The highest incidence is found in South American countries and the majority (>90%) are adenocarcinomas with the remainder of the squamous cell type.[144]

Risk factors and prevention
Similar to other bile duct tumors, any chronic inflammatory state that increases cell turnover predisposes to gallbladder carcinoma, and like many gastrointestinal tumors, there is an established dysplasia–carcinoma in situ leading to established carcinoma sequence.[145] Gallstones are the commonest cause of gallbladder carcinoma.[146-148] In addition, a heavily calcified gallbladder often referred to as a "*porcelain gallbladder*" and gallbladder polyps greater than 1 cm or multiple polyps increase the risk of gallbladder carcinoma.[91,149,150] There is also evidence that chronic infection with *Salmonella typhi* increases the risk of gallbladder cancer.[151]

Presentation and diagnosis

More than 75% of patients present with advanced malignancy, which is unresectable. Often patients complain of vague symptoms such as abdominal pain or biliary colic and weight loss. Jaundice as a presenting symptom is usually a poor prognostic index and is indicative of locally advanced, unresectable disease.[91,152] Any suspicious findings on ultrasonography such as asymmetrical wall thickening or intraluminal papillary projections, should alert the surgeon of the possibility of an underlying carcinoma and prompt further investigations usually in the form of a CT scan[153,154] and often, if liver invasion is suspected, an MRI scan.

Cancer management

Surgical resection offers the only possible cure for gallbladder carcinoma. The TNM staging is summarized in Table 8.4[131], and the T staging usually dictates the type of surgery performed and the nodal status predicts long-term survival. Over the years, increasingly aggressive surgical approach with local resection and up to and including an extended hemihepatectomy has vastly improved survival. Studies from high volume centers have demonstrated 83%, 63%, and 25% 5-year survival for stages II, III, and IV, respectively.[152] As expected, Tis and T1 tumors are usually diagnosed postlaparoscopic cholecystectomy and often that is all that is required to

Table 8.4 TNM staging for gallbladder cancer.[131]

Tumor (T)	Node (N)	Metastases (M)
TX: Primary tumor cannot be assessed	NX: Regional lymph nodes cannot be assessed	MX: Distant metastasis cannot be assessed
T0: No evidence of primary tumor	N0: No regional lymph node metastasis	M0: No distant metastasis
Tis: Carcinoma in situ	N1: Regional lymph node metastasis	M1: Distant metastasis
T1: Tumor invades lamina propria or muscle layer		
T1a: Tumor invades lamina propria		
T1b: Tumor invades the muscle layer		
T2: Tumor invades the perimuscular connective tissue; no extension beyond the serosa or into the liver		
T3: Tumor perforates the serosa (visceral peritoneum) and/or directly invades the liver and/or one other adjacent organ or structure, such as the stomach, duodenum, colon, or pancreas, omentum or extrahepatic bile ducts		
T4: Tumor invades main portal vein or hepatic artery or invades multiple extrahepatic organs or structures		
Stage 0: Tis, N0, M0		
Stage I: T1, N0, M0		
Stage Ii: T2, N0, M0		
Stage IIIA: T3, N0, M0		
Stage IIIB: Any T, N1, M0		
Stage IVA: T4, any N, M0		
Stage IVB: Any T, any N, M1		

achieve a cure rate approaching 100%.[155] T2 tumors usually require a wedge resection of adjacent liver with lymph node dissection in order to achieve a R0 resection and 5-year survival of 70%.[156] T3 tumors usually require a hemihepatectomy and/or bile duct excision as often just cystic duct clearance is inadequate. This approach has a 5-year survival approaching 30–50%.[152,157] T4 lesions are generally considered inoperable.

Neoadjuvant and adjuvant treatment of gallbladder cancer

One randomized controlled trial showed a survival benefit in patients offered postoperative adjuvant therapy versus no therapy.[158,159] However, there is lack of good quality evidence to suggest that patients with unresectable disease should be offered palliative oncological treatment.

Case Studies

Case 1

A 56-year-old gentleman presents with painless jaundice. An ultrasound shows dilated intra- and extrahepatic ducts and a possibility of a mass in the head of the pancreas. He underwent a CT scan (Figure 8.1) and a diagnosis of a tumor in the head of the pancreas was suspected. He underwent a staging laparoscopy and after an ERCP and stent placement (as there was a delay prior to his operation date), a successful Whipple's operation. He underwent adjuvant chemotherapy and is disease free 2 years postoperatively.

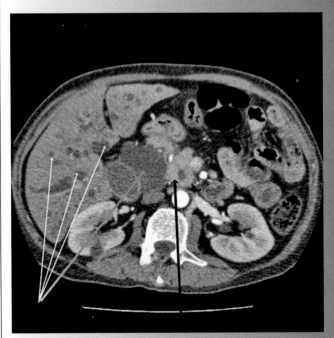

Figure 8.1 Dilated intrahepatic ducts ( ), dilated bile duct ( ), and mass in the head of the pancreas (→).

Case 2

A 52-year-old female presented with vague abdominal pain and weight loss. A CT scan of her abdomen revealed multiple cystic dilatations of her pancreatic duct (Figure 8.2). An ERCP confirmed a patulous ampulla extruding mucus and a diagnosis of IPMN was made. She successfully underwent a total pancreatectomy. Histology confirmed a completely excised IPMN. She is now a well-controlled insulin-dependent diabetic patient.

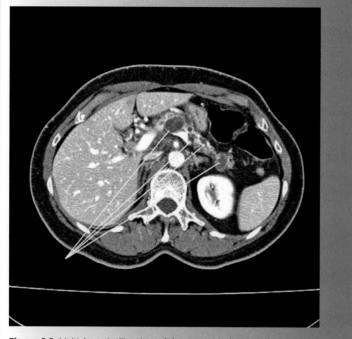

Figure 8.2 Multiple cystic dilatations of the pancreatic duct (→).

Key Points/Potential Pitfalls for Biliary Cancer

- Surgery offers the only chance of long-term cure in all biliary tree cancers
- All inoperable disease have a dismal prognosis
- More randomized controlled trials are required to determine the role of adjuvant therapy

Cholangiocarcinomas of the biliary tree:

- The extent of contralateral portal vein involvement and associated liver atrophy often determines resectability in advanced cases of hilar tumors
- Distal tumors often require a Whipple's operation
- Intrahepatic cholangiocarcinomas require thorough investigation to exclude a primary hepatocellular carcinoma or the possibility of secondary spread from elsewhere.

Gallbladder tumors:

- Duplex ultrasound scan followed by CT or MRI is required to assess resectability
- Extensive resection with negative resection margins and nodes confers the best prognosis

References

1. Jemal, A., Siegel, R., Xu, J., Ward, E. (2010) Cancer statistics, 2010. *CA Cancer J Clin*, **60(5)**, 277–300.
2. Cancer Research UK. Pancreatic Cancer Statistics-Key Facts.; 2010; Available at: http://info.cancerresearchuk.org/cancerstats/types/pancreas/.
3. Decker, G.A., Batheja, M.J., Collins, J.M. *et al.* Risk factors for pancreatic adenocarcinoma and prospects for screening. *Gastroenterol Hepatol (NY)*, **6(4)**, 246–254.
4. Gillen, S., Schuster, T., Meyer Zum Buschenfelde, C., Friess, H., Kleeff, J. Preoperative/neoadjuvant therapy in pancreatic cancer: a systematic review and meta-analysis of response and resection percentages. *PLoS Med*, **7(4)**, e1000267.
5. Yeo, C.J., Cameron, J.L., Lillemoe, K.D., Sitzmann, J.V., Hruban, R.H., Goodman, S.N. (1995) Pancreaticoduodenectomy for cancer of the head of the pancreas. 201 patients. *Ann Surg*, **221(6)**, 721–731; discussion 31–33.
6. Li, D., Xie, K., Wolff, R., Abbruzzese, J.L. (2004) Pancreatic cancer. *Lancet*, **363(9414)**, 1049–1057.
7. Almoguera, C., Shibata, D., Forrester, K., Martin, J., Arnheim, N., Perucho, M. (1988) Most human carcinomas of the exocrine pancreas contain mutant c-K-ras genes. *Cell*, **53(4)**, 549–554.
8. Hruban, R.H., van Mansfeld, A.D., Offerhaus, G.J., van Weering, D.H., Allison, D.C., Goodman, S.N. (1993) K-ras oncogene activation in adenocarcinoma of the human pancreas. A study of 82 carcinomas using a combination of mutant-enriched polymerase chain reaction analysis and allele-specific oligonucleotide hybridization. *Am J Pathol*, **143(2)**, 545–554.
9. Schutte, M., Hruban, R.H., Geradts, J., Maynard, R., Hilgers, W., Rabindran, S.K. (1997) Abrogation of the Rb/p16 tumor-suppressive pathway in virtually all pancreatic carcinomas. *Cancer Research*, **57(15)**, 3126–3130.
10. Caldas, C., Hahn, S.A., da Costa, L.T., Redston, M.S., Schutte, M., Seymour, A.B. (1994) Frequent somatic mutations and homozygous deletions of the p16 (MTS1) gene in pancreatic adenocarcinoma. *Nat Genet*, **8(1)**, 27–32.
11. Weyrer, K., Feichtinger, H., Haun, M., Weiss, G., Ofner, D., Weger, A.R. (1996) p53, Ki-ras, and DNA ploidy in human pancreatic ductal adenocarcinomas. *Lab Invest*, **74(1)**, 279–289.
12. Ruggeri, B.A., Huang, L., Berger, D., Chang, H., Klein-Szanto, A.J., Goodrow, T. (1997) Molecular pathology of primary and metastatic ductal pancreatic lesions: analyses of mutations and expression of the p53, mdm-2, and p21/WAF-1 genes in sporadic and familial lesions. *Cancer*, **79(4)**, 700–716.
13. Cubilla, A.L., Fitzgerald, P.J. (1976) Morphological lesions associated with human primary invasive nonendocrine pancreas cancer. *Cancer Research*, **36(7, Pt 2)**, 2690–2698.
14. Hruban, R.H., Adsay, N.V., Albores-Saavedra, J., Compton, C., Garrett, E.S., Goodman, S.N. (2001) Pancreatic intraepithelial neoplasia: a new nomenclature and classification system for pancreatic duct lesions. *Am J Surg Pathol*, **25(5)**, 579–586.
15. Winter, J.M., Maitra, A., Yeo, C.J. (2006) Genetics and pathology of pancreatic cancer. *HPB (Oxford)*, **8(5)**, 324–336.
16. Luttges, J., Schlehe, B., Menke, M.A., Vogel, I., Henne-Bruns, D., Kloppel, G. (1999) The K-ras mutation pattern in pancreatic ductal adenocarcinoma

usually is identical to that in associated normal, hyperplastic, and metaplastic ductal epithelium. *Cancer*, **85(8)**, 1703–1710.

17. Khan, I.Z., Conlon, K.C.P. (2009) Pancreatic adenocarcinoma. In: O.J. Garden (ed), *Hepatobiliary and Pancreatic Surgery*, pp. 283–298. Elsevier.

18. Goggins, M., Hruban, R.H., Kern, S.E. (2000) BRCA2 is inactivated late in the development of pancreatic intraepithelial neoplasia: evidence and implications. *Am J Pathol*, **156(5)**, 1767–1771.

19. Wilentz, R.E., Iacobuzio-Donahue, C.A., Argani, P., McCarthy, D.M., Parsons, J.L., Yeo, C.J. (2000) Loss of expression of Dpc4 in pancreatic intraepithelial neoplasia: evidence that DPC4 inactivation occurs late in neoplastic progression. *Cancer Research*, **60(7)**, 2002–2006.

20. Iodice, S., Gandini, S., Maisonneuve, P., Lowenfels, A.B. (2008) Tobacco and the risk of pancreatic cancer: a review and meta-analysis. *Langenbecks Arch Surg*, **393(4)**, 535–545.

21. Hassan, M.M., Bondy, M.L., Wolff, R.A., Abbruzzese, J.L., Vauthey, J.N., Pisters, P.W. (2007) Risk factors for pancreatic cancer: case-control study. *Am J Gastroenterol*, **102(12)**, 2696–2707.

22. Risch, H.A. (2003) Etiology of pancreatic cancer, with a hypothesis concerning the role of N-nitroso compounds and excess gastric acidity. *J Natl Cancer Inst*, **95(13)**, 948–960.

23. Stevens, R.J., Roddam, A.W., Beral, V. (2007) Pancreatic cancer in type 1 and young-onset diabetes: systematic review and meta-analysis. *Br J Cancer*, **96(3)**, 507–509.

24. Huxley, R., Ansary-Moghaddam, A., Berrington de Gonzalez, A., Barzi, F., Woodward, M. (2005) Type-II diabetes and pancreatic cancer: a meta-analysis of 36 studies. *Br J Cancer*, **92(11)**, 2076–2083.

25. Bansal, P., Sonnenberg, A. (1995) Pancreatitis is a risk factor for pancreatic cancer. *Gastroenterology*, **109(1)**, 247–251.

26. Malka, D., Hammel, P., Maire, F., Rufat, P., Madeira, I., Pessione, F. (2002) Risk of pancreatic adenocarcinoma in chronic pancreatitis. *Gut*, **51(6)**, 849–852.

27. Tersmette, A.C., Petersen, G.M., Offerhaus, G.J., Falatko, F.C., Brune, K.A., Goggins, M. (2001) Increased risk of incident pancreatic cancer among first-degree relatives of patients with familial pancreatic cancer. *Clin Cancer Res*, **7(3)**, 738–744.

28. Giardiello, F.M., Brensinger, J.D., Tersmette, A.C., Goodman, S.N., Petersen, G.M., Booker, S.V. (2000) Very high risk of cancer in familial Peutz-Jeghers syndrome. *Gastroenterology*, **119(6)**, 1447–1453.

29. Salovaara, R., Loukola, A., Kristo, P., Kaariainen, H., Ahtola, H., Eskelinen, M. (2000) Population-based molecular detection of hereditary nonpolyposis colorectal cancer. *J Clin Oncol*, **18(11)**, 2193–2200.

30. Lynch, H.T., Voorhees, G.J., Lanspa, S.J., McGreevy, P.S., Lynch, J.F. (1985) Pancreatic carcinoma and hereditary nonpolyposis colorectal cancer: a family study. *Br J Cancer*, **52(2)**, 271–273.

31. Rieder, H., Bartsch, D.K. (2004) Familial pancreatic cancer. *Fam Cancer*, **3(1)**, 69–74.

32. Vasen, H.F., Gruis, N.A., Frants, R.R., van Der Velden, P.A., Hille, E.T., Bergman, W. (2000) Risk of developing pancreatic cancer in families with familial atypical multiple mole melanoma associated with a specific 19 deletion of p16 (p16-Leiden). *Int J Cancer*, **87(6)**, 809–811.

33. Risch, H.A., McLaughlin, J.R., Cole, D.E., Rosen, B., Bradley, L., Fan, I. (2006) Population BRCA1 and BRCA2 mutation frequencies and cancer

penetrances: a kin-cohort study in Ontario, Canada. *J Natl Cancer Inst*, **98(23)**, 1694–1706.

34. van Asperen, C.J., Brohet, R.M., Meijers-Heijboer, E.J., Hoogerbrugge, N., Verhoef, S., Vasen, H.F. (2005) Cancer risks in BRCA2 families: estimates for sites other than breast and ovary. *J Med Genet*, **42(9)**, 711–719.

35. Lowenfels, A.B., Maisonneuve, P., DiMagno, E.P., Elitsur, Y., Gates, L.K. Jr., Perrault, J. (1997) Hereditary pancreatitis and the risk of pancreatic cancer. International Hereditary Pancreatitis Study Group. *J Natl Cancer Inst*, **89(6)**, 442–446.

36. Bakkevold, K.E., Arnesjo, B., Kambestad, B. (1992) Carcinoma of the pancreas and papilla of Vater: presenting symptoms, signs, and diagnosis related to stage and tumour site. A prospective multicentre trial in 472 patients. Norwegian Pancreatic Cancer Trial. *Scand J Gastroenterol*, **27(4)**, 317–325.

37. Morris-Stiff, G., Teli, M., Jardine, N., Puntis, M.C. (2009) CA19-9 antigen levels can distinguish between benign and malignant pancreaticobiliary disease. *Hepatobiliary Pancreat Dis Int*, **8(6)**, 620–626.

38. Goonetilleke, K.S., Siriwardena, A.K. (2007) Systematic review of carbohydrate antigen (CA 19-9) as a biochemical marker in the diagnosis of pancreatic cancer. *Eur J Surg Oncol*, **33(3)**, 266–270.

39. Nazli, O., Bozdag, A.D., Tansug, T., Kir, R., Kaymak, E. (2000) The diagnostic importance of CEA and CA 19-9 for the early diagnosis of pancreatic carcinoma. *Hepatogastroenterology*, **47(36)**, 1750–1752.

40. Safi, F., Schlosser, W., Falkenreck, S., Beger, H.G. (1996) CA 19-9 serum course and prognosis of pancreatic cancer. *Int J Pancreatol*, **20(3)**, 155–161.

41. Marrelli, D., Caruso, S., Pedrazzani, C., Neri, A., Fernandes, E., Marini, M. (2009) CA19-9 serum levels in obstructive jaundice: clinical value in benign and malignant conditions. *Am J Surg*, **198(3)**, 333–339.

42. Hidalgo, M. (2010) Pancreatic cancer. *N Engl J Med*, **362(17)**, 1605–1617.

43. Edge, S.B., Compton, C.C. (2010) The American Joint Committee on Cancer: the 7th edition of the AJCC cancer staging manual and the future of TNM. *Ann Surg Oncol*, **17(6)**, 1471–1474.

44. Tseng, J.F., Tamm, E.P., Lee, J.E., Pisters, P.W., Evans, D.B. (2006) Venous resection in pancreatic cancer surgery. *Best Pract Res Clin Gastroenterol*, **20(2)**, 349–364.

45. Jimenez, R.E., Warshaw, A.L., Rattner, D.W., Willett, C.G., McGrath, D., Fernandez-del Castillo, C. (2000) Impact of laparoscopic staging in the treatment of pancreatic cancer. *Arch Surg*, **135(4)**, 409–414; discussion 14–15.

46. Sewnath, M.E., Birjmohun, R.S., Rauws, E.A., Huibregtse, K., Obertop, H., Gouma, D.J. (2001) The effect of preoperative biliary drainage on postoperative complications after pancreaticoduodenectomy. *J Am Coll Surg*, **192(6)**, 726–734.

47. Povoski, S.P., Karpeh, M.S. Jr., Conlon, K.C., Blumgart, L.H., Brennan, M.F. (1999) Association of preoperative biliary drainage with postoperative outcome following pancreaticoduodenectomy. *Ann Surg*, **230(2)**, 131–142.

48. Whipple, A.O., Parsons, W.B., Mullins, C.R. (1935) Treatment of carcinoma of the ampulla of Vater. *Ann Surg*, **102(4)**, 763–779.

49. McPhee, J.T., Hill, J.S., Whalen, G.F., Zayaruzny, M., Litwin, D.E., Sullivan, M.E. (2007) Perioperative mortality for pancreatectomy: a national perspective. *Ann Surg*, **246(2)**, 246–253.

50. Berger, A.C., Garcia, M. Jr., Hoffman, J.P., Regine, W.F., Abrams, R.A., Safran, H. (2008) Postresection CA 19-9 predicts overall survival in patients with pancreatic cancer treated with adjuvant chemoradiation: a prospective validation by RTOG 9704. *J Clin Oncol*, **26(36)**, 5918–5922.

51. Lieberman, M.D., Kilburn, H., Lindsey, M., Brennan, M.F. (1995) Relation of perioperative deaths to hospital volume among patients undergoing pancreatic resection for malignancy. *Ann Surg*, **222(5)**, 638–645.

52. Dennison, A.R., Maddern, G.J. (2010) Pancreas. In: A.R. Dennison, G.J. Maddern (eds), *Operative Solutions in Hepatobiliary and Pancreatic Surgery*, pp. 1–87. Oxford University Press.

53. Connor, S. (2009) Non-adenocarcinoma of the pancreas. In: O.J. Garden (ed), *Hepatobiliary and Pancreatic Surgery*, pp. 299–312. Elsevier.

54. Evans, D.B., Varadhachary, G.R., Crane, C.H., Sun, C.C., Lee, J.E., Pisters, P.W. (2008) Preoperative gemcitabine-based chemoradiation for patients with resectable adenocarcinoma of the pancreatic head. *J Clin Oncol*, **26(21)**, 3496–3502.

55. Varadhachary, G.R., Wolff, R.A., Crane, C.H., Sun, C.C., Lee, J.E., Pisters, P.W. (2008) Preoperative gemcitabine and cisplatin followed by gemcitabine-based chemoradiation for resectable adenocarcinoma of the pancreatic head. *J Clin Oncol*, **26(21)**, 3487–3495.

56. Kalser, M.H., Ellenberg, S.S. (1985) Pancreatic cancer. Adjuvant combined radiation and chemotherapy following curative resection. *Arch Surg*, **120(8)**, 899–903.

57. Roy, R., Maraveyas, A. (2010) Chemoradiation in pancreatic adenocarcinoma: a literature review. *Oncologist*, **15(3)**, 259–269.

58. Neoptolemos, J.P., Dunn, J.A., Stocken, D.D., Almond, J., Link, K., Beger, H. (2001) Adjuvant chemoradiotherapy and chemotherapy in resectable pancreatic cancer: a randomised controlled trial. *Lancet*, **358(9293)**, 1576–1585.

59. Neoptolemos, J.P., Stocken, D.D., Friess, H., Bassi, C., Dunn, J.A., Hickey, H. (2004) A randomized trial of chemoradiotherapy and chemotherapy after resection of pancreatic cancer. *N Engl J Med*, **350(12)**, 1200–1210.

60. Neoptolemos, J.P., Stocken, D.D., Bassi, C., Ghaneh, P., Cunningham, D., Goldstein, D. (2010) Adjuvant chemotherapy with fluorouracil plus folinic acid vs gemcitabine following pancreatic cancer resection: a randomized controlled trial. *JAMA*, **304(10)**, 1073–1081.

61. Regine, W.F., Winter, K.A., Abrams, R.A., Safran, H., Hoffman, J.P., Konski, A. (2008) Fluorouracil vs gemcitabine chemotherapy before and after fluorouracil-based chemoradiation following resection of pancreatic adenocarcinoma: a randomized controlled trial. *JAMA*, **299(9)**, 1019–1026.

62. Moertel, C.G., Frytak, S., Hahn, R.G., O'Connell, M.J., Reitemeier, R.J., Rubin, J. (1981) Therapy of locally unresectable pancreatic carcinoma: a randomized comparison of high dose (6000 rads) radiation alone, moderate dose radiation (4000 rads +5-fluorouracil), and high dose radiation + 5-fluorouracil: The Gastrointestinal Tumor Study Group. *Cancer*, **48(8)**, 1705–1710.

63. Minsky, B.D., Hilaris, B., Fuks, Z. (1988) The role of radiation therapy in the control of pain from pancreatic carcinoma. *J Pain Symptom Manage*, **3(4)**, 199–205.

64. Chauffert, B., Mornex, F., Bonnetain, F., Rougier, P., Mariette, C., Bouche, O. (2008) Phase III trial comparing intensive induction chemoradiotherapy (60 Gy, infusional 5-FU and intermittent cisplatin) followed by maintenance

gemcitabine with gemcitabine alone for locally advanced unresectable pancreatic cancer. Definitive results of the 2000-01 FFCD/SFRO study. *Ann Oncol*, **19(9)**, 1592–1599.

65. Ohhashi, K., Murakami, Y., Takekoshi, T. (1982) Four cases of mucin producing cancer of pancreas on specific findings of the papilla of Vater. *Prog Dig Endosc*, **20**, 348–351.

66. Longnecker, D.S., Hruban, R.H. (2000) Intraductal papillary-mucinous neoplasms of the pancreas. In: S.R. Hamilton, A.L., (ed), *WHO Classification of Tumors Pathology and Genetics of Tumours of Digestive System*, pp. 237–240. IARC Press, Lyon.

67. Jang, J.Y., Kim, S.W., Ahn, Y.J., Yoon, Y.S., Choi, M.G., Lee, K.U. (2005) Multicenter analysis of clinicopathologic features of intraductal papillary mucinous tumor of the pancreas: is it possible to predict the malignancy before surgery? *Ann Surg Oncol*, **12(2)**, 124–132.

68. Sarr, M.G., Kendrick, M.L., Nagorney, D.M., Thompson, G.B., Farley, D.R., Farnell, M.B. (2001) Cystic neoplasms of the pancreas: benign to malignant epithelial neoplasms. *Surg Clin North Am*, **81(3)**, 497–509.

69. Obara, T., Maguchi, H., Saitoh, Y., Itoh, A., Arisato, S., Ashida, T. (1993) Mucin-producing tumor of the pancreas: natural history and serial pancreatogram changes. *Am J Gastroenterol*, **88(4)**, 564–569.

70. Tanaka, M., Kobayashi, K., Mizumoto, K., Yamaguchi, K. (2005) Clinical aspects of intraductal papillary mucinous neoplasm of the pancreas. *J Gastroenterol*, **40(7)**, 669–675.

71. Morana, G., Guarise, A. (2006) Cystic tumors of the pancreas. *Cancer Imaging*, **6**, 60–71.

72. Sohn, T.A., Yeo, C.J., Cameron, J.L., Hruban, R.H., Fukushima, N., Campbell, K.A. (2004) Intraductal papillary mucinous neoplasms of the pancreas: an updated experience. *Ann Surg*, **239(6)**, 788–797; discussion 97–99.

73. Tanaka, M., Chari, S., Adsay, V., Fernandez-del Castillo, C., Falconi, M., Shimizu, M. (2006) International consensus guidelines for management of intraductal papillary mucinous neoplasms and mucinous cystic neoplasms of the pancreas. *Pancreatology*, **6(1–2)**, 17–32.

74. Fujino, Y., Suzuki, Y., Yoshikawa, T., Ajiki, T., Ueda, T., Matsumoto, I. (2006) Outcomes of surgery for intraductal papillary mucinous neoplasms of the pancreas. *World J Surg*, **30(10)**, 1909–1914; discussion 15.

75. Salvia, R., Crippa, S., Falconi, M., Bassi, C., Guarise, A., Scarpa, A. (2007) Branch-duct intraductal papillary mucinous neoplasms of the pancreas: to operate or not to operate? *Gut*, **56(8)**, 1086–1090.

76. Wada, K., Kozarek, R.A., Traverso, L.W. (2005) Outcomes following resection of invasive and noninvasive intraductal papillary mucinous neoplasms of the pancreas. *Am J Surg*, **189(5)**, 632–636; discussion 7.

77. D'Angelica, M., Brennan, M.F., Suriawinata, A.A., Klimstra, D., Conlon, K.C. (2004) Intraductal papillary mucinous neoplasms of the pancreas: an analysis of clinicopathologic features and outcome. *Ann Surg*, **239(3)**, 400–408.

78. Eloubeidi, M.A., Hawes, R.H. (2000) Mucinous tumors of the exocrine pancreas. *Cancer Control*, **7(5)**, 445–451.

79. Zamboni, G., Scarpa, A., Bogina, G., Iacono, C., Bassi, C., Talamini, G. (1999) Mucinous cystic tumors of the pancreas: clinicopathological features, prognosis, and relationship to other mucinous cystic tumors. *Am J Surg Pathol*, **23(4)**, 410–422.

80. Thompson, L.D., Becker, R.C., Przygodzki, R.M., Adair, C.F., Heffess, C.S. (1999) Mucinous cystic neoplasm (mucinous cystadenocarcinoma of low-grade malignant potential) of the pancreas: a clinicopathologic study of 130 cases. *Am J Surg Pathol*, **23(1)**, 1–16.
81. Procacci, C., Biasiutti, C., Carbognin, G., Accordini, S., Bicego, E., Guarise, A. (1999) Characterization of cystic tumors of the pancreas: CT accuracy. *J Comput Assist Tomogr*, **23(6)**, 906–912.
82. Halfdanarson, T.R., Rubin, J., Farnell, M.B., Grant, C.S., Petersen, G.M. (2008) Pancreatic endocrine neoplasms: epidemiology and prognosis of pancreatic endocrine tumors. *Endocr Relat Cancer*, **15(2)**, 409–427.
83. Kimura, W., Kuroda, A., Morioka, Y. (1991) Clinical pathology of endocrine tumors of the pancreas. Analysis of autopsy cases. *Dig Dis Sci*, **36(7)**, 933–942.
84. Debas, H.T., Mulvihill, S.J. (1994) Neuroendocrine gut neoplasms. Important lessons from uncommon tumors. *Arch Surg*, **129(9)**, 965–971; discussion 71–72.
85. Tomassetti, P., Migliori, M., Lalli, S., Campana, D., Tomassetti, V., Corinaldesi, R. (2001) Epidemiology, clinical features and diagnosis of gastroenteropancreatic endocrine tumours. *Ann Oncol*, **12(Suppl 2)**, S95–S99.
86. Yubin, L., Chihua, F., Zhixiang, J., Jinrui, O., Zixian, L., Jianghua, Z. (2008) Surgical management and prognostic factors of hilar cholangiocarcinoma: experience with 115 cases in China. *Ann Surg Oncol*, **15(8)**, 2113–2119.
87. Abbas, G., Lindor, K.D. (2009) Cholangiocarcinoma in primary sclerosing cholangitis. *J Gastrointest Cancer*, **40(1–2)**, 19–25.
88. Gatto, M., Bragazzi, M.C., Semeraro, R., Napoli, C., Gentile, R., Torrice, A. (2010) Cholangiocarcinoma: update and future perspectives. *Dig Liver Dis*, **42(4)**, 253–260.
89. Welzel, T.M., McGlynn, K.A., Hsing, A.W., O'Brien, T.R., Pfeiffer, R.M. (2006) Impact of classification of hilar cholangiocarcinomas (Klatskin tumors) on the incidence of intra- and extrahepatic cholangiocarcinoma in the United States. *J Natl Cancer Inst*, **98(12)**, 873–875.
90. Klatskin, G. (1965) Adenocarcinoma of the hepatic duct at its bifurcation within the porta hepatis. An unusual tumor with distinctive clinical and pathological features. *Am J Med*, **38**, 241–256.
91. Maithel, S.K., Jarnagin, W.R. (2010) Malignant lesions of the biliary tract. In: O.J. Garden (ed), *Hepatobiliary and Pancreatic Surgery*, pp. 219–242. Elsevier.
92. Weinbren, K., Mutum, S.S. (1983) Pathological aspects of cholangiocarcinoma. *J Pathol*, **139(2)**, 217–238.
93. Yamamoto, J., Kosuge, T., Shimada, K., Takayama, T., Yamasaki, S., Ozaki, H. (1993) Intrahepatic cholangiocarcinoma: proposal of new macroscopic classification. *Nippon Geka Gakkai Zasshi*, **94(11)**, 1194–1200.
94. Pitt, H.A., Dooley, W.C., Yeo, C.J., Cameron, J.L. (1995) Malignancies of the biliary tree. *Curr Probl Surg*, **32(1)**, 1–90.
95. Bergquist, A., Ekbom, A., Olsson, R., Kornfeldt, D., Loof, L., Danielsson, A. (2002) Hepatic and extrahepatic malignancies in primary sclerosing cholangitis. *J Hepatol*, **36(3)**, 321–327.
96. Burak, K., Angulo, P., Pasha, T.M., Egan, K., Petz, J., Lindor, K.D. (2004) Incidence and risk factors for cholangiocarcinoma in primary sclerosing cholangitis. *Am J Gastroenterol*, **99(3)**, 523–526.

97. Khan, S.A., Thomas, H.C., Davidson, B.R., Taylor-Robinson, S.D. (2005) Cholangiocarcinoma. *Lancet*, **366(9493)**, 1303–1314.

98. Boberg, K.M., Bergquist, A., Mitchell, S., Pares, A., Rosina, F., Broome, U. (2002) Cholangiocarcinoma in primary sclerosing cholangitis: risk factors and clinical presentation. *Scand J Gastroenterol*, **37(10)**, 1205–1211.

99. Charatcharoenwitthaya, P., Enders, F.B., Halling, K.C., Lindor, K.D. (2008) Utility of serum tumor markers, imaging, and biliary cytology for detecting cholangiocarcinoma in primary sclerosing cholangitis. *Hepatology*, **48(4)**, 1106–1117.

100. Levy, C., Lymp, J., Angulo, P., Gores, G.J., Larusso, N., Lindor, K.D. (2005) The value of serum CA 19-9 in predicting cholangiocarcinomas in patients with primary sclerosing cholangitis. *Dig Dis Sci*, **50(9)**, 1734–1740.

101. Abdalla, E.K., Forsmark, C.E., Lauwers, G.Y., Vauthey, J.N. (1999) Monolobar Caroli's disease and cholangiocarcinoma. *HPB Surg*, **11(4)**, 271–276; discussion 6–7.

102. de Vries, J.S., de Vries, S., Aronson, D.C., Bosman, D.K., Rauws, E.A., Bosma, A. (2002) Choledochal cysts: age of presentation, symptoms, and late complications related to Todani's classification. *J Pediatr Surg*, **37(11)**, 1568–1573.

103. Voyles, C.R., Smadja, C., Shands, W.C., Blumgart, L.H. (1983) Carcinoma in choledochal cysts. Age-related incidence. *Arch Surg*, **118(8)**, 986–988.

104. Miyazaki, M., Takada, T., Miyakawa, S., Tsukada, K., Nagino, M., Kondo, S. (2008) Risk factors for biliary tract and ampullary carcinomas and prophylactic surgery for these factors. *J Hepatobiliary Pancreat Surg*, **15(1)**, 15–24.

105. Tashiro, S., Imaizumi, T., Ohkawa, H., Okada, A., Katoh, T., Kawaharada, Y. (2003) Pancreaticobiliary maljunction: retrospective and nationwide survey in Japan. *J Hepatobiliary Pancreat Surg*, **10(5)**, 345–351.

106. Su, C.H., Shyr, Y.M., Lui, W.Y., P'Eng, F.K. (1997) Hepatolithiasis associated with cholangiocarcinoma. *Br J Surg*, **84(7)**, 969–973.

107. Rizzi, P.M., Ryder, S.D., Portmann, B., Ramage, J.K., Naoumov, N.V., Williams, R. (1996) p53 Protein overexpression in cholangiocarcinoma arising in primary sclerosing cholangitis. *Gut*, **38(2)**, 265–268.

108. Sturm, P.D., Baas, I.O., Clement, M.J., Nakeeb, A., Johan, G., Offerhaus, A. (1998) Alterations of the p53 tumor-suppressor gene and K-ras oncogene in perihilar cholangiocarcinomas from a high-incidence area. *Int J Cancer*, **78(6)**, 695–698.

109. Wattanasirichaigoon, S., Tasanakhajorn, U., Jesadapatarakul, S. (1998) The incidence of K-ras codon 12 mutations in cholangiocarcinoma detected by polymerase chain reaction technique. *J Med Assoc Thai*, **81(5)**, 316–323.

110. Terada, T., Ashida, K., Endo, K., Horie, S., Maeta, H., Matsunaga, Y. (1998) c-erbB-2 protein is expressed in hepatolithiasis and cholangiocarcinoma. *Histopathology*, **33(4)**, 325–331.

111. Vatanasapt, V., Tangvoraphonkchai, V., Titapant, V., Pipitgool, V., Viriyapap, D., Sriamporn, S. (1990) A high incidence of liver cancer in Khon Kaen Province, Thailand. *Southeast Asian J Trop Med Public Health*, **21(3)**, 489–494.

112. Shin, H.R., Lee, C.U., Park, H.J., Seol, S.Y., Chung, J.M., Choi, H.C. (1996) Hepatitis B and C virus, *Clonorchis sinensis* for the risk of liver cancer: a case-control study in Pusan, Korea. *Int J Epidemiol*, **25(5)**, 933–940.

113. Zhou, Y.M., Yin, Z.F., Yang, J.M., Li, B., Shao, W.Y., Xu, F. (2008) Risk factors for intrahepatic cholangiocarcinoma: a case-control study in China. *World J Gastroenterol*, **14(4)**, 632–635.

114. El-Serag, H.B., Engels, E.A., Landgren, O., Chiao, E., Henderson, L., Amaratunge, H.C. (2009) Risk of hepatobiliary and pancreatic cancers after hepatitis C virus infection: a population-based study of U.S. veterans. *Hepatology*, **49(1)**, 116–123.

115. Lipshutz, G.S., Brennan, T.V., Warren, R.S. (2002) Thorotrast-induced liver neoplasia: a collective review. *J Am Coll Surg*, **195(5)**, 713–718.

116. Ito, Y., Kojiro, M., Nakashima, T., Mori, T. (1988) Pathomorphologic characteristics of 102 cases of thorotrast-related hepatocellular carcinoma, cholangiocarcinoma, and hepatic angiosarcoma. *Cancer*, **62(6)**, 1153–1162.

117. Khan, S.A., Davidson, B.R., Goldin, R., Pereira, S.P., Rosenberg, W.M., Taylor-Robinson, S.D. (2002) Guidelines for the diagnosis and treatment of cholangiocarcinoma: consensus document. *Gut*, **51(Suppl 6)**, VI1–VI19.

118. Patel, A.H., Harnois, D.M., Klee, G.G., LaRusso, N.F., Gores, G.J. (2000) The utility of CA 19-9 in the diagnoses of cholangiocarcinoma in patients without primary sclerosing cholangitis. *Am J Gastroenterol*, **95(1)**, 204–207.

119. Sakamoto, E., Nimura, Y., Hayakawa, N., Kamiya, J., Kondo, S., Nagino, M. (1998) The pattern of infiltration at the proximal border of hilar bile duct carcinoma: a histologic analysis of 62 resected cases. *Ann Surg*, **227(3)**, 405–411.

120. Ebata, T., Watanabe, H., Ajioka, Y., Oda, K., Nimura, Y. (2002) Pathological appraisal of lines of resection for bile duct carcinoma. *Br J Surg*, **89(10)**, 1260–1267.

121. Sharma, M.P., Ahuja, V. (1999) Aetiological spectrum of obstructive jaundice and diagnostic ability of ultrasonography: a clinician's perspective. *Trop Gastroenterol*, **20(4)**, 167–169.

122. Cho, E.S., Park, M.S., Yu, J.S., Kim, M.J., Kim, K.W. (2007) Biliary ductal involvement of hilar cholangiocarcinoma: multidetector computed tomography versus magnetic resonance cholangiography. *J Comput Assist Tomogr*, **31(1)**, 72–78.

123. Lee, S.S., Kim, M.H., Lee, S.K., Kim, T.K., Seo, D.W., Park, J.S. (2002) MR cholangiography versus cholangioscopy for evaluation of longitudinal extension of hilar cholangiocarcinoma. *Gastrointest Endosc*, **56(1)**, 25–32.

124. Manfredi, R., Barbaro, B., Masselli, G., Vecchioli, A., Marano, P. (2004) Magnetic resonance imaging of cholangiocarcinoma. *Semin Liver Dis*, **24(2)**, 155–164.

125. Manfredi, R., Masselli, G., Maresca, G., Brizi, M.G., Vecchioli, A., Marano, P. (2003) MR imaging and MRCP of hilar cholangiocarcinoma. *Abdom Imaging*, **28(3)**, 319–325.

126. Choi, J.Y., Kim, M.J., Lee, J.M., Kim, K.W., Lee, J.Y., Han, J.K. (2008) Hilar cholangiocarcinoma: role of preoperative imaging with sonography, MDCT, MRI, and direct cholangiography. *AJR Am J Roentgenol*, **191(5)**, 1448–1457.

127. Freeman, M.L. (2002) Adverse outcomes of ERCP. *Gastrointest Endosc*, **56(6, Suppl)**, S273–S282.

128. Chung, Y.E., Kim, M.J., Park, Y.N., Choi, J.Y., Pyo, J.Y., Kim, Y.C. (2009) Varying appearances of cholangiocarcinoma: radiologic-pathologic correlation. *Radiographics*, **29(3)**, 683–700.

129. Buc, E., Lesurtel, M., Belghiti, J. (2008) Is preoperative histological diagnosis necessary before referral to major surgery for cholangiocarcinoma? *HPB (Oxford)*, **10(2)**, 98–105.

130. Bismuth, H., Nakache, R., Diamond, T. (1992) Management strategies in resection for hilar cholangiocarcinoma. *Ann Surg*, **215(1)**, 31–38.
131. Sobin, L., Gospodarowicz, M., Wittekind, C (eds). (2010) *TNM Classification of Malignant Tumours*, 7th ed. Blackwell Publishing, Oxford.
132. Jarnagin, W.R., Fong, Y., DeMatteo, R.P., Gonen, M., Burke, E.C., Bodniewicz, B.J. (2001) Staging, resectability, and outcome in 225 patients with hilar cholangiocarcinoma. *Ann Surg*, **234(4)**, 507–517; discussion 17–19.
133. Ohtsuka, M., Ito, H., Kimura, F., Shimizu, H., Togawa, A., Yoshidome, H. (2002) Results of surgical treatment for intrahepatic cholangiocarcinoma and clinicopathological factors influencing survival. *Br J Surg*, **89(12)**, 1525–1531.
134. Isaji, S., Kawarada, Y., Taoka, H., Tabata, M., Suzuki, H., Yokoi, H. (1999) Clinicopathological features and outcome of hepatic resection for intrahepatic cholangiocarcinoma in Japan. *J Hepatobiliary Pancreat Surg*, **6(2)**, 108–116.
135. Valverde, A., Bonhomme, N., Farges, O., Sauvanet, A., Flejou, J.F., Belghiti, J. (1999) Resection of intrahepatic cholangiocarcinoma: a Western experience. *J Hepatobiliary Pancreat Surg*, **6(2)**, 122–127.
136. Hasegawa, S., Ikai, I., Fujii, H., Hatano, E., Shimahara, Y. (2007) Surgical resection of hilar cholangiocarcinoma: analysis of survival and postoperative complications. *World J Surg*, **31(6)**, 1256–1263.
137. DeOliveira, M.L., Cunningham, S.C., Cameron, J.L., Kamangar, F., Winter, J.M., Lillemoe, K.D. (2007) Cholangiocarcinoma: thirty-one-year experience with 564 patients at a single institution. *Ann Surg*, **245(5)**, 755–762.
138. Fong, Y., Blumgart, L.H., Lin, E., Fortner, J.G., Brennan, M.F. (1996) Outcome of treatment for distal bile duct cancer. *Br J Surg*, **83(12)**, 1712–1715.
139. Wade, T.P., Prasad, C.N., Virgo, K.S., Johnson, F.E. (1997) Experience with distal bile duct cancers in U.S. Veterans Affairs hospitals: 1987-1991. *J Surg Oncol*, **64(3)**, 242–245.
140. Weber, S.M., DeMatteo, R.P., Fong, Y., Blumgart, L.H., Jarnagin, W.R. (2002) Staging laparoscopy in patients with extrahepatic biliary carcinoma. Analysis of 100 patients. *Ann Surg*, **235(3)**, 392–399.
141. Kiesslich, T., Wolkersdorfer, G., Neureiter, D., Salmhofer, H., Berr, F. (2009) Photodynamic therapy for non-resectable perihilar cholangiocarcinoma. *Photochem Photobiol Sci*, **8(1)**, 23–30.
142. Baisden, J.M., Kahaleh, M., Weiss, G.R., Sanfey, H., Moskaluk, C.A., Yeaton, P. (2008) Multimodality treatment with helical tomotherapy intensity modulated radiotherapy, capecitabine, and photodynamic therapy is feasible and well tolerated in patients with hilar cholangiocarcinoma. *Gastrointest Cancer Res*, **2(5)**, 219–224.
143. Kuvshinoff, B.W., Armstrong, J.G., Fong, Y., Schupak, K., Getradjman, G., Heffernan, N. (1995) Palliation of irresectable hilar cholangiocarcinoma with biliary drainage and radiotherapy. *Br J Surg*, **82(11)**, 1522–1525.
144. Lazcano-Ponce, E.C., Miquel, J.F., Munoz, N., Herrero, R., Ferrecio, C., Wistuba, I.I. (2001) Epidemiology and molecular pathology of gallbladder cancer. *CA Cancer J Clin*, **51(6)**, 349–364.
145. Albores-Saavedra, J., de Jesus Manrique, J., Angeles-Angeles, A., Henson, D.E. (1984) Carcinoma in situ of the gallbladder. A clinicopathologic study of 18 cases. *Am J Surg Pathol*, **8(5)**, 323–333.

146. Henson, D.E., Albores-Saavedra, J., Corle, D. (1992) Carcinoma of the gallbladder. Histologic types, stage of disease, grade, and survival rates. *Cancer*, **70(6)**, 1493–1497.

147. Strom, B.L., Soloway, R.D., Rios-Dalenz, J.L., Rodriguez-Martinez, H.A., West, S.L., Kinman, J.L. (1995) Risk factors for gallbladder cancer. An international collaborative case-control study. *Cancer*, **76(10)**, 1747–1756.

148. Okamoto, M., Okamoto, H., Kitahara, F., Kobayashi, K., Karikome, K., Miura, K. (1999) Ultrasonographic evidence of association of polyps and stones with gallbladder cancer. *Am J Gastroenterol*, **94(2)**, 446–450.

149. Yeh, C.N., Jan, Y.Y., Chao, T.C., Chen, M.F. (2001) Laparoscopic cholecystectomy for polypoid lesions of the gallbladder: a clinicopathologic study. *Surg Laparosc Endosc Percutan Tech*, **11(3)**, 176–181.

150. Stephen, A.E., Berger, D.L. (2001) Carcinoma in the porcelain gallbladder: a relationship revisited. *Surgery*, **129(6)**, 699–703.

151. Caygill, C.P., Hill, M.J., Braddick, M., Sharp, J.C. (1994) Cancer mortality in chronic typhoid and paratyphoid carriers. *Lancet*, **343(8889)**, 83–84.

152. Bartlett, D.L., Fong, Y., Fortner, J.G., Brennan, M.F., Blumgart, L.H. (1996) Long-term results after resection for gallbladder cancer. Implications for staging and management. *Ann Surg*, **224(5)**, 639–646.

153. Kalra, N., Suri, S., Gupta, R., Natarajan, S.K., Khandelwal, N., Wig, J.D. (2006) MDCT in the staging of gallbladder carcinoma. *AJR Am J Roentgenol*, **186(3)**, 758–762.

154. Jang, J.Y., Kim, S.W., Lee, S.E., Hwang, D.W., Kim, E.J., Lee, J.Y. (2009) Differential diagnostic and staging accuracies of high resolution ultrasonography, endoscopic ultrasonography, and multidetector computed tomography for gallbladder polypoid lesions and gallbladder cancer. *Ann Surg*, **250(6)**, 943–949.

155. Shirai, Y., Yoshida, K., Tsukada, K., Muto, T. (1992) Inapparent carcinoma of the gallbladder. An appraisal of a radical second operation after simple cholecystectomy. *Ann Surg*, **215(4)**, 326–331.

156. de Aretxabala, X.A., Roa, I.S., Burgos, L.A., Araya, J.C., Villaseca, M.A., Silva, J.A. (1997) Curative resection in potentially resectable tumours of the gallbladder. *Eur J Surg*, **163(6)**, 419–426.

157. Chijiiwa, K., Tanaka, M. (1994) Carcinoma of the gallbladder: an appraisal of surgical resection. *Surgery*, **115(6)**, 751–756.

158. Rajagopalan, V, Daines, W.P., Grossbard, M.L., Kozuch, P. (2004) Gallbladder and biliary tract carcinoma: a comprehensive update, Part 1. *Oncology (Williston Park)*, **18(7)**, 889–896.

159. Daines, W.P., Rajagopalan, V, Grossbard, M.L., Kozuch, P. (2004) Gallbladder and biliary tract carcinoma: a comprehensive update, Part 2. *Oncology (Williston Park)*, **18(8)**, 1049–1059; discussion 60, 65–66, 68.

9 Gastrointestinal Endocrine Cancer

Mohid Shakil Khan and Martyn Caplin
Royal Free Hospital, London, UK

> ## Key Points
>
> - Neuroendocrine tumors (NETs) are heterogeneous and management depends on the site of primary.
> - Metastatic NETs can be nonfunctional or functional: carcinoid syndrome with midgut NETs and various secretory syndromes with pancreatic NETs.
> - The biology of NETs and prognosis is reliably predicted by grade, which affects management choice.
> - First-line therapy for most metastatic/advanced NETs are somatostatin analogs if demonstrated on OctreoScan™ (or Gallium-68 PET); or chemotherapy with some pancreatic NETs.
> - Various options exist for further therapy including peptide receptor targeted therapy, transarterial hepatic embolization, chemotherapy, and new small molecules.

> ## Key Web Links
>
> http://www.enets.org/guidelines_tnm_classifications.html
>
> http://royalfree.nhs.uk/NET/
>
> http://www.ukinets.org.uk/
>
> http://www.net-cme.net
>
> http://www.bsg.org.uk/clinical-guidelines/liver/guidelines-for-the-management-of-gastroenteropancreatic-neuroendocrine-including-carcinoid-tumours.html

Epidemiology

Neuroendocrine tumors (NETs) are malignant transformations of cells of the diffuse neuroendocrine system (DNES), which comprises a variety of neuroendocrine cells scattered throughout the body. The original name,

Handbook of Gastrointestinal Cancer, First Edition. Edited by Janusz Jankowski and Ernest Hawk.
© 2013 John Wiley & Sons, Ltd. Published 2013 by John Wiley & Sons, Ltd.

"carcinoid" (carcinoma-like), proposed by Oberndorfer in 1907,[1] is often paired with primary site, for example, ileal carcinoid, gastric carcinoid, but this is now an outdated term.

Commonly thought to be rare, incidence rates in the 1980s reported fewer than 2 per 100,000 per year.[2] Recent data, however, suggests an incidence of 5.25 per 100,000.[3] This increase, particularly in gastroenteropancreatic NETs (GEP-NETs), probably reflects changes in detection, better pathological expertise and awareness, incidental findings on imaging/endoscopy rather than increasing burden, since GEP-NETs were found in up to 1% of necropsies,[4] more than expected.

NETs are a heterogeneous group of tumors arising from midgut, pancreas, stomach, lungs, or colorectum, exhibiting diverse biological behavior from relatively indolent to highly aggressive cancers. Given heterogeneity in survival, it is not surprising that recent prevalence rates have been reported as up to 35 per 100,000, more common than that of most gastrointestinal cancers including hepatobiliary, esophageal, and pancreatic carcinomas.[3]

Survival data for NETs are difficult to interpret from historical studies due to heterogeneity in terms of type and grade of NET and difficulties in formulating globally accepted classification systems. Overall 5-year survival of all NET cases in the largest series to date was 67.2% with the surveillance, epidemiology, and end results (SEER) data reporting mean 5-year survival of 58.4% across 49,012 patients with NETs.[5]

Survival varies depending on grade and site of tumor. Pancreatic NET 5-year survival from the SEER registry was only 37.6%, but within this group, survival heterogeneity existed. Survival ranged from 30% for somatostatinomas to 95% for insulinomas at 5 years. Five-year survival for other GEP-NETs were 68.1% for midgut NETs, 64.7% for gastric NETs, 81.3% for appendix NETs, and 88.6% for rectal NETs.

Recent data have shown that 20% of patients with NETs develop other cancers, one-third of which arise in the gastrointestinal tract.[5]

Diagnosis

GEP-NETs can be asymptomatic, diagnosed incidentally on imaging, but may produce specific symptoms. These symptoms may relate to physical compression or obstruction of viscera by the tumor (pain, nausea, vomiting) or particularly in the case of NETs, related to secretion of hormones. The syndromes described below are typically seen in patients with secretory pancreatic tumors (Table 9.1).

"Carcinoid syndrome," characterized by diarrhea and flushing, is commonly a result of metastases to the liver, usually from a midgut NET, with release of hormones (serotonin and other vasoactive compounds) directly into the systemic circulation. In addition, midgut NETs may be associated with desmoplasia manifesting as intestinal (Figure 9.1), ureteric obstruction, or even heart failure associated with cardiac valve fibrosis (Figures 9.2 and 9.3). NETs are often diagnosed with advanced disease after numerous years of misdiagnosis with, for example, irritable bowel syndrome.

Table 9.1 Syndromes associated with pancreatic NETs.

Tumor	Symptoms	Malignancy
Insulinoma	Confusion, sweating, dizziness, weakness, unconsciousness, relief with eating	10% of patients develop metastases
Gastrinoma	Zollinger–Ellison syndrome of severe peptic ulceration and diarrhea	Metastases develop in 60% of patients; likelihood correlated with size of primary
Glucagonoma	Necrolytic migratory erythema, weight loss, diabetes mellitus, stomatitis, diarrhea	Metastases develop in 60% or more patients
VIPoma	Werner–Morrison syndrome of profuse watery diarrhea with marked hypokalemia	Metastases develop in up to 70% of patients; majority found at presentation
Somatostatinoma	Cholelithiasis, weight loss, diarrhea, and steatorrhea. Diabetes mellitus	Metastases likely in about 50% of patients
Nonsyndromic pancreatic neuroendocrine tumor	Symptoms from pancreatic mass and/or liver metastases	Metastases develop in up to 50% of patients

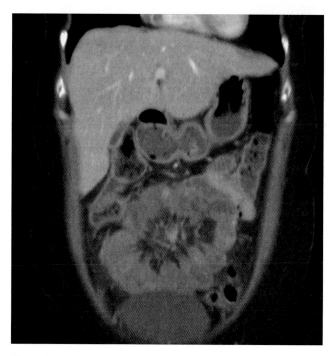

Figure 9.1 CT scan demonstrating midgut neuroendocrine tumor: mesenteric mass with surrounding desmoplasia and tethering of small intestine with dilated fluid-filled small bowel loops.

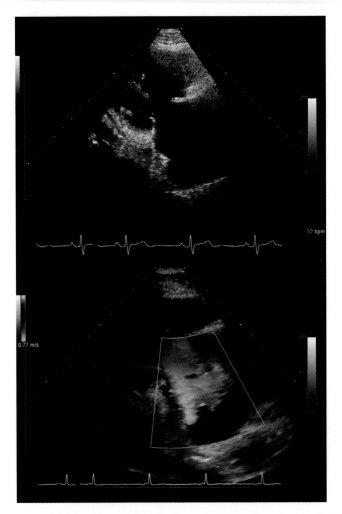

Figure 9.2 Echocardiogram demonstrating carcinoid heart disease involving the tricuspid valve. *Above*: parasternal right ventricular inflow view demonstrating fixed, thickened, and retracted tricuspid valve leaflets and associated chordae. *Below*: Color Doppler showing free-flowing, severe tricuspid regurgitation through non-coapting valve leaflets into a dilated right atrium.

The diagnosis is therefore based on clinical symptoms, hormone profile, radiological and nuclear medicine imaging, and histological confirmation. The gold standard in diagnosis is detailed histopathology and this should be obtained whenever possible.

Blood and urine investigations

In addition to general hematological and biochemical tests such as full blood count, parathyroid hormone (PTH), thyroid function tests (TFTs), calcitonin, prolactin, CEA, α-fetoprotein, and β-human chorionic

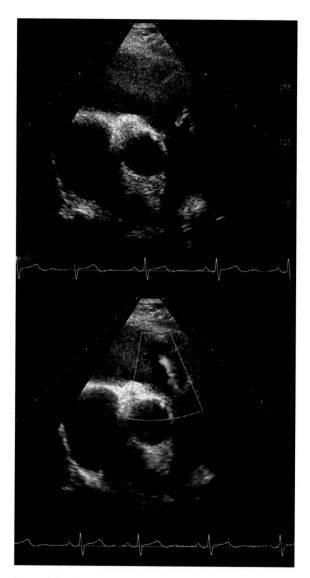

Figure 9.3 Echocardiogram demonstrating carcinoid heart disease involving the pulmonary valve. *Above*: parasternal short-axis view of the pulmonary valve demonstrating fixed, thickened, and retracted valve leaflets that fail to coapt, resulting in the valve remaining in a semi-open position. *Below*: color Doppler showing a severe jet of pulmonary regurgitation in diastole.

gonadotrophin, there are a number of specific biochemical tests. Measurement of circulating and urinary peptides and amines in patients with NETs can assist in making the initial diagnosis and may provide prognostic and predictive information.

The most commonly used and clinically useful "general" NET-circulating marker is plasma chromogranin A (CgA).[6,7] It is raised in many

NETs with a sensitivity and specificity ranging from 27% to 95% depending on the type of assay used.[8,9] It is also useful as a prognostic marker: patients with a CgA greater than 5000 µg/L have a 5-year survival of only 22% compared with 63% for patients with CgA less than 5000 µg/L.[10]

Fasting hormones should be evaluated in pancreatic NETs in order identify the syndromes in Table 9.1. Further dynamic testing, including prolonged fast (insulinoma) or secretin test (gastrinoma), should be performed depending on the syndrome suspected. Intrinsic factor and parietal cell antibodies are positive in gastric NETs associated with atrophic gastritis.

Twenty-four-hour urinary 5-hydroxy-indoleacetic acid (5-HIAA) is a product of serotonin metabolism, often raised in midgut NETs, particularly if symptoms of carcinoid syndrome are present. Care must be taken when evaluating urinary 5-HIAA as certain foods taken just prior to, or during collection, can alter results. Banana, avocado, aubergine, pineapple, plums, walnut, paracetamol, fluorouracil, methysergide, naproxen, and caffeine may cause false-positive results. Levodopa, aspirin, adrenocorticotrophic hormone (ACTH), methyldopa, and phenothiazines may give false-negative results.

Radiology and endoscopy

Primary midgut NETs may be difficult to identify on imaging as they are often small. Frequently, however, a lymph node metastasis with surrounding desmoplasia, a "mesenteric mass," can be demonstrated. Pancreatic NETs and some NET liver metastases can be diagnosed on CT or MRI due to their hypervascular nature, especially with several contrast-enhancement phases.[11] MRI may be useful in characterizing small liver metastases, and also in young patients requiring repeated imaging.

Gastric NETs are often found incidentally at upper gastrointestinal endoscopy as polyps in the stomach fundus or body (with associated atrophic gastritis and hypergastrinemia in Type-I gastric NETs). Gastric, duodenal, rectal, and colonic NETs are diagnosed at endoscopy with CT utilized to detect regional and distant metastases for staging in these cases. However, MRI or endorectal ultrasound may be of more benefit in the latter two to ascertain local invasion. Endoscopic ultrasound (EUS) can be performed to assess local invasion of gastric and duodenal NETs and for identifying and aspirating pancreatic lesions for tissue diagnosis. EUS is a useful diagnostic investigation in patients with suspected pancreatic NETs (mean sensitivity 90%).[12,13] Its sensitivity may be less with extra-pancreatic gastrinomas (80% of gastrinomas in MEN1 are found in the duodenum) for which an upper gastrointestinal endoscopy and CT/MRI should be performed.[14]

For clinical and research purposes, observing or monitoring response to therapy can be assessed by RECIST (Response Evaluation Criteria in Solid Tumors).

Nuclear medicine imaging

NETs express somatostatin receptors (SSTRs), which led to the development of radiolabeled somatostatin analogs (SSA) for diagnosis and

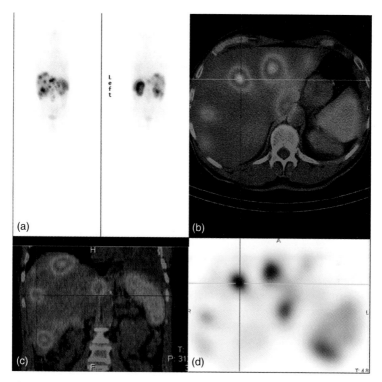

Figure 9.4 Whole body OctreoScan™ supplemented with SPECT/CT of liver and upper abdomen demonstrating focal uptake of tracer in liver lesions on whole body coronal image (a), SPECT/CT trans-axial (b) and coronal slices (c) and OctreoScan™ axial image (d).

therapy. There are five SSTR subtypes (SSTR1–5) with SSTR2 and SSTR5 expressed in at least 80% and 77% of gastrointestinal NETs, respectively.[15,16] With the exception of insulinomas (only 50% express SSTR2), somatostatin scintigraphy (with Octreoscan™) is the mainstay of staging and may assist in localizing primary lesions in GEP-NETs[17,18] (Figure 9.4).

Unlike adenocarcinomas, PET–CT with 18-fluorodeoxyglucose ([18F]FDG) is not very useful, but it can assess the extent of high-grade NETs or other lesions suggestive of coexistent cancers.[19] Increasing use of PET with compounds such as [68]Gallium-DOTA-Octreotate and ^{68}Ga-DOTA-Octreotide and more recently ^{68}Ga-DOTANOC have been found to be sensitive for NETs due to detection of more SSTR subtypes and enhanced affinity compared with OctreoScan™.[19] These characterize metastases, assess extent of disease, and locate primary lesions (Figure 9.9).

Frequently, patients present with metastases without an obvious primary. Investigations for localizing the primary site may include EUS; CT of chest (bronchial carcinoid), abdomen, and pelvis; endoscopy (colonoscopy, gastroscopy, video capsule enteroscopy); and nuclear medicine imaging. In one series, primary tumors were localized in 81–96% of cases using radiological and nuclear medicine imaging.[20]

Pathology

Historically, prognostic classifications in NETs have proven difficult due to complexity of different classification systems. NETs should be classified according to the tumor node metastasis classification system proposed by the European Neuroendocrine Tumor Society (ENETS) for foregut, midgut, and hindgut NETs[21,22] that have proved valid and applicable.[23–25] Alternatively, the World Health Organization (WHO) 2010 classification may be used.[26]

Classification is made according to site of primary tumor, size, invasion to muscularis propria, and histological grade. The latter is particularly useful prognostically. It uses mitotic count per 10 high power fields (HPF) or the Ki-67 proliferation index to group NETs into:

- low (G1) (<2 mitoses/10 HPF or Ki-67 ≥2%);
- intermediate (G2) (2–20 mitoses/10 HPF or Ki-67 3–20%);
- high (G3) (>20 mitoses/10 HPF or ≥20%).

Ki-67 proliferation index should be assessed in 2000 tumor cells in areas where the highest nuclear labeling is observed and mitoses in at least 40 HPF.

Five-year survival rates for pancreatic NETs are 94%, 63%, and 14% for low-, intermediate-, and high-grade tumors, respectively.[27] For midgut NETs, the figures are 95%, 82%, and 51%, respectively.[24]

All suspected NET samples should undergo immunostaining with a panel of antibodies to general neuroendocrine markers.[28] These include PGP9.5, synaptophysin, CgA, and MIB-1 (to generate Ki-67 index). High-grade tumors indicate a poorly differentiated endocrine carcinoma, showing significantly reduced CgA expression while maintaining intense staining for synaptophysin. Where a syndrome of hormone excess is present, the tumor can also be confirmed as the source using antibodies to the specific hormone(s).

Prevention

There is no evidence to date to suggest measures that can be taken to prevent NETs. However, in a case-control study, a family history of cancer was a significant risk factor for all NETs and a history of diabetes mellitus for gastric NETs.[29] Smoking and alcohol consumption were not associated with NET development.

Cancer management

General objectives

Wherever possible, in localized cases, surgery should be attempted to obtain curative resection. In some cases with liver metastases, where the primary is resectable, resection of the liver metastases +/− ablation of nonresectable lesions may be considered as a curative approach.

Metastases are often present at the time of diagnosis, where curative resection is usually not possible, and when surgery is undertaken, it can be considered palliative in view of residual disease. The aim of treatment

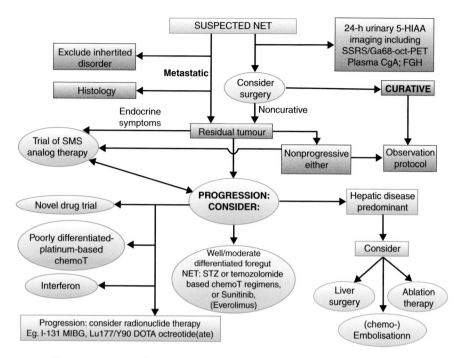

Figure 9.5 Algorithm for the management of patients with NETs. 5-HIAA, 5-hydroxyindole acetic acid; SSRS, somatostatin receptor scintigraphy; CgA, chromogranin A; STZ, streptozocin; MIBG, metaiodobenzylguanidine; chemoT, chemotherapy; Ga68-oct PET, Gallium68-DOTA-Octreotate positron emission topography. (Adapted from Ramage et al.[47] with permission from BMJ Publishing Group Limited.)

is thus to control tumor growth, prolong survival, and improve symptoms (including those from excess hormone secretion) and quality of life. Treatment choice depends on site of primary, grade, comorbidities, patient tolerability, and availability of options. Management should be guided by guidelines produced by the ENETS.[30–32]

In low- and intermediate-grade metastatic midgut NETs, SSAs are the mainstay of treatment. Until recently, these were only indicated in functioning midgut NETs with "carcinoid syndrome," but recent evidence suggests that their use can be extended to nonfunctioning midgut NETs to prolong progression-free survival (PFS).[33] For well-differentiated pancreatic NETs, chemotherapy is often the first-line choice of therapy with good evidence of efficacy[34] and it is the first-line treatment for poorly differentiated or high grade NETs. All therapeutic options should be discussed within a multidisciplinary team. A general algorithm is shown in Figure 9.5.

Surgery

Emergency surgery
Patients with midgut NETs may often present in the emergency situation with intestinal obstruction caused by peritumoral fibrosis.

After emergency laparotomy, the subsequent diagnosis of midgut NET is made on the surgical specimen. However, the tumor may be deemed unresectable and an intestinal bypass procedure performed. Following definitive histopathology, a limited small bowel resection for an obstructing tumor can be followed at a later date by elective surgery to remove further small intestine or nodal disease.

Another common emergency situation may arise whereby patients presenting with appendicitis have their NET diagnosed on the surgical specimen after appendicectomy is performed. Further management may be required as explained later. Rarely, a hindgut NET may present with large bowel obstruction with emergency resection and Hartmann's procedure. Similarly, the diagnosis of NET is made on the surgical specimen.

When a functioning tumor is diagnosed before surgery, there is a risk of carcinoid crisis when the tumor is operated upon. This should be prevented by the administration of continuous intravenous Octreotide at a dose of 50 µg/hour for 12 hours prior to and at least 48 hours after surgery.[35] Similarly, prophylaxis with glucose infusion for insulinoma surgery, proton pump inhibitor, and Octreotide for gastrinomas may be required.

Stomach

There are three types of gastric NET that are usually found incidentally as polyps during upper gastrointestinal endoscopy. Management is dependent on the type as suggested by the ENETS guidelines.[36]

Type-I gastric NETs are associated with hypergastrinemia and chronic atrophic gastritis. They present as polyps resulting from the hypergastrinemia causing hyperplasia and proliferation of enterochromaffin-like cells (ECL cells). Their metastatic potential is very low and in the majority of cases <10 mm; only annual endoscopic surveillance is required with serial mucosal biopsies taken due to the risk of gastric adenocarcinomas developing from intestinal metaplasia.[37] In larger tumors of 10–20 mm, EUS is required to assess depth of invasion. Endoscopic resection is recommended for up to 6 polyps not involving the muscularis propria. For other patients with polyps over 20 mm, local surgical tumor resection should be considered with antral resection to avoid repeated gastrin stimulation of gastric ECL cells. This is effective in 80% of Type-I tumors.[38]

Type-II gastric NETs are caused by hypergastrinemia due to Zollinger–Ellison syndrome almost exclusively in multiple endocrine neoplasia (MEN) Type I.[39] These can be more aggressive especially in those greater than 20 mm. Endoscopic or local resection may be required as with Type-I gastric NETs. Consideration should be taken to search for and resect the gastrin-secreting primary tumor. Annual endoscopic surveillance is recommended with mucosal resection of polyps over 10 mm.

Type-III gastric NETs are more aggressive. Local endoscopic or surgical excision may be appropriate for lesions <20 mm with management of larger lesions similar to that for gastric adenocarcinomas—partial or total gastrectomy with lymph node dissection. EUS in addition to CT/MRI is important in staging.

Midgut

Midgut NETs are usually over 2 cm at diagnosis, having invaded the muscularis propria and frequently metastasized to regional lymph nodes. For those with localized NETs of the jejunum–ileum, surgery should be curative. Resection of the primary, either through open or laparoscopic approach, should adhere to oncological principles and should involve lymph node clearance, aiming to preserve vascular supply and limit intestinal resection.[40] At laparotomy, the small intestine should be explore for a second primary that can occur in 30%. There is a lack of positive phase III studies in an adjuvant situation.

In patients with limited liver metastases, curative resection involving removal of the primary, regional lymph nodes, and resectable liver metastases is possible in up to 20% of patients.[40,41] Further evidence of surgery for liver metastases is given in Section "Liver metastases."

In the presence of unresectable metastases or unresectable small intestinal NET, resection of jejunal-ileal NETs should be considered to prevent future intestinal obstruction or ischemic complications due to the desmoplastic reaction or compression of the mesenteric vein due to tumor mass.[30] Surgery should be performed according to oncological principles and may include resection of nodal metastases with associated desmoplasia. This has been reported to increase survival benefit from 69 to 130 months.[42] Commonly, the associated desmoplasia may preclude tumor resection, and in these cases, bypass procedures should be undertaken to prevent obstructive symptoms. Palliative or cytoreductive surgery can be considered in patients in whom 90% of the tumor load can be removed safely. This may involve resection of the primary with locoregional metastases or intra-abdominal debulking or synchronous resection of primary and liver metastases.[43]

Pancreas

Whipple pancreaticoduodenectomy, distal, or even total pancreatectomy may be appropriate in functioning and nonfunctioning pancreatic NETs. Localized tumors >2 cm should have aggressive surgery and resection of nearby organs if required.[44] With tumors <2 cm, surgical cure needs to balanced with postoperative complications and morbidity due to lack of evidence. Small, easily accessible tumors can be treated with enucleation or middle pancreatectomy. The laparoscopic approach may be considered in expert hands for insulinomas and small nonfunctioning tumors in the body or tail. Resection of locally advanced nonfunctioning pancreatic NETs may prolong survival with a 5-year survival up to 80%.[45]

With regard to metastatic nonfunctioning pancreatic NETs, resection of the primary fails to improve survival but may reduce symptoms in hormonally active primary tumors.[45]

Patients with MEN1 often have multiple small NETs throughout the pancreas and gastrinoma patients throughout the duodenum. However, fit patients with sporadic gastrinomas with resectable disease should be considered for surgical exploration for cure.

Surgery for liver metastases is discussed in Section "Liver metastases."

Colorectum

Surgical management of colonic NETs is similar to colonic adenocarcinomas due to aggressive behavior. Since most invade the muscularis propria and are greater than 2 cm in diameter, colectomy and oncological resection of lymph drainage is recommended.[46] This may also be indicated to prevent intestinal obstruction or ischemic complications especially if there is desmoplastic reaction in proximal colonic lesions similar to that of classical midgut NETs. Liver metastases are managed as discussed in Section "Liver metastases" and this is where management differs from colonic adenocarcinomas.

Rectal NETs often present incidentally as polyps at endoscopy with low risk of metastases (3%) in those with a diameter <10 mm. Muscularis propria invasion, size, and high Ki-67 are indicators of aggressive behavior. When rectal NETs are between 10 and 20 mm, outcome is unclear, but management should be guided by Ki-67 index and EUS. In general, those <20 mm with low Ki-67 can be removed by local resection at endoscopy or another transanal method. Lesions >20 mm commonly invade the muscularis propria and require total mesorectal excision due to higher metastatic potential.[47] Locoregional resection can be considered in metastatic disease to control local symptoms without any impact on survival. Adjuvant chemotherapy can be contemplated in poorly differentiated tumors with incomplete resection, but there is no evidence.

Appendix

Diagnosis of appendiceal NET is often made after histopathological assessment on an appendix resected after acute appendicitis. Right hemicolectomy (open or laparoscopic) with locoregional lymphadenectomy is usually indicated when the tumor is at the base of appendix, or ≥20 mm diameter, or shows >3 mm mesoappendiceal invasion, or histology suggests goblet cell (adenocarcinoid).[48] These patients require longer term follow-up, but prognosis is very good.

Mixed endocrine/exocrine tumors of the appendix, so-called goblet cell appendiceal NET, share histological properties of both adenocarcinoma and NET (6% of appendiceal NETs). They also have higher metastatic potential with 20% presenting with metastases compared with 2–5% of classical appendiceal NETs[49] Full staging with CT/MRI should be undertaken. Most metastases occur in lymph nodes or to ovaries conferring a poorer overall survival, median 12 months. Therefore, right hemicolectomy is recommended after an appendicectomy demonstrating goblet cell appendiceal NET.

Liver metastases

Management of liver metastases has to be taken into account prior to any therapy as these are frequently present at diagnosis. Liver surgery includes metastasis enucleation, segmental or wedge resection, hemihepatectomy, or extended hemihepatectomy. Intraoperative ultrasonography is essential in detecting all metastases. Surgery can be proposed in all patients with GEP-NETs regardless of the site of primary, although resection with metastatic hindgut NETs is rare. The minimum criteria for liver surgery with "curative intent" are (a) resectable well-differentiated liver disease with acceptable morbidity and <5% mortality, (b)absence of right heart insufficiency, (d) absence of extra-abdominal, and (e) absence of diffuse peritoneal carcinomatosis.[43] The primary tumor is also usually deemed resectable (or has been resected previously). Cardiac surgery, if required, should be planned 3 months prior to liver surgery for anticoagulation purposes.

Surgery can be undertaken together with resection of the primary with a curative intent in 10% of cases if confined to one lobe. With bilobar metastases, it may also be undertaken as a cytoreductive procedure to alleviate symptoms of carcinoid (or other functional) syndrome particularly if there is resistance to medical therapy. Radiofrequency ablation (RFA) can be performed either before or during surgery.[50]

With bilobar metastases, the difficulty is achieving adequate tumor resection while maintaining sufficient liver function. Options include 2-stage procedures (including branch portal vein ligation/embolization), repeated hepatectomies, or a combination of surgical resection and loco ablative methods.[51,52]

Postoperative 5-year survival rate is 61% or higher compared with 30–40% reported from noncontrolled studies with patients not resected, with perioperative mortality <5% in most reports.[43,53–57]

Total tumor hepatectomy with liver transplantation may be considered in a small group of patients with bilobar liver metastases without extra-hepatic disease in two situations: (a) with intent to cure and (b) to palliate from life-threatening hormonal disturbances.[58] In an analysis of all UK transplants for NETs, survival was 62% at 1 year and 23% at 5 years, similar to other series. However, these include cases from many years ago with inferior imaging technology to present day and some cases were undoubtedly transplanted with extrahepatic disease. Various other series have shown good initial outcomes but poor long-term cure rates with very low 5-year disease-free survival. Survival is better with metastatic midgut NETs compared with metastatic pancreatic NETs. Currently, orthotopic transplant should only be considered in exceptional circumstances with a comprehensive assessment to exclude extrahepatic disease, while the issues of perioperative morbidity and ethical distribution of donor organs are contemplated.

Biotherapy

Somatostatin analogs
The foundation of NET therapy, especially in functional midgut NETs, is based on long-acting SSA. They alleviate symptoms in carcinoid syndrome, stabilize tumor growth, and improve quality of life.

SSAs bind to SSTRs, and upon ligand activation, there is inhibition of the release of many hormones and impairment of hormonally mediated exocrine function. By this mechanism, SSAs abrogate flushing and secretory diarrhea in patients with carcinoid syndrome with NETs expressing SSTRs.[59]

Short-acting Octreotide, with a high affinity for SSTR2 and SSTR5, is administered by subcutaneous injection (or intravenous infusion) with subcutaneous dosing starting at 50–100 μg two to three times daily to a maximum daily dose of 3000 μg. Similar efficacy is found between Octreotide and another short-acting SSA, lanreotide.[60] Short-acting SSAs are indicated in testing tolerability, immediate relief of carcinoid syndromic symptoms, stabilization prior to converting to long-acting therapy, rescue therapy of breakthrough symptoms despite long-acting SSAs, and perioperatively for prevention and treatment of carcinoid crises.

The development of long-acting depot formulations, Octreotide LAR[61] and Lanreotide Autogel,[62] has allowed clinically practical administration of these drugs by intramuscular and deep subcutaneous routes every 28 days. Biochemical response rates with an inhibition of hormone production are seen in 30–70% with symptom control in the majority of patients.[63] Escalation of dose is often required over time for symptom control due to poorly understood "tachyphylaxis." When symptoms recur on SSA therapy, options include dose escalation, a reduction in interval between administrations, switching to an alternate SSA, or other therapies as stated later.

Recently, it has been confirmed that SSAs have an antitumor role in nonfunctioning small intestinal tumors. Data derived from the PROMID phase III study has shown that long-term administration inhibits tumor growth in midgut NETs with low-volume metastatic disease, with time to progression twice as long as with placebo.[33] Tumor growth inhibition is more likely in midgut compared with foregut tumors, but the results of Lanreotide Autogel in nonfunctioning pancreatic NETs are awaited.

Other benefits of SSAs may include prevention of the advancement of carcinoid heart disease and intestinal fibrosis, but studies are conflicting.[64]

Few side effects have been reported with SSAs and these include fat malabsorption, gallstones, gall bladder dysfunction, vitamin A and D malabsorption, headaches, diarrhea, dizziness, and hypo/hyperglycemia.

Interferon-α

Interferon-α was introduced as a treatment for GEP-NETs in the early 1980s and exerts antiproliferation, antisecretory, and antiangiogenic effects. The usual dose employed is 3–5 million units subcutaneously, three to five times a week. Symptomatic and biochemical responses have been noted in approximately 50% of patients with disease stabilization in 60–80% at a follow-up of 4 years. However, significant tumor reduction only occurs in 10–15%.[65] Limitations include side effects including flu-like symptoms, bone marrow suppression, thyroid disorders, psychiatric phenomenon, and chronic fatigue syndrome. Therefore, it may be considered as second-line therapy. Prospective randomized trials have not demonstrated any benefit with combined interferon and SSA.[66] Longer acting weekly pegylated interferons have been used with anecdotally at least similar efficacy and interferon-gamma has been tested in phase II studies with similar effect.[67]

Chemotherapy

Systemic chemotherapy is widely used but its precise role is not known due to studies including various grades, sites, and inconsistent response criteria. Thus there is no standard regimen. Systemic chemotherapy has been the standard treatment for pancreatic NETs based on original data with an objective response of 69%[68] with streptozocin (STZ) and 5-fluorouracil (5-FU). The main indication for STZ + 5-FU or DOX includes well-differentiated malignant pancreatic NETs. A recent series (*n* = 79) combined 5-FU, cisplatin, and STZ (FCiSt) in chemo-naive patients with metastatic or locally advanced NETs.[34] Response rates were 38% for pancreatic and 25% for nonpancreatic sites with median time to progression 9.1 months and median overall survival 31.5 months with an acceptable toxicity profile and an advantageous 1-day outpatient administration.

Regarding functioning pancreatic NETs, response rates with 5-FU, STZ, and DOX in islet cell tumors vary between 40% and 70%.[69]

The use of chemotherapy in midgut and hindgut NETs has a much lower response rate, with <20% of patients deriving benefit, which may only last 6–8 months with STZ/FU/DOX, cyclophosphamide regimens.[70] A recent retrospective analysis found monotherapy with the alkylating agent, temozolomide, achieved radiological response in 14% and stable disease in 53%.[71] It is generally well tolerated with minimal side effects including leucopenia, nausea, and abdominal pain. Its response rate and duration of effect are similar to those of other established regimens.

Poorly differentiated or anaplastic NETs are more aggressive and etoposide and cisplatin combinations have been used to induce response rates of over 50% albeit with short median survival rates and significant toxicity.[72]

Rare functioning tumors

VIPomas (Werner–Morrison syndrome): Rehydration is always indicated. Patients with this rare life-threatening syndrome frequently respond dramatically to small doses of SSA with cessation of diarrhea.[73] The dose of the drug may be titrated against VIP levels with normalization of levels being the target. VIPomas resistant has demonstrated response to oral glucocorticoids, although this approach has not been proven.

Glucagonomas: It has been reported that SSAs improve symptoms, although there is no indication for the drugs if the patient has no syndrome. The characteristic rash of necrolytic migratory erythema may also be improved.

Gastrinomas: The syndrome is adequately controlled with high-dose proton pump inhibitor drugs, and although some groups advise adding SSAs, there is no definite added benefit.

Insulinomas: Diazoxide has been shown to be effective in controlling hypoglycemic symptoms in patients with insulinoma.[74] This treatment therefore should be considered in patients not cured by surgery or unsuitable for surgery. Administration of SSAs in patients with a positive OctreoScan™ may be beneficial, but only 50% of insulinomas have Type-II SSTRs. Patients may require additional therapy, for example, chemotherapy or radionuclide receptor therapy.

Other drugs: Ondansetron has been used for general symptom control in the carcinoid syndrome and can be useful. Cyproheptadine is still occasionally used for resistant carcinoid syndrome. Pancreatic enzyme supplements for pancreatic insufficiency or cholestyramine for bile salt malabsorption are often used to control diarrhea, which may be especially troublesome after intestinal resection. Pancreatic insufficiency can also occur with octreotide/lanreotide therapy. In patients with glucagonoma, zinc therapy can be used to prevent further skin lesions and prophylactic anticoagulation (for the high incidence of thrombosis) is considered.

Peptide receptor radionuclide therapy

Peptide receptor radionuclide therapy (PRRT) involves directing radioactivity internally to the tumor site delivered by a radionuclide coupled to a tumor-targeting molecule. This involves substitution of the gamma emitting diagnostic imaging radionuclide by a therapeutic beta (Auger) emitting therapy radionuclide, for example, $^{131-}$I-MIBG instead of $^{123-}$I-MIBG, $^{90-}$Yttrium or $^{177-}$Lutetium instead of $^{111-}$Indium-octreotide or ^{68}Gallium octreotate. They are reserved for those tumors expressing the receptor of interest on nuclear medicine imaging with avid uptake of $^{123-}$I-MIBG or $^{111-}$In-octreotide scintigraphy (or ^{68}Gallium Octreotate PET). The aim of radionuclide therapy is to induce DNA damage to target cells resulting in apoptosis together with damage of tumor cells by spread of radiation or toxic metabolites.

Current evidence for PRRT mainly comes from nonblinded, nonrandomized trials with varying activities and protocols with stabilization in up to 78% but partial responses only up to 20%. Patients may require a period of admission in relative isolation, consequently treating patients who have a high dependency on nursing or daily care may not be appropriate. Long-acting SSA should be stopped 6 weeks prior to radiolabeled SSA therapy.

Embolization and ablative methods

Embolization of hepatic artery branches is indicated for those with multiple nonresectable and hormone-secreting tumors. The intention is to reduce tumor bulk and thus hormone output that may improve quality of life and survival. It can be effective in both symptom control and as an antiproliferative treatment.

Symptomatic response is achieved in 40–80%, biochemical response in 50–60% with overall 5-year survival 50–60% postembolization.[75] Particle and chemoembolization are the most common forms. Obliterating agents include polyvinyl chloride, lipoidal, and gel-foam powder. Ischemia may increase the sensitivity to chemotherapeutic agents, hence the rationale behind transarterial chemoembolization utilizing concomitant doxorubicin or cisplatin.[76] Contraindications to embolization include complete portal vein obstruction, hepatic insufficiency, biliary reconstruction, and severe carcinoid heart disease. Mortality has been quoted as 2–6% with adverse events in 8–17%, the most common being postembolization syndrome (nausea, fever, abdominal pain). Rates are improved in more recent series.

Octreotide therapy should be used prophylactically as with perioperative prophylaxis in syndromic patients. Some units use prophylactic antibiotics and allopurinol predosing to prevent tumor lysis syndrome. Adequate hydration and analgesics are recommended.

RFA has been used in reducing tumor size in liver metastases from colorectal and hepatocellular cancers. Randomized trials are lacking in NET metastases, but series indicate that patients with bilobar metastases less than 5 in number with diameter less than 5 cm may benefit in terms of symptom relief and in achieving local control of the metastases. It may also be considered in combination with resection with a better survival rate than with RFA alone.[77]

RFA (percutaneous or laparoscopic) is a low-risk procedure with a mortality rate of 0.5%.[55] However, NETs, in comparison with colorectal cancer metastases, often have multiple tiny metastases and destruction of the largest lesion may not reduce hormone secretion; thus, it may be necessary to ablate at least 90% of visible tumor. It becomes increasingly difficult to fully eradicate tumors >3 cm.

Emerging therapies

Sunitinib, an oral tyrosine kinase inhibitor, initially has shown promising results. In phase II studies in midgut NETs, median time to progression was 10.2 months, 68% achieving stable disease.[78] The recent phase III study of Sunitinib versus placebo in slowly progressing pancreatic NETs ($n = 171$) was halted due to the interim analysis showing significant benefit with PFS 11.4 months for Sunitinib versus 5.5 months with placebo.[79]

In a key paper, Yao *et al.* published the results of RADIANT 1 (*RAD*001 *In Advanced Neuroendocrine Tumors*-1), a phase II study, evaluating the mTOR inhibitor, Everolimus, alone versus everolimus and Octreotide in patients with advanced pancreatic NETs who had progressed on first-line chemotherapy. In the combined treatment arm, median PFS was 17 months compared with 9.7 months with everolimus alone.[80] Similarly, in the phase III study, RADIANT-2, in patients with progressing NETs with symptoms of carcinoid syndrome, everolimus and octreotide prolonged PFS compared to placebo and octreotide (median PFS 16.4 vs 11.3 months).[81] Results from RADIANT-3 have recently demonstrated prolonged PFS with median PFS of 11.0 months with everolimus compared with 4.6 months with placebo alone in advanced pancreatic NETs.[82]

Pasireotide (SOM 230) is a newer multiligand SST analog with high affinity to SSTR1, 2, 3, and 5 receptors. Preclinical evidence and early phase II trial data indicate promise in controlling symptoms of metastatic carcinoid tumors refractory or resistant to SSA.[83]

Coexpression of dopamine and SST receptors has been demonstrated in NETs.[16,84] New SST–dopamine chimeric compounds such as BIM-23A387 have shown promising results in *in vitro* and clinical studies are ongoing.[85]

Surveillance

Once a patient with advanced NET is undergoing or has had treatment, surveillance with imaging (CT/MRI) and biochemical markers should be performed 6-monthly although evidence is lacking. Similarly, after curative resection, patients should undergo surveillance due to the indolent nature of NETs.

Family screening

The risk of NET in an individual with one affected first-degree relative has been estimated to be approximately four times that of the general population, increasing to twelve times with two affected first-degree relatives.[86] Although GEP-NETs are usually sporadic, familial syndromes including von Hippel–Lindau (vHL), tuberous sclerosis, MEN-1 syndrome, and neurofibromatosis (NF-1) may be associated with pancreatic and proximal intestinal NETs.

MEN-1 is an autosomal dominant disorder classically consisting of primary hyperparathyroidism (95%), pancreatic NETs (25–75%), and pituitary tumors (25–30%).[87]

All pancreatic and midgut NETs should be tested for serum calcium, PTH, vitamin D, and prolactin. If PTH is raised in the absence of vitamin D deficiency or there is hyperprolactinemia, genetic testing for MEN1 should be undertaken as well as referral for formal endocrine testing. Relatives of patients with MEN1 should have genetic testing.

In those relatives <40 years old found to carry a mutation of the menin gene, PTH, pituitary biochemical testing, fasting gut hormones, and insulinoma assessment should be undertaken with imaging of the pituitary, pancreas, and adrenals.[88] If normal, biochemical screening should be undertaken every 12 months and imaging every 24–36 months. In those carriers >40 years old, similar assessments should be undertaken with additional assessment for gastrinomas and acromegaly. If abnormalities are found, these should be investigated further.

NF-1 is an autosomal dominant disorder where loss of heterozygosity of NF-1 gene results in mTOR activation and tumor development.[89] It is usually diagnosed clinically and characterized by café au lait spots, cutaneous neurofibromas, optic gliomas, and iris hamartomas.

vHL syndrome is caused by mutations in the vHL tumor suppressor gene (3p25–26) involved in regulating hypoxia-induced cell proliferation and angiogenesis. Clinical features include retinal or central hemangioblastomas, clear cell renal carcinomas, pheochromocytomas, and pancreatic cysts. Pancreatic NETs occur in 15%, so this should be screened for in cases.[90]

Key Patient Consent Issues

- When consenting for resection of a midgut NET, talk about risk of needing a stoma.
- When considering PRRT, mention renal failure and bone marrow suppression.

- Transarterial hepatic embolization can result in liver failure, iatrogenic dissection, bleeding, and renal failure, so discuss these.
- Discuss the side effects of FCiSt chemotherapy—hand–foot syndrome, nail changes, hair thinning, neuropathy, hearing loss, risk of leukemia.
- Biobanking of NET tissue is vital to advancement of knowledge, so attempt to consent for this wherever possible.

Case Studies

Case 1

Mr. X is a 47-year-old gentleman with no significant medical or family history. He presented with 5 years of cutaneous flushing and a year of diarrhea with symptoms of intermittent subacute small intestinal obstruction. He developed exertional dyspnea that prompted him to seek medical attention. An echocardiogram demonstrated plaques on tricuspid and pulmonary valves and CT demonstrated an ileal tumor with lymph node involvement and bilobar liver metastases. Liver biopsy confirmed a well-differentiated NET with Ki-67 of 1% and an OctreoScan™ demonstrated avid uptake in primary lesion, liver, and bone metastases (Figure 9.6). Urinary 5-HIAA was elevated at 630 µmol/24 hours (normal 0–42) and plasma CgA was >1000 pmol/L (normal <60). He was commenced on Octreotide LAR 30 mg 4-weekly, which improved symptoms of diarrhea and flushing.

For cardiac valve disease, he underwent tricuspid and pulmonary valve replacement (under intravenous octreotide cover) with histology of a mediastinal node also confirming NET. After good recovery, resection of the ileal primary (with cholecystectomy) was undertaken, which relieved obstructive symptoms and he remained on SSAs and vitamin B compound. Unfortunately, restaging 6 months postoperatively showed progression of liver and nodal metastases (Figure 9.7) and the patient developed breakthrough symptoms of flushing. He was thus considered for therapy with intravenous ^{90}Yttrium-DOTA-Octreotate and received three doses of 3.06, 3.28, and 3.61 Gigabecquerels (GBq) at 3 monthly intervals. At 6 months after therapy, flushing is experienced less often and he has stable radiological disease.

This case demonstrates that carcinoid heart disease needs to be addressed prior to treatment of the midgut NET in order to improve outcome. It also demonstrates that resection of the primary improves symptoms as well as outcome. Finally, SSAs are first-line treatment of carcinoid syndrome with consideration of other therapies such as PRRT when there is progressive disease or breakthrough syndromic symptoms.

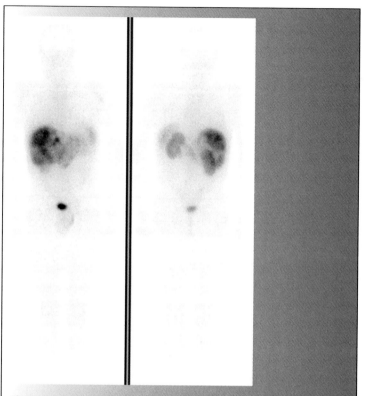

Figure 9.6 OctreoScan™ of Case 1 demonstrating uptake of tracer in known tumor sites (bilobar liver metastases).

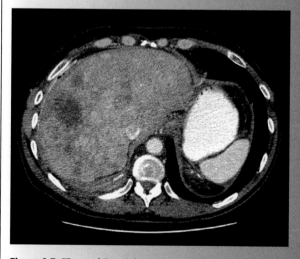

Figure 9.7 CT scan of Case 1 demonstrating bilobar liver metastases.

Case 2

Mrs. Y, 52 years old, was initially diagnosed with a pancreatic adenocarcinoma after presenting to her local team with biliary obstruction and a pancreatic mass on CT (Figure 9.8). Laparoscopic staging unfortunately demonstrated gastric lymph nodes, the histology of which was reported as metastatic adenocarcinoma. She initially received cisplatin/5-fluorouracil and gemcitabine a year later following progression. She underwent repeated biliary stenting due to repeated cholangitis but needed hepatico-jejunostomy with cholecystectomy.

As she was well 4 years after diagnosis, review of the histology was undertaken and she was referred to a specialist hepatobiliary center where the diagnosis was considered to be a well-differentiated pancreatic intermediate-grade NET (Ki-67 5%). [68]Gallium-DOTA-Octreotate PET images demonstrated uptake within the pancreatic mass and lymph nodes (Figure 9.9). Due to radiological stability after previous chemotherapy, she was monitored with CT imaging but progressed 7 years after diagnosis when local infiltration of the ampulla caused gastrointestinal bleeding, responding to laser therapy. Six cycles of 5-fluorouracil, cisplatin, and streptozocin (FCiSt) was given. She was commenced on Lanreotide Autogel as part of a clinical

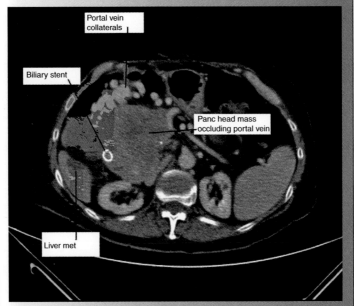

Portal vein collaterals

Biliary stent

Panc head mass occluding portal vein

Liver met

Figure 9.8 CT scan of Case 2 demonstrating hypervascular pancreatic head mass occluding superior mesenteric vein with prominent portal vein collaterals, patent biliary stent, and liver metastasis.

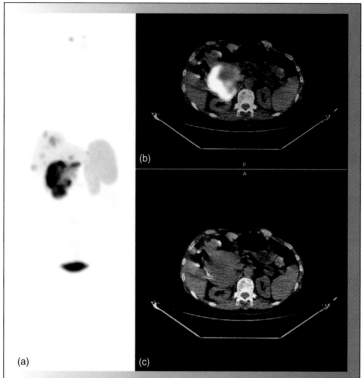

(b)

(a)

(c)

Figure 9.9 [68]Gallium-DOTA-Octreotate PET imaging supplemented with CT demonstrating uptake of tracer in large pancreatic mass, liver metastases, and dura (meningioma) on whole body image (a) and transaxial slices (b, c).

trial but developed steatorrhea that responded to pancreatic enzyme supplementation (Creon). She currently is in follow-up 14 years after diagnosis.

This case demonstrates the importance of reviewing histology and a multidisciplinary approach in NET management. Chemotherapy should be considered as first-line therapy in intermediate-grade pancreatic NETs. It also demonstrates the common adverse effect of steatorrhea with SSAs.

Potential Pitfalls

- Consider repeat review of histology when NETs are being considered or there is neuroendocrine differentiation.
- With functioning midgut NETs, be aware of carcinoid heart disease and screen with NT-proBNP and echocardiogram.

- Obstructive symptoms may reflect desmoplasia requiring dietetic and surgical management.
- Survival is variable but quality of life may be impaired; thus, consider NETs as a chronic illness.
- Not all diarrhea is carcinoid syndrome relate; consider bacterial overgrowth, bile salt malabsorption, steatorrhea, or VIPoma
- Carcinoid syndrome symptoms are usually experienced with liver or lung metastases from a midgut NET or serotonin-secreting pancreatic NET (where urinary 5-HIAA is elevated).
- When operating, consider cholecystectomy as SSAs can predispose to cholelithiasis.
- Consider resection of the primary lesion even if metastases are present, especially with midgut NETs.

References

1. Modlin, I.M., Shapiro, M.D., Kidd, M. (2004) Siegfried Oberndorfer: origins and perspectives of carcinoid tumors. *Hum Pathol*, **35(12)**, 1440–1451.
2. Buchanan, K.D., Johnston, C.F., O'Hare MM. *et al.* (1986) Neuroendocrine tumors. A European view. *Am J Med*, **81(6B)**, 14–22.
3. Yao, J.C., Hassan, M., Phan, A. *et al.* (2008) One hundred years after "carcinoid": epidemiology of and prognostic factors for neuroendocrine tumors in 35,825 cases in the United States. *J Clin Oncol*, **26(18)**, 3063–3072.
4. Berge, T., Linell, F. (1976) Carcinoid tumours. Frequency in a defined population during a 12-year period. *Acta Pathol Microbiol Scand A*, **84(4)**, 322–330.
5. Modlin, I.M., Lye, K.D., Kidd, M. (2003) A 5-decade analysis of 13,715 carcinoid tumors. *Cancer*, **97(4)**, 934–959.
6. Seregni, E., Ferrari, L., Bajetta, E. *et al.* (2001) Clinical significance of blood chromogranin A measurement in neuroendocrine tumours. *Ann Oncol*, **12(Suppl 2)**, S69–S72.
7. Tomassetti, P., Migliori, M., Simoni, P. *et al.* (2001) Diagnostic value of plasma chromogranin A in neuroendocrine tumours. *Eur J Gastroenterol Hepatol*, **13(1)**, 55–58.
8. Stridsberg, M., Eriksson, B., Oberg, K. *et al.* (2003) A comparison between three commercial kits for chromogranin A measurements. *J Endocrinol*, **177(2)**, 337–341.
9. Campana, D., Nori, F., Piscitelli, L. *et al.* (2007) Chromogranin A: is it a useful marker of neuroendocrine tumors? *J Clin Oncol*, **25(15)**, 1967–1973.
10. Janson, E.T., Holmberg, L., Stridsberg, M. *et al.* (1997) Carcinoid tumors: analysis of prognostic factors and survival in 301 patients from a referral center. *Ann Oncol*, **8(7)**, 685–690.
11. Sundin, A., Vullierme, M.P., Kaltsas, G. *et al.* (2009) ENETS Consensus Guidelines for the Standards of Care in Neuroendocrine Tumors: radiological examinations. *Neuroendocrinology*, **90(2)**, 167–183.
12. Zimmer, T., Ziegler, K., Bader, M. *et al.* (1994) Localisation of neuroendocrine tumours of the upper gastrointestinal tract. *Gut*, **35(4)**, 471–475.

13. Zimmer, T., Ziegler, K., Liehr, R.M. *et al.* (1994) Endosonography of neuroendocrine tumors of the stomach, duodenum, and pancreas. *Ann N Y Acad Sci*, **733**, 425–436.
14. Zimmer, T., Scherubl, H., Faiss, S. *et al.* (2000) Endoscopic ultrasonography of neuroendocrine tumours. *Digestion*, **62(Suppl 1)**, 45–50.
15. Reubi, J.C., Kvols, L., Krenning, E. *et al.* (1990) Distribution of somatostatin receptors in normal and tumor tissue. *Metabolism*, **39(9, Suppl 2)**, 78–81.
16. Srirajaskanthan, R., Watkins, J., Marelli, L. *et al.* (2009) Expression of somatostatin and dopamine 2 receptors in neuroendocrine tumours and the potential role for new biotherapies. *Neuroendocrinology*, **89(3)**, 308–314.
17. Krenning, E.P., Kwekkeboom, D.J., Bakker, W.H. *et al.* (1993) Somatostatin receptor scintigraphy with [111In-DTPA-D-Phe1]- and [123I-Tyr3]-octreotide: the Rotterdam experience with more than 1000 patients. *Eur J Nucl Med*, **20(8)**, 716–731.
18. Lebtahi, R., Cadiot, G., Sarda, L. *et al.* (1997) Clinical impact of somatostatin receptor scintigraphy in the management of patients with neuroendocrine gastroenteropancreatic tumors. *J Nucl Med*, **38(6)**, 853–858.
19. Khan, S., Lloyd, C., Szyszko, T. *et al.* (2008) PET imaging in endocrine tumours. *Minerva Endocrinol*, **33(2)**, 41–52.
20. Corleto, V.D., Panzuto, F., Falconi, M. *et al.* (2001) Digestive neuroendocrine tumours: diagnosis and treatment in Italy. A survey by the Oncology Study Section of the Italian Society of Gastroenterology (SIGE). *Dig Liver Dis*, **33(3)**, 217–221.
21. Rindi, G., Kloppel, G., Alhman, H. *et al.* (2006) TNM staging of foregut (neuro)endocrine tumors: a consensus proposal including a grading system. *Virchows Arch*, **449(4)**, 395–401.
22. Rindi, G., Kloppel, G., Couvelard, A. *et al.* (2007) TNM staging of midgut and hindgut (neuro) endocrine tumors: a consensus proposal including a grading system. *Virchows Arch*, **451(4)**, 757–762.
23. Pape, U.F., Jann, H., Muller-Nordhorn, J. *et al.* (2008) Prognostic relevance of a novel TNM classification system for upper gastroenteropancreatic neuroendocrine tumors. *Cancer*, **113(2)**, 256–265.
24. Jann, H., Roll, S., Couvelard, A. *et al.* (2011) Neuroendocrine tumors of midgut and hindgut origin: tumor-node-metastasis classification determines clinical outcome. *Cancer*, **117(15)**, 3332–3341.
25. Ekeblad, S., Skogseid, B., Dunder, K. *et al.* (2008) Prognostic factors and survival in 324 patients with pancreatic endocrine tumor treated at a single institution. *Clin Cancer Res*, **14(23)**, 7798–77803.
26. Bosman, F.T., Carneiro, F., Hruban, R.H. *et al.* (2010) *WHO Classification of Tumours of the Digestive System*. IARC, Lyon.
27. Scarpa, A., Mantovani, W., Capelli, P. *et al.* (2010) Pancreatic endocrine tumors: improved TNM staging and histopathological grading permit a clinically efficient prognostic stratification of patients. *Mod Pathol*, **23(6)**, 824–833.
28. Kloppel, G., Couvelard, A., Perren, A. *et al.* (2009) ENETS Consensus Guidelines for the Standards of Care in Neuroendocrine Tumors: towards a standardized approach to the diagnosis of gastroenteropancreatic neuroendocrine tumors and their prognostic stratification. *Neuroendocrinology*, **90(2)**, 162–166.
29. Hassan, M.M., Phan, A., Li, D. *et al.* (2008) Risk factors associated with neuroendocrine tumors: A U. S.-based case-control study. *Int J Cancer*, **123(4)**, 867–873.

30. Eriksson, B., Kloppel, G., Krenning, E. *et al.* (2008) Consensus guidelines for the management of patients with digestive neuroendocrine tumors–well-differentiated jejunal-ileal tumor/carcinoma. *Neuroendocrinology*, **87(1)**, 8–19.

31. Falconi, M., Plockinger, U., Kwekkeboom, D.J. *et al.* (2006) Well-differentiated pancreatic nonfunctioning tumors/carcinoma. *Neuroendocrinology*, **84(3)**, 196–211.

32. Ahlman, H., Nilsson, O., McNicol, A.M. *et al.* (2008) Poorly-differentiated endocrine carcinomas of midgut and hindgut origin. *Neuroendocrinology*, **87(1)**, 40–46.

33. Rinke, A., Muller, H.H., Schade-Brittinger, C. *et al.* (2009) Placebo-controlled, double-blind, prospective, randomized study on the effect of octreotide LAR in the control of tumor growth in patients with metastatic neuroendocrine midgut tumors: a report from the PROMID Study Group. *J Clin Oncol*, **27(28)**, 4656–4663.

34. Turner, N.C., Strauss, S.J., Sarker, D. *et al.* (2010) Chemotherapy with 5-fluorouracil, cisplatin and streptozocin for neuroendocrine tumours. *Br J Cancer*, **102(7)**, 1106–1112.

35. Roy, R.C., Carter, R.F., Wright, P.D. (1987) Somatostatin, anaesthesia, and the carcinoid syndrome. Peri-operative administration of a somatostatin analogue to suppress carcinoid tumour activity. *Anaesthesia*, **42(6)**, 627–632.

36. Ruszniewski, P., Delle Fave, G., Cadiot, G. *et al.* (2006) Well-differentiated gastric tumors/carcinomas. *Neuroendocrinology*, **84(3)**, 158–164.

37. Borch, K., Ahren, B., Ahlman, H. *et al.* (2005) Gastric carcinoids: biologic behavior and prognosis after differentiated treatment in relation to type. *Ann Surg*, **242(1)**, 64–73.

38. Ahlman, H. (1999) Surgical treatment of carcinoid tumours of the stomach and small intestine. *Ital J Gastroenterol Hepatol*, **31(Suppl 2)**, S198–S201.

39. Solcia, E., Capella, C., Fiocca, R. *et al.* (1990) Gastric argyrophil carcinoidosis in patients with Zollinger-Ellison syndrome due to type 1 multiple endocrine neoplasia. A newly recognized association. *Am J Surg Pathol*, **14(6)**, 503–513.

40. Ahlman, H., Wangberg, B., Jansson, S. *et al.* (2000) Interventional treatment of gastrointestinal neuroendocrine tumours. *Digestion*, **62(Suppl 1)**, 59–68.

41. Frilling, A., Rogiers, X., Malago, M. *et al.* (1998) Treatment of liver metastases in patients with neuroendocrine tumors. *Langenbecks Arch Surg*, **383(1)**, 62–70.

42. Soreide, O., Berstad, T., Bakka, A. *et al.* (1992) Surgical treatment as a principle in patients with advanced abdominal carcinoid tumors. *Surgery*, **111(1)**, 48–54.

43. Steinmuller, T., Kianmanesh, R., Falconi, M. *et al.* (2008) Consensus guidelines for the management of patients with liver metastases from digestive (neuro)endocrine tumors: foregut, midgut, hindgut, and unknown primary. *Neuroendocrinology*, **87(1)**, 47–62.

44. Norton, J.A., Kivlen, M., Li M. *et al.* (2003) Morbidity and mortality of aggressive resection in patients with advanced neuroendocrine tumors. *Arch Surg*, **138(8)**, 859–866.

45. Solorzano, C.C., Lee, J.E., Pisters, P.W. *et al.* (2001) Nonfunctioning islet cell carcinoma of the pancreas: survival results in a contemporary series of 163 patients. *Surgery*, **130(6)**, 1078–1085.

46. Ramage, J.K., Goretzki, P.E., Manfredi, R. *et al.* (2008) Consensus guidelines for the management of patients with digestive neuroendocrine tumours: well-differentiated colon and rectum tumour/carcinoma. *Neuroendocrinology*, **87(1)**, 31–39.

47. Ramage, J.K., Davies, A.H., Ardill, J. *et al.* (2005) Guidelines for the management of gastroenteropancreatic neuroendocrine (including carcinoid) tumours. *Gut*, **54(Suppl 4)**, iv1–iv16.

48. Moertel, C.G., Weiland, L.H., Nagorney, D.M. *et al.* (1987) Carcinoid tumor of the appendix: treatment and prognosis. *N Engl J Med*, **317(27)**, 1699–1701.

49. Toumpanakis, C., Standish, R.A., Baishnab, E. *et al.* (2007) Goblet cell carcinoid tumors (adenocarcinoid) of the appendix. *Dis Colon Rectum*, **50(3)**, 315–322.

50. O'Toole, D., Maire, F., Ruszniewski, P. (2003) Ablative therapies for liver metastases of digestive endocrine tumours. *Endocr Relat Cancer*, **10(4)**, 463–468.

51. Kianmanesh, R., Sauvanet, A., Hentic, O. *et al.* (2008) Two-step surgery for synchronous bilobar liver metastases from digestive endocrine tumors: a safe approach for radical resection. *Ann Surg*, **247(4)**, 659–665.

52. Jaeck, D., Oussoultzoglou, E., Bachellier, P. *et al.* (2001) Hepatic metastases of gastroenteropancreatic neuroendocrine tumors: safe hepatic surgery. *World J Surg*, **25(6)**, 689–692.

53. Wangberg, B., Westberg, G., Tylen, U. *et al.* (1996) Survival of patients with disseminated midgut carcinoid tumors after aggressive tumor reduction. *World J Surg*, **20(7)**, 892–899; discussion 99.

54. Sarmiento, J.M., Que, F.G. (2003) Hepatic surgery for metastases from neuroendocrine tumors. *Surg Oncol Clin N Am*, **12(1)**, 231–242.

55. Nave, H., Mossinger, E., Feist, H. *et al.* (2001) Surgery as primary treatment in patients with liver metastases from carcinoid tumors: a retrospective, unicentric study over 13 years. *Surgery*, **129(2)**, 170–175.

56. McMichael, J.W., Roghanian, A., Jiang, L. *et al.* (2005) The antimicrobial antiproteinase elafin binds to lipopolysaccharide and modulates macrophage responses. *Am J Respir Cell Mol Biol*, **32(5)**, 443–452.

57. Pederzoli, P., Falconi, M., Bonora, A. *et al.* (1999) Cytoreductive surgery in advanced endocrine tumours of the pancreas. *Ital J Gastroenterol Hepatol*, **31(Suppl 2)**, S207–S212.

58. Pfitzmann, R., Benscheidt, B., Langrehr, J.M. *et al.* (2007) Trends and experiences in liver retransplantation over 15 years. *Liver Transpl*, **13(2)**, 248–257.

59. Kvols, L.K., Moertel, C.G., O'Connell, M.J. *et al.* (1986) Treatment of the malignant carcinoid syndrome. Evaluation of a long-acting somatostatin analogue. *N Engl J Med*, **315(11)**, 663–666.

60. O'Toole, D., Ducreux, M., Bommelaer, G. *et al.* (2000) Treatment of carcinoid syndrome: a prospective crossover evaluation of lanreotide versus octreotide in terms of efficacy, patient acceptability, and tolerance. *Cancer*, **88(4)**, 770–776.

61. Toumpanakis, C., Garland, J., Marelli, L. *et al.* (2009) Long-term results of patients with malignant carcinoid syndrome receiving octreotide LAR. *Aliment Pharmacol Ther*, **30(7)**, 733–740.

62. Khan, M.S., El-Khouly, F., Davies, P. *et al.* (2011) Long term results of treatment of malignant carcinoid syndrome with lanreotide autogel. *Aliment Pharmacol Ther*, **34(2)**, 235–242.

63. Modlin, I.M., Pavel, M., Kidd, M. *et al.* (2010) Review article: somatostatin analogues in the treatment of gastroenteropancreatic neuroendocrine (carcinoid) tumours. *Aliment Pharmacol Ther*, **31**(2), 169–188.
64. Modlin, I.M., Shapiro, M.D., Kidd, M. (2004) Carcinoid tumors and fibrosis: an association with no explanation. *Am J Gastroenterol*, **99**(12), 2466–2478.
65. Oberg, K. (2000) Interferon in the management of neuroendocrine GEP-tumors: a review. *Digestion*, **62**(**Suppl 1**), 92–97.
66. Arnold, R., Rinke, A., Klose, K.J. *et al.* (2005) Octreotide versus octreotide plus interferon-alpha in endocrine gastroenteropancreatic tumors: a randomized trial. *Clin Gastroenterol Hepatol*, **3**(8), 761–771.
67. Stuart, K., Levy, D.E., Anderson, T. *et al.* (2004) Phase II study of interferon gamma in malignant carcinoid tumors (E9292): a trial of the Eastern Cooperative Oncology Group. *Invest New Drugs*, **22**(1), 75–81.
68. Moertel, C.G., Lefkopoulo, M., Lipsitz, S. *et al.* (1992) Streptozocin-doxorubicin, streptozocin-fluorouracil or chlorozotocin in the treatment of advanced islet-cell carcinoma. *N Engl J Med*, **326**(8), 519–523.
69. Bajetta, E., Ferrari, L., Procopio, G. *et al.* (2002) Efficacy of a chemotherapy combination for the treatment of metastatic neuroendocrine tumours. *Ann Oncol*, **13**(4), 614–621.
70. O'Toole, D., Hentic, O., Corcos, O. *et al.* (2004) Chemotherapy for gastro-enteropancreatic endocrine tumours. *Neuroendocrinology*, **80**(**Suppl 1**), 79–84.
71. Ekeblad, S., Sundin, A., Janson, E.T. *et al.* (2007) Temozolomide as monotherapy is effective in treatment of advanced malignant neuroendocrine tumors. *Clin Cancer Res*, **13**(10), 2986–2991.
72. Mitry, E., Baudin, E., Ducreux, M. *et al.* (1999) Treatment of poorly differentiated neuroendocrine tumours with etoposide and cisplatin. *Br J Cancer*, **81**(8), 1351–1355.
73. Soga, J., Yakuwa, Y. (1998) VIPoma/diarrheagenic syndrome: a statistical evaluation of 241 reported cases. *J Exp Clin Cancer Res*, **17**(4), 389–400.
74. Gill, G.V., Rauf, O., MacFarlane, I.A. (1997) Diazoxide treatment for insulinoma: a national UK survey. *Postgrad Med J*, **73**(864), 640–641.
75. Marrache, F., Vullierme, M.P., Roy, C. *et al.* (2007) Arterial phase enhancement and body mass index are predictors of response to chemoembolisation for liver metastases of endocrine tumours. *Br J Cancer*, **96**(1), 49–55.
76. Drougas, J.G., Anthony, L.B., Blair, T.K. *et al.* (1998) Hepatic artery chemoembolization for management of patients with advanced metastatic carcinoid tumors. *Am J Surg*, **175**(5), 408–412.
77. Abdalla, E.K., Vauthey, J.N., Ellis, L.M. *et al.* (2004) Recurrence and outcomes following hepatic resection, radiofrequency ablation, and combined resection/ablation for colorectal liver metastases. *Ann Surg*, **239**(6), 818–825; discussion 25–27.
78. Kulke, M.H., Lenz, H.J., Meropol, N.J. *et al.* (2008) Activity of sunitinib in patients with advanced neuroendocrine tumors. *J Clin Oncol*, **26**(20), 3403–3410.
79. Raymond, E., Dahan, L., Raoul, J.L. *et al.* (2011) Sunitinib malate for the treatment of pancreatic neuroendocrine tumors. *N Engl J Med*, **364**(6), 501–513.
80. Yao, J.C., Lombard-Bohas, C., Baudin, E. *et al.* (2010) Daily oral everolimus activity in patients with metastatic pancreatic neuroendocrine tumors after failure of cytotoxic chemotherapy: a phase II trial. *J Clin Oncol*, **28**(1), 69–76.

81. Pavel, M., Hainsworth, J., Baudin, E. *et al.* (2011) Everolimus plus octreotide long-acting repeatable for the treatment of advanced neuroendocrine tumors associated with carcinoid syndrome (RADIANT-2): a randomised, placebo-controlled, phase 3 study. *The Lancet*, **378(9808)**, 2005–2012.

82. Yao, J.C., Shah, M.H., Ito, T. *et al.* (2011) Everolimus for advanced pancreatic neuroendocrine tumors. *N Engl J Med*, **364(6)**, 514–523.

83. Schmid, H.A. (2008) Pasireotide (SOM230): development, mechanism of action and potential applications. *Mol Cell Endocrinol*, **286(1–2)**, 69–74.

84. Kouvaraki, M.A., Ajani, J.A., Hoff, P. *et al.* (2004) Fluorouracil, doxorubicin, and streptozocin in the treatment of patients with locally advanced and metastatic pancreatic endocrine carcinomas. *J Clin Oncol*, **22(23)**, 4762–4771.

85. Kidd, M., Drozdov, I., Joseph, R. *et al.* (2008) Differential cytotoxicity of novel somatostatin and dopamine chimeric compounds on bronchopulmonary and small intestinal neuroendocrine tumor cell lines. *Cancer*, **113(4)**, 690–700.

86. Hemminki, K., Li, X. (2001) Incidence trends and risk factors of carcinoid tumors: a nationwide epidemiologic study from Sweden. *Cancer*, **92(8)**, 2204–2210.

87. Duh, Q.Y., Hybarger, C.P., Geist, R. *et al.* (1987) Carcinoids associated with multiple endocrine neoplasia syndromes. *Am J Surg*, **154(1)**, 142–148.

88. Thakker, R.V. (2010) Multiple endocrine neoplasia type 1 (MEN1). *Best Pract Res Clin Endocrinol Metab*, **24(3)**, 355–370.

89. Hough, D.R., Chan, A., Davidson, H. (1983) Von Recklinghausen's disease associated with gastrointestinal carcinoid tumors. *Cancer*, **51(12)**, 2206–2208.

90. Griffiths, D.F., Williams, G.T., Williams, E.D. (1987) Duodenal carcinoid tumours, phaeochromocytoma and neurofibromatosis: islet cell tumour, phaeochromocytoma and the von Hippel-Lindau complex: two distinctive neuroendocrine syndromes. *Q J Med*, **64(245)**, 769–782.

10 Gastrointestinal Lymphoma

Eliza A. Hawkes, Andrew Wotherspoon, and David Cunningham
Royal Marsden Hospital, London and Surrey, UK

Key Points

- Primary gastrointestinal (GI) tract lymphoma is relatively rare and encompasses many subtypes. In contrast, the GI tract is the most common extranodal site to be involved with advanced lymphoma. Correct histological diagnosis is essential for prognostic evaluation and to guide optimum management and follow-up.
- Initial staging investigations of lymphoma include computed tomography (CT) of the neck, chest, abdomen, pelvis; bone marrow biopsy; full blood count and film; lactate dehydrogenase (LDH); uric acid; assessment of organ function; and positron emission tomography (PET) scan plus endoscopy and endoscopic ultrasound (EUS) where indicated.
- GI tract lymphoma is generally treated with chemotherapy regimens used for nodal counterparts of identical histological subtype. The only exception is localized extranodal marginal zone lymphoma of mucosa-associated lymphoid tissue (MALT lymphoma) in the stomach, which should initially be treated with *Helicobacter pylori* eradication. Radiotherapy can be utilized in localized disease. Surgery plays a very limited role in the treatment of lymphoma, and decisions regarding its use in individual cases should be agreed by a multidisciplinary team.

Key Web Links

www.lymphomas.org.uk
The UK Lymphoma Association

www.llresearch.org.uk
UK Leukaemia and Lymphoma Research

http://www.cancer.gov/cancertopics/pdq/treatment/adult-non-hodgkins/patient
The American National Cancer Institute Web site (Non-Hodgkin Lymphoma)

Handbook of Gastrointestinal Cancer, First Edition. Edited by Janusz Jankowski and Ernest Hawk.
© 2013 John Wiley & Sons, Ltd. Published 2013 by John Wiley & Sons, Ltd.

Potential Pitfalls

- Accurate diagnosis can be difficult to obtain and may require repeat procedures in order to obtain adequate tissue specimens.
- Certainty of the diagnosis is vital due to the prominent role of chemotherapy or radiotherapy rather than surgery as a first-line treatment strategy in localized disease.
- Staging investigations differ considerably from other malignancies of the GI tract; therefore, early referral to a lymphoma specialist is essential.
- Routine follow-up varies depending on lymphoma subtype. Specific procedural requirements for endoscopy must be relayed to the endoscopist, particularly with MALT lymphoma (gastric mapping) to ensure adequate assessment of disease.

Introduction

The term "gastrointestinal (GI) lymphoma" is generally reserved for primary extranodal lymphomas that arise in the GI tract; however, involvement of the GI tract by lymphoma has been described with all histological subtypes. GI lymphoma is the most common form of primary extranodal lymphoma, accounting for 30–40% of cases. The most common site of disease is the stomach (60–70% of cases) followed by small bowel, ileocecal region, duodenum, colon, and rectum.[1,2] The most common histologies are diffuse large B-cell lymphoma (DLBCL) and extranodal marginal zone lymphoma of mucosa-associated lymphoid tissue (MALT lymphoma). Other GI-specific lymphomas, although rare, include enteropathy-associated T-cell lymphoma (EATL) and immunoproliferative small intestinal disease (IPSID). Less common extranodal lymphomas of the GI tract are mantle cell lymphoma (MCL); follicular lymphoma (FL); peripheral T-cell lymphoma, which present far more commonly as nodal disease; and Burkitt lymphoma (BL) (Figure 10.1, Tables 10.1 and 10.2).

A wide geographical variability in incidence exists, with the highest rates in the Middle East. Of interest, the most common disease site in Middle Eastern countries is the small intestine, rather than the stomach.[3] A 13-fold higher incidence of gastric MALT lymphoma in north-east Italy compared with Britain has also been described.[4] This variability probably arises due to the different prevalence of etiological factors such as *Helicobacter pylori* (*H. pylori*) infection (associated with MALT lymphoma) in north-east Italy.

Presentation is often with nonspecific symptoms that develop at a rate determined by the aggressiveness of the underlying lymphoma pathology. Dyspepsia, abdominal pain and/or bloating, change in bowel habit, hemorrhage, and, rarely, perforation or obstruction are seen. Classical B symptoms are less common than nodal lymphoma, with weight loss usually secondary to the abdominal symptoms rather than

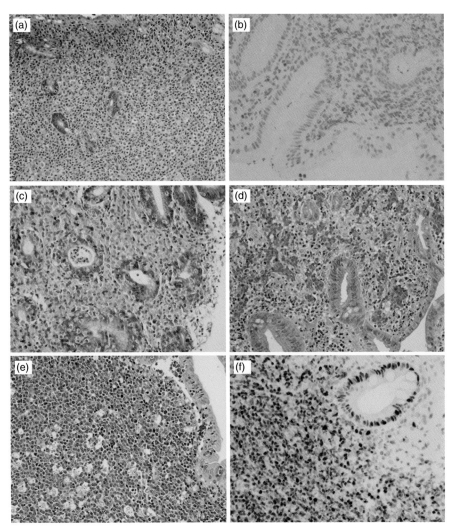

Figure 10.1 Histological images of primary GI lymphomas: (a) MALT lymphoma; (b) MALT lymphoma-*Helicobacter pylori* immunostaining; (c) EATL Type I duodenum; (d) DLBCL colon; (e) Burkitt lymphoma colon; (f) MCL colon-CyclinD1 immunostaining.

Table 10.1 Common primary gastrointestinal non-Hodgkin's lymphoma.

B cell
Extranodal marginal zone lymphoma of mucosa-associated lymphoid tissue (MALT lymphoma)
Immunoproliferative small intestinal disease
Diffuse large B-cell lymphoma—not otherwise specified
Mantle cell lymphoma
Follicular lymphoma
Burkitt lymphoma
T cell
Enteropathy-associated T-cell lymphoma

Table 10.2 Common immunophenotypic features of common GI lymphomas.

Lymphoma subtype	CD2	CD3	CD5	CD7	CD8	CD10	CD19	CD20	CD23	CD43	CD56	MUM1	BCL6	Cyclin D1	SOX11	TIA-1	Molecular biology
MALT lymphoma	-	-	-	-	-	-	+++	+++	-	+/-	-	+++	-	-	-	-	t(11;18)
DLBCL	-	-	-	-	-	+(GCB)	+++	+++	-/+	+	-	++(ABC)	++(GCB)	-	-	-	BCL6
Mantle cell lymphoma	-	-	+++	-	-	-	+++	+++	+	+++	-	-	-	+++	+++	-	t(11;14)
Follicular lymphoma	-	-	-	-	-	+	+++	+++	+	-	-	+	+++	-	-	-	t(14;18)
CLL	-	-	+++	-	-	-	+++	+++	+++	+++	-	-	+++	-	-	-	
Burkitt lymphoma	-	-	-	-	-	+++	+++	+++	+	++	-	+	+++	-	+	-	t(8;14)
EATL	+++	+++	-	+++	+(Type II)	-	-	-	-	+	+?(Type II)	-	-	-	-	+++	

+++, >90% cases; ++, >50% cases; +, 10–50% cases; −, <10% cases; ABC, activated B-cell type; GCB, germinal center B-cell type; NA, not applicable; TIA-1, T cell-restricted intracellular antigen.

as a direct result of the lymphoma. Physical examination uncommonly yields specific findings. However, a palpable abdominal mass, peripheral lymphadenopathy, hepatomegaly or splenomegaly, and features of autoimmune or immunodeficiency disorders should be excluded.

Extranodal marginal zone lymphoma of mucosa-associated lymphoid tissue

Epidemiology

MALT lymphoma is an indolent B-cell non-Hodgkin lymphoma (NHL) first described as a separate entity in 1983 by Isaacson and Wright.[5] Accounting for 8% of all NHL, approximately one-third of MALT lymphomas originate in the stomach.[6] MALT lymphoma arises from marginal zone B cells that have undergone postfollicular differentiation following chronic antigenic stimulation secondary to persistent infection or autoimmune disease. In the stomach, it is strongly associated with *H. pylori* infection with 90–95% of patients with gastric MALT lymphoma showing evidence of concurrent or previous infection,[7,8] compared with 50% of the global population.[9]

Other infections that have been linked to MALT lymphoma in nongastric locations include *Chlamydia psittaci* (ocular adnexa), *Borrelia burgdorferi* (skin), and *Campylobacter jejuni* (small bowel). An association with autoimmune diseases is also described including Sjögren's syndrome (salivary gland MALT lymphoma), Hashimoto's autoimmune thyroiditis (thyroid MALT lymphoma), and polymyalgia rheumatica. Uncertainty remains as to whether lymphoma outcomes differ in this population.[10,11] No inherited component has been identified.

The median age at presentation is 61 years[12] and prognosis is generally considered good. Poor prognostic features include non-GI or distant nodal involvement, poor WHO performance status, bulky tumor, high beta-2 microglobulin level, high lactate dehydrogenase (LDH), low serum albumin, and anemia.[13] Five-year survival ranges from 80% to 95%, despite progression-free survival (PFS) being comparably short in those with advanced stage or poor prognostic features.[13-16]

Diagnosis and staging

MALT lymphoma is often multifocal disease in the organ of origin and is frequently macroscopically indistinguishable from other disease processes in the GI tract.[17] Endoscopy is key to diagnosing MALT lymphoma, with multiple biopsies of the visible lesions required, as well as samples of macroscopically normal tissue, termed "gastric mapping."

Histologically, there is expansion of the marginal zone compartment with development of sheets of neoplastic small lymphoid cells (Figure 10.1a). The morphology of the neoplastic cells is variable with small mature lymphocytes, cells resembling centrocytes (centrocyte-like cells), or marginal zone/monocytoid B cells. Plasmacytoid or plasmacytic differentiation is frequent. Lymphoid follicles are ubiquitous to MALT lymphoma but may be indistinct as they are often overrun or colonized by the neoplastic cells. Large transformed B cells are present scattered among the small cell population. If these large cells are present in clusters or sheets, a diagnosis of associated large B-cell lymphoma should be considered. A characteristic feature of MALT lymphoma is the presence of neoplastic cells within epithelial structures with associated destruction of the glandular architecture to form lymphoepithelial lesions.

MALT lymphoma may be difficult to distinguish from reactive infiltrates, and in some cases, multiple endoscopies are required before a confident diagnosis is reached. The Wotherspoon score, which grades the presence of histological features associated with MALT lymphoma, is useful in expressing confidence in diagnosis at presentation (Table 10.3).[18]

Immunohistochemistry can be used to help distinguish MALT lymphoma from other small B-cell NHLs. B-cell-associated antigens such as CD19, CD20, CD22, and CD79a are usually expressed. In contrast to small lymphocytic lymphoma and MCL, staining for CD5 is usually negative, and these lymphomas can be further distinguished with CD23 (positive in small lymphocytic lymphoma) and CyclinD1 (positive in MCL).

Immunoglobulin genes are rearranged and B-cell monoclonality is present in almost all cases, and PCR analysis may be useful where diagnosis remains ambiguous although caution is advised as a proportion (probably up to 3%) of gastritis cases may give a clonal pattern. Cytogenetic translocations seen in MALT lymphoma include translocation t(11;18)(q21;q21), t(14;18)(q32;q21), and occasionally t(1;14)(p22;q32). Each of these has a final common pathway resulting in aberrant activation of NFκB. Trisomies 3 and 18 have been described. When present, t(11;18) is usually the sole cytogenetic abnormality found and this translocation is almost never seen in cases that transform to more aggressive large cell lymphoma.[21] Testing for t(11;18) is important, as evidence suggests that it is associated with more advanced, invasive tumors and with lymphomas that are less likely to respond to *H. pylori* eradication.[22] The t(11;18) is present in 25–40% of gastric cases; however, higher frequencies are seen in MALT lymphoma of the lung, while it is rare in MALT lymphomas of the thyroid, ocular adnexa, and skin.[23,24]

Due to the causal relationship between *H. pylori* infection and MALT lymphoma, identification of the infection is mandatory. Histological examination of GI biopsies yields a sensitivity of 95% with five biopsies,[25] but these should be from sites uninvolved by lymphoma and the identification of the organism may be compromised by areas of extensive intestinal metaplasia (Figure 10.1b). As proton-pump inhibition can suppress infection, any treatment with this class of drug should be ceased 2 weeks prior to biopsy retrieval. Serology should be performed if histology is negative, to detect suppressed or recently treated infections.[26,27]

Table 10.3 Histological scores for response assessment in gastric MALT lymphoma.

Wotherspoon histological score for diagnosis[18]		
Grade	Description	Histological features
0	Normal	Scattered plasma cells in LP. No lymphoid follicles
1	Chronic active gastritis	Small clusters of lymphocytes in lamina propria. No lymphoid follicles. No LELs
2	Chronic active gastritis with florid lymphoid follicle formation	Prominent lymphoid follicles with surrounding mantle zone and plasma cells. No LELs
3	Suspicious lymphoid infiltrate in LP, probably reactive	Lymphoid follicles surrounded by small lymphocytes that infiltrate diffusely in LP and occasionally into epithelium
4	Suspicious lymphoid infiltrate in LP, probably lymphoma	Lymphoid follicles surrounded by CCL cells that infiltrate diffusely in LP and into epithelium in small groups
5	Low-grade B-cell lymphoma of MALT	Presence of dense diffuse infiltrate of CCL cells in LP with prominent LELs
GELA grading system for posttreatment evaluation[83]		
GELA category	Histology	
CR (complete histological response)	Absent or scattered plasma cells and small lymphoid cells in the LP. No LELs. Normal or empty LP and/or fibrosis	
pMRD (probable minimal residual disease)	Aggregates of lymphoid cells or lymphoid nodules in the LP/muscularis mucosa and/or submucosa. No LELs. Empty LP and/or fibrosis	
rRD (responding residual disease)	Dense, diffuse, or nodular extending around glands in the LP Focal or no LELs focal empty LP and/or fibrosis	
NC (no change)	Dense, diffuse, or nodular LELs present (may be absent). No changes	

CCL, centrocyte like; LEL, lymphoepithelial lesions; LP, lamina propria.

The Ann Arbor staging system[28] (Table 10.4), originally designed for Hodgkin's lymphoma, has been adapted for NHL to assist in determining prognosis and management. However, its prognostic value is significantly

Table 10.4 Ann Arbor staging system for lymphoma.[30]

Stage	Extent of tumour spread
I	Single anatomical lymph node region (I) Or single extralymphatic site (IE)[a]
II	≥2 lymph node regions or lymphatic structures (II) and/or an extralymphatic site (IIE) on the same side of the diaphragm
III	Lymph node regions above and below the diaphragm (III) and/or an extralymphatic site (IIIE) above and below the diaphragm
IV	Widespread involvement of ≥1 extralymphatic organs or tissues, +/– lymphatic involvement.

Notes: Each stage is further divided according to absence (A) or presence (B) of "B" symptoms, which include fever (>38°C), night sweats, or weight loss >10% of total body weight <6 months prior to diagnosis, which are attributed to the lymphoma. For example, a patient with stage IA lymphoma has no "B" symptoms, whereas Stage IIB has at least one "B" symptom present.
The presence of splenic involvement is denoted by the label "S" after the stage (e.g., Stage IIIS or Stage IIIES if there is both splenic and extranodal involvement).
[a]The label "E" generally refers to extranodal disease that can be encompassed within a single radiation field.

limited in MALT lymphoma with GI tract localization at presentation, as depth of gastric wall invasion is an important predictive factor for response to *H. pylori* eradication therapy. Musshoff originally suggested a modified Ann Arbor system,[29] which was then further modified in 1994 to the Lugano system,[19] which is still used today. The "TNMB" or Paris staging system[20] has been proposed to more accurately incorporate tumor depth and local spread; however, it is variably used in clinical practice (Table 10.5).

As MALT lymphoma has a predisposition to preferentially spread to other extranodal sites, staging investigations must include clinical examination of the oropharynx, thyroid, and Waldeyer's ring. Referral for ophthalmologic examination and imaging of the salivary glands should be considered to ascertain involvement of other extranodal sites. Computed tomography (CT) imaging of the neck, chest, abdomen, and pelvis, as well as bone marrow aspirate and trephine examining for distant spread; endoscopic ultrasound (EUS) for gastric MALT to assess depth and local nodal involvement; and hematological and biochemical parameters including full blood count, LDH, and beta-2 microglobulin should all be performed. Positron emission tomography (PET) is not recommended routinely as MALT lymphoma is often PET negative.

Investigation for associated autoimmune diseases such as Sjögren's syndrome and autoimmune thyroiditis should also be considered.

Treatment

Historically, surgical treatment of localized disease was adopted with high cure rates. Distal partial gastrectomy was frequently associated with stump recurrence after a disease-free interval and total gastrectomy resulted in significant long-term morbidity. With the advent of stomach conserving therapies with similar outcomes, the role of surgery is restricted to the treatment of rare complications such as perforation or bleeding that cannot be controlled endoscopically.[30]

Following the recognition of the association of gastric MALT lymphoma with *H. pylori* infection, it was established that early-stage gastric disease could be cured by *H. pylori* eradication, which is now the mainstay of therapy. Fifty to 95% of cases achieve complete response (CR) with *H. pylori* treatment.[18,31] *H. pylori* eradication therapy consists of proton-pump inhibitor (PPI) plus clarithromycin-based triple therapy with amoxicillin or metronidazole for 14 days. Increasing clarithromycin-resistant strains has led to the recommendation that this drug is avoided in areas where resistant strains are prevalent. In these areas, and when second-line therapy is required, quadruple therapy with PPI, colloidal bismuth, tetracycline, and metronidazole is recommended and this is effective even in areas with high prevalence of metronidazole-resistant strains.

A urea breath test should be performed approximately 2 months after treatment and at least 2 weeks after withdrawal of PPI therapy to confirm eradication. The time to remission can be 12 months or longer in some cases. The rates of relapse are reasonably high in some series (22% gastric, up to 48% systemic).[32,33] It is recommended that patients be followed up closely with repeat endoscopy, gastric mapping biopsies, and EUS.

Due to the usually localized nature of this disease and the requirements of biopsy to diagnose a response, the standard response criteria for lymphoma[34] based on radiological imaging results are difficult to apply. However, repeat CT imaging is recommended. Endoscopic evaluation of response is imperative in localized disease, with histological assessment of posteradication biopsies being crucial to the planning of further management. Assessment of sequential biopsies using the GELA grading system gives useful information in this regard with clear indication of the quality of response over time.[31] Many patients will have residual lymphoid aggregates in the gastric mucosa following complete endoscopic resolution of the lesion, termed probable minimal residual disease in the GELA scheme. These frequently harbor occasional clonal B cells but are of no clinical significance, as long-term follow-up has shown that they usually remain unchanged or show regression over time. The presence of these small clonal populations in residual lymphoid aggregates mean molecular follow-up by PCR has no role in the clinical setting. In the absence of further evolution of disease, either histologically or macroscopically, no further intervention is required. In some patients, histologically detected relapse may develop. This may be associated with recrudescence of *H. pylori* in which case further eradication may result in further remission. In a proportion of cases, small histologically detected relapses have been shown to regress on subsequent biopsies without further therapy and hence a "watch and wait" policy may be adopted.

Overall 30–40% of patients will not respond to *H. pylori* eradication.[8] The probability of response to *H. pylori* eradication appears to be related in part to the depth of mural invasion and to local nodal involvement, with the more invasive cases less likely to respond. Failure to respond the eradication therapy alone has also been shown to be related to the presence of t(11;18) with cases harboring the translocation unlikely to respond.

Extra-gastric MALT lymphomas have, in some cases, been shown to respond to antibiotic-related therapies. While this is unlikely to be due to *H. pylori* itself, it is possible that other microbial factors could be involved in the pathogenesis of the lymphomas at these sites with eradication of these organisms having a similar effect on the lymphoma.

For those requiring further management, there is no consensus on standard treatment. Published data are largely restricted to phase II trials and retrospective series. One small prospective randomized trial has compared surgery, radiotherapy, and chemotherapy and demonstrated equivalent 10-year event-free survival (EFS) with surgery and radiotherapy but improved EFS with chemotherapy. No difference in overall survival (OS) with any of the treatments was reported.[30]

Radiotherapy is a valid option for MALT lymphoma; however, it is not universally used. It provides local control and potential cure in localized gastric stage IE and II_1E disease with 5-year EFS of 75–90% reported in retrospective studies.[35-37] However, the irradiation field is potentially large as it must include the whole stomach, which can vary greatly in size and shape. Irradiation techniques have improved considerably in the last 20 years, including treating the patient in a fasting state, decreasing the irradiated field and required dose. The moderate dose of 30 Gray (Gy) of involved-field radiotherapy administered in 15 fractions (doses) can be associated with tolerable toxicity and adequate outcomes. Hence, radiotherapy is an acceptable approach for local disease where antibiotic therapy has failed, or is not indicated; however, its use in individuals is determined by the radiation field. Evidence also suggests that radiotherapy can be utilized to control localized relapses outside the original radiation field.[30]

MALT lymphoma is exquisitely chemotherapy sensitive. Chemotherapy is reserved for those with disseminated disease at presentation or lack of response to local treatment. Rituximab, the anti-CD20 chimeric antibody, is a key component of therapy. Responses vary from 55% to 77% with monotherapy and 100% in combination with chemotherapy.[38-43] Oral alkylating agents such as cyclophosphamide or chlorambucil have been administered for a median duration of 12 months with high rates of disease control (CR up to 75%) but appear not to be active in t(11;18) disease.[44,45] The purine nucleoside analogs fludarabine and cladribine also demonstrate activity,[42,46] the latter conferring a CR rate of 84% (100% in those with gastric primaries) in a small study.[47] A pivotal study of rituximab plus chlorambucil compared with chlorambucil alone (IELSG-19 study, $n = 227$) demonstrated a significantly higher CR rate (78% vs. 65%; $p = 0.017$) and 5-year EFS (68% vs. 50%; $p = 0.024$) over chlorambucil alone. However, 5-year OS was not improved (88% in both arms).[48] First-line treatment of choice is generally rituximab in combination with single alkylating agents or fludarabine, or a combination of all three drugs. The final results of this study, including the later addition of a rituximab-alone arm, are pending.

Immunoproliferative small intestinal disease

IPSID is a subtype of MALT lymphoma occurring only in the small intestine, which was previously called alpha-heavy chain disease, due to the expression of monotypic truncated Ig α-chain in the absence of associated light-chain expression, or Mediterranean lymphoma because of its distinct geographical distribution with cases occurring almost exclusively in the Middle East, areas bordering the Mediterranean sea, and Cape region of South Africa. It has recently been associated with *C. jejuni* infection.[49,50] As opposed to "Western" MALT lymphoma of the intestine, which occurs predominantly in elderly patients, the median age at diagnosis of IPSID is 25–30.[51] There is no one gender preponderance.

Clinical manifestations include malabsorption, diarrhea, abdominal pain with obstruction, and, in more advanced disease, ascites. Involvement of peripheral nodes, the spleen, bone marrow, or other organs is uncommon except in advanced disease.[52,53] Diagnosis is made via endoscopy or laparotomy, with solitary primary lesions occurring in most cases. The histological features are similar to MALT lymphoma of other sites; however, these usually demonstrate prominent plasmacytic differentiation.[54] The serum contains detectable alpha-heavy chain proteins in 20–90% of patients. IPSID does not harbor the t(11;18) translocation seen in other MALT lymphomas.[24,53,55,56]

Treatment recommendations are based on small series in the literature but include antibiotics such as tetracycline and metronidazole for early-stage disease and anthracycline-based chemotherapy in addition to antibiotics for advanced disease.[55,57,58] Total abdominal irradiation has been reported to achieve remissions. Surgery is reserved for mechanical obstructions in the treatment setting, but can be necessary to obtain a diagnosis.

Enteropathy-associated T-cell lymphoma

Epidemiology
Enteropathy-associated T-cell lymphoma (EATL) is a rare, aggressive intestinal T-cell lymphoma arising in the intraepithelial T lymphocytes (IELs) comprising less than 1% of NHL.[6] Eighty to ninety percent of EATL (Type I) is associated with celiac disease (CD), with Type II EATL occurring sporadically with differing morphological and immunophenotypic features, suggesting a possible separate disease entity.[54] It was initially believed that the malabsorption associated with EATL was a consequence of the intestinal lymphoma, but subsequently proven that

malabsorption (CD) was the preceding condition leading to lymphoma.[59,60] The term EATL was first used in 1986.[61]

While the strong association with CD exists, the precise etiology is still uncertain. CD is an immune-mediated enteropathy triggered by exposure to gluten in the diet. Consumption of gluten causes villous atrophy and inflammation in the small bowel mucosa. It is more common in northern Europeans, affecting up to 1% of Caucasians, hence the rates of EATL in these locations is slightly higher.[62] Only 2–5% of patients with CD develop intestinal lymphoma, of which 65% have a T-cell immunophenotype.[63,64] Of interest, patients with CD additionally have a higher risk of other NHL such as DLBCL, anaplastic large cell lymphoma, and peripheral T-cell lymphomas than the normal population.[65–67] Dermatitis herpetiformis is an immunologic skin condition characterized by gluten sensitivity, which is similarly associated with increased risk of lymphoma and responds to a gluten-free diet. The majority of patients who develop EATL are diagnosed with adult-onset CD just preceding or at the time of the lymphoma diagnosis, with only a small proportion having a documented history of childhood CD, and in these cases, the disease has often been poorly controlled.

Refractory CD (RCD) occurs when clinical and histological features persist despite adherence to a gluten-free diet. A proportion of RCD cases is associated with a monoclonal T-cell proliferation and shows an aberrant phenotype with downregulation of CD8 expression. Approximately half of the patients with RCD develop EATL; hence, it is considered a precursor condition.

Median age at onset of EATL is in the seventh decade and there is a slightly higher rate in males (64%) despite CD being more common in females. Presenting symptoms of EATL include abdominal pain, weight loss, diarrhea, and bowel obstruction or intestinal perforation, the last one being relatively common. Patients can be considerably malnourished, with poor performance status and immunological compromise at the time of diagnosis, often with the complications associated with intestinal perforation necessitating surgical procedures, which contributes to the dismal prognosis in this disease. Approximately 80% of those who respond to treatment relapse and the reported 5-year survival is 11–20%.[68,69] Due to the paucity of data, definitive prognostic features have not been well defined. In larger studies of intestinal lymphomas as a whole, perforation, multiple primary sites, high-grade histology, and advanced stage have all been reported as adverse prognosticators.[70] In EATL, stage is important with a 5-year disease-specific survival of more than 60% for limited disease, yet 25% in advanced disease patients.[71,72]

Diagnosis and staging

Histological diagnosis is often obtained at the time of emergency laparotomy due to the high rate of intestinal perforation at presentation. In those not requiring surgery, biopsies can be obtained using double-balloon enteroscopy. EATL can be a multifocal disease occurring most commonly in the jejunum and ileum with duodenal, stomach, or colonic involvement rare (Figure 10.1c). In contrast to B-cell lymphomas, which are usually polypoid or annular lesions in the distal or terminal ileum, macroscopic appearance is that of ulcerating mucosal lesions invading the intestinal wall. Adjacent tissue classically shows villous atrophy and crypt hyperplasia with increased lamina propria lymphocytes and plasma cells. Type I and Type II have distinct histologic and immunophenotypic features. Morphology can be varied, but tumor cells are mostly monotonous medium-to-large sized cells with round or angulated vesicular nuclei, prominent nucleoli, and moderate-to-abundant pale-staining cytoplasm. Occasionally, pleomorphic multinucleated cells that resemble that of anaplastic large cell lymphoma are seen. Type II EATL comprises monomorphic, small-to-medium sized neoplastic cells with only a rim of pale cytoplasm. There is distinct absence of inflammatory infiltrate and less necrosis than with Type I. However, villous atrophy, crypt hyperplasia, and intraepithelial lymphocytosis are evident in the adjacent tissue of both. Immunophenotypically, EATL tumor cells are usually CD3+, CD5−, CD7+, CD4−, CD8+/−, mucosal homing receptor CD103+, CD30+, and TCRβ+/− and contain cytotoxic molecules such as TIA-1 (T-cell restricted intracellular antigen), perforin, granzyme A, and granzyme M. In contrast, the Type II form is CD8+, NK antigen CD56+, and TCRβ+. The adjacent intraepithelial lymphocytes are often identical to that of the lymphoma.[54]

There is clonal rearrangement of the TCR gene in the majority of cases. Genetic association with the human leukocyte antigen (HLA) class II HLADQ2/8 is strong, unsurprising given the link seen in CD, and the absence of this has a high negative predictive value for diagnosis. More than 90% of Type I EATL have the *HLADQA1*0501* and *DQB1*0201* genotype. Deletions in the 16q12.1 chromosome and segmental amplifications of 9q31.3-qter are seen in 58–70% of EATL, which can assist in distinguishing from nodal peripheral T-cell lymphoma. Type I EATL tends to harbor gains in 1q and 5q, while Type II more frequently displays 8q24 *(MYC)* amplifications.

Staging is once again performed using the adapted Ann Arbor systems shown in Table 10.5. The need for accurate staging prior to treatment has been debated, as all patients receive chemotherapy regardless of stage, often urgently, and the invasive investigations can cause significant delay; however, stage is the main prognostic factor. Physical examination for Waldeyer's ring involvement and complete hematological and biochemical investigations should be performed. CT scan, bone marrow aspirate, and trephine and PET scan assess extent of disease. PET has been shown in one small study of 38 patients to discriminate between RCD and EATL being more sensitive (100% vs. 87%) and specific (90% vs. 53%) than CT at establishing sites of lymphoma.[73] Evaluation of the GI tract is mandatory in those able to tolerate the procedures, due to the multifocal nature of EATL. Gastroscopy and colonoscopy, as well as video capsule enteroscopy, barium meal, or double-balloon enteroscopy, should be performed to assess the entire GI tract.

Table 10.5 Lugano[19] and Paris[20] staging systems for gastrointestinal lymphomas.

Lugano staging	Paris staging	Extent of tumor spread
Stage I	T1–3 N0 M0	Tumor confined to GI tract
I$_1$	T1 N0 M0	(Single primary site or multiple noncontiguous
I$_2$	T2-T3 N0 M0	lesions)
		Infiltration limited to mucosa and/or submucosa
		Tumor extends into muscularis propria and/or subserosa and/or serosa
Stage II	T1–3 N0–2 M0	Tumor extending into abdomen from primary
II$_1$	T1–3 N1 M0	GI site (nodal involvement)
II$_2$	T1–3 N2 M0	Local
		Perigastric nodes in gastric lymphoma
		Mesenteric in small and large bowel lymphoma
		Distant
		Mesenteric in gastric lymphoma
		Para-aortic, paracaval, pelvic, inguinal
Stage IIE	T4N0–2M0	Penetration of serosa with involvement of adjacent organs/tissues
		(Enumerate actual site of involvement, e.g., IIE$_{(pancreas)}$, IIE$_{(large\ intestine)}$)
		Where there is both nodal involvement and penetration into adjacent organs, stage should be denoted using both subscript and E, e.g., II$_1$E$_{(pancreas)}$
Stage IV	T1–4 N3M0	GI tract lesion with supradiaphragmatic or
	T1–4 N0–3 M1–2	extra-abdominal nodal involvement
	B1	Disseminated extranodal involvement
		(M1 = noncontiguous separate site in GI tract,
		M2 = noncontiguous other organs)
		Bone marrow involved

Treatment

No one standard approach in the treatment of EATL has been determined. Despite the role of surgery diminishing in other GI lymphomas, resection of lesions at high risk of perforation is recommended prior to commencement of chemotherapy, to avoid fatal perforation during immunosuppressive treatment. Radiotherapy can be considered for bulky lesions; however, risk of perforation must also be assessed prior to instituting this modality.

No prospective data exist for chemotherapy; however, combination chemotherapy is recommended due to the poor outcomes. In one retrospective study of 31 patients, 7 underwent surgery alone and 24 received combination chemotherapy, all but 1 with anthracycline-based regimens. Disappointingly, less than 50% completed treatment due to complications, and although response rate was 58%, 5-year disease-free survival was only 3.2%. In a second series, 66% (23/35) of patients completed CHOP-like chemotherapy with 32% achieving remission. However, median survival was only 7.1 months.[74]

More recently, chemotherapy with consolidation autologous stem-cell transplant (ASCT) has been attempted with some promising results.[75] Twenty-six patients from one institution received one cycle of CHOP followed by IVE/MTX (ifosfamide, vincristine, etoposide, methotrexate): 14 of these then underwent ASCT with melphalan, total body irradiation, or BEAM (carmustine, etoposide, arabinoside, and melphalan) conditioning regimens. Five-year PFS and OS were both significantly higher than in the historical control group who received CHOP-like regimens (PFS: 52% vs. 22%, $p = 0.01$; OS: 60% vs. 22%, $p = 0.003$).[74] One smaller conflicting study reported three of four patients relapsing within a few months of ASCT, yet different induction chemotherapy was used.[76] Retrospective data for allogeneic stem cell transplant exists for relapsed or refractory NHL; however, the study contained a heterogeneous group of patients with only 11 peripheral T-cell lymphomas and, therefore, would not be considered a standard treatment option in EATL.[77]

Alemtuzumab, a novel monoclonal antibody targeting CD52, has activity in T-cell lymphoma, with a more favorable toxicity profile than that of combination chemotherapy.[78] One study evaluated alemtuzumab plus CHOP (CHOP-C) in advanced peripheral T-cell lymphoma with promising results; however, again, EATL was not represented in this population.[79] Only lymphomas that express CD52 respond to alemtuzumab; therefore, testing of CD52 cell surface marker should be performed prior to considering this experimental treatment.[80]

In addition to the treatment of the lymphoma, nutritional supplementation and aggressive prevention and treatment of infection are imperative. Those with CD should be maintained on a gluten-free diet.

Diffuse large B-cell lymphoma

Epidemiology

DLBCL is the most common B-cell NHL, comprising 31% of all NHL and 40–70% of all gastric lymphomas.[12,81,82] While the stomach is the most common site for GI DLBCL, it can also occur in the terminal ileum, and rarely in the colon or rectum. It is an aggressive lymphoma, arising *de novo*, or a coexistent pathology with MALT lymphoma in the stomach in which a transformation event is thought to have occurred. Whether the DLBCL is a transformation of MALT lymphoma or arises due to a similar underlying causative factor is uncertain. While certain histological features can distinguish between the two presentations, natural history and management are similar.

Median age of presentation is 50–60 years with a slight male predominance. No risk factors have been clearly identified; however, there is evidence that immunodeficiency increases likelihood of DLBCL in extranodal sites such as the GI tract,[1] initially described in congenital immunodeficiency diseases and transplant settings, but more recently in HIV-positive patients. *H. pylori* is detected in 35% of DLBCL of the stomach, but the majority of these are in lesions with simultaneous MALT lymphoma suggesting that it is the MALT lymphoma transforming to a DLBCL rather than *H. pylori* infection as a causative agent.[84]

DLBCL is a curable disease and prognosis is estimated using the international prognostic index (IPI) (Table 10.6) with 5-year survival rates in low-risk and high-risk patients of 73% and 26%, respectively.[85] Current clinical parameters identifying poor prognosis include advanced stage or age, elevated serum LDH, poor performance status, and higher number of extranodal sites. A high proliferation rate, as determined by the Ki67 index, has been reported to confer a worse survival in some studies, but data are conflicting.

Diagnosis and staging
Histological diagnosis is usually obtained from endoscopic or percutaneous biopsies. It is characterized by a diffuse growth pattern of large B lymphoid cells with a nuclear size more than twice the size of a normal lymphocyte (Figure 10.1d). The cells usually have abundant eosinophilic cytoplasm and nuclei that contain nucleoli. The cells may resemble centroblasts, immunoblasts, or plasmablasts or a combination of these appearances.

Table 10.6 International Prognostic Index.[85]

International Prognostic Index			
Age >60			
Elevated serum lactate dehydrogenase			
ECOG performance status ≥2			
Ann Arbor stage III or IV			
>1 extranodal disease site			
(One point each for the above characteristics)			
IPI score	Risk group	5-year OS (%)	CR rate (%)
0 or 1	Low	73	87
2	Low intermediate	51	67
3	High intermediate	43	55
4 or 5	High risk	26	44
Age-adjusted IPI for patients over 60			
(One point for each of the above characteristics apart from age and extranodal sites)			
aa-IPI Score	Risk group	5-year OS (%)	CR rate (%)
0	Low	56	91
1	Low intermediate	44	71
2	High intermediate	37	56
3	High	21	36

Immunophenotyping is used to diagnose and categorize DLBCL. The malignant cells express pan B-cell markers including CD19, CD20, CD79a, CD30, and CD5 (<10% of cases). Surface and cytoplasmic immunoglobulin is present in 50–75% of cases. Staining for Ki67 can be used to detect the proliferation fraction, which ranges from 40% to >90%. In nodal DLBCL, the disease can be divided into germinal-center B-cell like (GCB) and non-germinal-center B-cell like (non-GCB) subgroups and both can be seen in the GI tract.

No single genetic mutation is diagnostic of DLBCL, but somatic hypermutations of the *PIMI, MYC, RHOH/TTF (ARHH)*, and *PAX5* genes have been described in >50% of cases. The most common translocation is in the *BCL6* gene at 3q27; additionally, the *BCL2* gene t(14:18), which is prominent in FL, can be present, particularly in the GCB subgroup, each occurring at a frequency of 20–30%. Gene expression profiling has identified differences between GCB and activated B-cell-like DLBCL with the latter featuring gains in 3q and 9p as well as *NFkB* activation but GCB demonstrating *BCL2* rearrangement, *REL* amplification, 12q12, and t(14;18).[54] Correlation between gene expression profiling and immunohistochemical assessment is variable.

Staging investigations are similar to those recommended in systemic nodal DLBCL. CT scan of the neck, chest, abdomen, and pelvis plus bone marrow trephine and aspirate should be performed. As most DLBCL is PET-avid (Figure 10.2a), an FDG-PET scan should be part of baseline and posttreatment evaluation. Blood tests include full blood count and film, LDH, beta-2 microglobulin, cytomegalovirus and Epstein–Barr virus (EBV) serology, HIV, and hepatitis B and C viral serology in high-risk groups. Assessment for adequate organ function prior to chemotherapy includes urea and electrolytes, liver function, and cardiac evaluation in high-risk patients.

Due to the limited accuracy with which the Ann Arbor staging predicts prognosis in this group, the IPI[85] (Table 10.6) was developed and validated in DLBCL as well as other subtypes to more precisely predict outcomes.

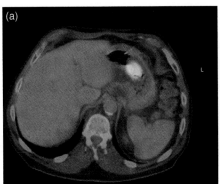
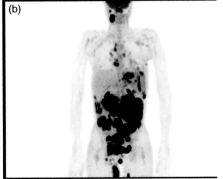

Figure 10.2 PET images of GI lymphoma: (a) PET-CT fused axial image of gastric DLBCL; (b) PET image of abdominal Burkitt lymphoma. (Images kindly provided by Dr. Gary Cook and Dr. Bhupinder Sharma.)

It incorporates a score calculated from stage, age, LDH, and performance status, all of which must therefore be part of baseline assessment.

While the role of EUS is well established in staging of gastric adenocarcinomas and MALT lymphoma, it remains controversial in DLBCL of the stomach and therefore cannot currently be recommended.

Treatment

Regardless of site of disease, the standard first-line treatment for DLBCL has remained anthracycline-based chemotherapy such as CHOP (cyclophosphamide, doxorubicin, vincristine, prednisolone) for many decades. The relatively recent addition of the anti-CD20 antibody rituximab significantly improved survival across all subgroups with overall long-term cure rates of 50–60%.[86–89] Intensification of this regimen has thus far shown no improved benefit. In cases of relapse, 40% are cured with combination chemotherapy followed by high-dose consolidative therapy and autologous stem cell transplant.[90] Multiple second-line combination regimens have demonstrated similar efficacy and successful stem-cell mobilization. However, none have been compared directly in a randomized-control setting; therefore, no universal standard chemotherapy exists for this indication. Results from allogeneic transplant are poor; therefore, it is not routinely recommended in this disease.

Central nervous system involvement is relatively rare with DLBCL; however, it has a poor outcome. In high-risk disease, prophylactic intrathecal chemotherapy is administered with R-CHOP to reduce the risk of central nervous system relapse following a reported reduction in CNS events with the addition of intrathecal methotrexate.[91] However, its role has been questioned since the introduction of rituximab.[92]

Radiotherapy alone yields poor results in DLBCL but can be used as consolidative therapy following chemotherapy. In localized disease, three cycles of R-CHOP is often followed by involved-field radiotherapy, rather than the standard six to eight cycles of chemotherapy delivered in disseminated disease.[93,94]

Few studies have evaluated treatment in primary GI DLBCL as a separate entity. However, in two small series of localized gastric DLBCL, 5-year EFS was >95% with both three cycles of CHOP and six cycles of R-CHOP chemotherapy, though a direct comparison was not made.[95,96]

Unlike T-cell lymphomas, luminal perforation associated with DLBCL is rare; hence, surgery plays a very limited role in the management of GI DLBCL and must only be considered as an adjunct to systemic therapy in individual cases.

Other lymphoma subtypes involving the GI tract

Although collectively rare, several additional subtypes of lymphoma manifest as primary GI disease and warrant brief discussion. Overall, histopathological features, staging, and management of these lymphomas mirror that of systemic disease.

Burkitt lymphoma

BL is an aggressive B-cell lymphoma most often presenting at extranodal sites. The infiltrate is composed of medium-sized, monomorphic cells with basophilic cytoplasm (Figure 10.1e). Proliferation rates are >95%, as determined by Ki67 staining. As apoptosis of the tumor cells is a frequent event, macrophages absorb the dead cells leading to a "starry sky" appearance on low-power viewing of the tumor. Deregulation of C-MYC as a result of a translocation on chromosome 8 is characteristic (usually t(8;14)(q24;q32)).[54] Division into three variants, endemic BL, immunodeficiency-associated BL, and sporadic BL, is based on clinical features, morphology, and tumor biology. Both endemic and sporadic BL carry a male predominance (2–3:1).

Endemic BL is the most common childhood malignancy in central Africa and worldwide, geographically corresponding to regions with endemic malaria. More than 95% of endemic BLs contain EBV genome. Fifty percent present with involvement of the facial bones and peak incidence is age 4–7 years.[54]

Immunodeficiency-associated BL is seen in the HIV-positive population, often as an AIDS-defining illness, yet rarely in other immunodeficient states. EBV is positive in 30–90% of cases. Plasmacytoid differentiation is a more common histopathologic feature in this variant. The introduction of highly-active antiretroviral therapy has improved the outcome in these patients; however, overall outcomes remain poor compared with the other variants of BL.[97,98]

Sporadic BL represents 30–50% of childhood lymphomas in Europe and the United States, but only 1–2% of adult lymphomas. In the adult population, median age at presentation is 30 years.[99] Only 20–30% are EBV positive. In contrast to endemic BL, facial involvement is rare, with an abdominal mass, the major feature in most cases, usually involving the ileocaecal region of the gut, the ovaries, and the mesenteric or retroperitoneal lymph nodes.

Due to the rapid doubling time of BL, 70% of patients present with advanced disease, and often local tumor bulk developing over several weeks (Figure 10.2b). Poor prognostic features include bone marrow or CNS disease, tumor size >10 cm, and elevated LDH. The unique St Jude/Murphy staging system has been developed from Ann Arbor to incorporate the higher extranodal burden of disease, yet this system incorrectly distinguishes Burkitt leukemia as a separate disease entity.[100] Short-duration, high-intensity chemotherapy (such as CODOX-M-IVAC) with aggressive CNS prophylaxis renders 80–90% of localized disease cured and 60–80% in advanced disease; therefore, it is the primary treatment in this disease.[101–103] Patients must be closely monitored for tumor lysis syndrome, and prophylactic measures against this with intravenous hydration, allopurinol, and rasburicase are routine. Transfusion support, administration of granulocyte colony-stimulating factor, and antimicrobial prophylaxis are all utilized in clinical practice to reduce treatment-related morbidity and mortality with these intense regimens.

Mantle cell lymphoma (lymphomatous polyposis)

MCL accounts for only 5–8% of all NHL. Primary GI MCL is even rarer, comprising only 4–9% of GI B-cell lymphomas, yet microscopic involvement of the GI tract in aggressive systemic disease has been reported in up to 88% of patients.[104] MCL is classified as an incurable indolent lymphoma; however, it has one of the worst NHL prognoses, with a 5-year survival of only 27%.[105] MCL of the GI tract often presents as "multiple lymphomatous polyposis," where segments of the GI tract are lined with malignant polyps, although this is not unique to MCL. A specific indolent subtype of MCL has been identified, presenting as leukemic disease with minimal nodal involvement. Evidence of specific clinicopathologic and genomic features is emerging. Median age of MCL diagnosis is 60 years and 76% of patients are male. Eighty-four percent of patients present with stage IV disease.[106] Symptoms of primary GI MCL are most commonly abdominal. A specific MCL-IPI score ("MIPI") to assess prognosis in advanced disease has been proposed, which stratifies patients into three risk categories according to four factors: age, performance status, LDH, and leukocyte count.[106] Routine staging procedures are as per DLBCL; however, due to limited information on utility of PET scanning, this should still be considered investigational. Endoscopy is not routinely performed as results rarely impact on therapeutic decisions in advanced disease. However, this may assist in early-stage disease and in confirming CRs.

MCL is composed of small-to-medium sized monomorphic malignant B cells, closely resembling centrocytes, which replace the normal mantle zone pattern. Four morphological variants are described with the blastoid and pleomorphic variants being clinically more aggressive. The proliferation fraction, measured by number of mitotic figures or Ki67 index, has prognostic association. The hallmark feature of MCL is the presence of a t(11;14)(q13;q32) causing Cyclin-D1 overexpression, which identified MCL as a separate disease entity for the first time in the 1990s (Figure 10.1f). More recently, overexpression of the transcription factor *SOX11* has been identified as a diagnostic marker of Cyclin-D1-positive and Cyclin-D1-negative MCL. SOX11 is useful in differentiating Cyclin-D1-negative MCL from other indolent NHL.[107] The absence of this marker is a characteristic feature of the indolent subtype carrying an excellent prognosis compared with conventional MCL (5-year OS 78% vs. 36%, respectively; $p = 0.001$).[108] This subtype also often harbors a mutation of the variable region of the expressed immunoglobulin heavy chain gene.[108] Typically, there is no transformation of MCL to large cell lymphomas.[54]

No one standard treatment exists across all groups of patients due to the paucity of prospective data. Despite aggressive chemotherapeutic management, CR rates are low and remissions are short. The active chemotherapy regimens are those used in other B-cell lymphomas: fludarabine based (FCM, FC) or anthracycline based (CHOP). The addition of rituximab improves CR rates, and a meta-analysis study demonstrated superior survival compared with chemotherapy alone (HR for death, 0.60; 95% CI, 0.37–0.98).[109] Based on studies with historical controls, consolidation of a first remission with autologous or allogeneic transplant is an accepted practice in younger patients; a randomized study demonstrated improved PFS; however, OS results are not mature.[110] Results of a recent phase III randomised study has confirmed R-CHOP chemotherapy followed by 2 years of maintenance rituximab to be the new standard of care in older patients not suitable for transplant.[111] Newer targeted agents such as mTOR inhibitors (temsirolimus), proteosome inhibitors (bortezomib), and immunomodulatory drugs (lenalidomide) have expanded treatment options, but their role in the management paradigm remains under evaluation.

Follicular lymphoma

FL is an indolent lymphoma, the second most common subtype of NHL worldwide, accounting for 20% of all new lymphoma cases. Involvement of the GI tract is usually in the context of widespread nodal disease; however, it can rarely be the primary site of disease, particularly the duodenum.[112,113] Median age at diagnosis is 59 years with a male-to-female ratio of 1:1.7.[81]

Nodal FL is generally advanced at the time of presentation with only 26–33% stage I–II at time of diagnosis, and 40–70% of cases presenting with bone marrow involvement.[6] It is regarded as incurable and the clinical course is heterogeneous, with 15% of patients dying within 2 years of diagnosis but a median survival of approximately 10 years. The rate of transformation to high-grade lymphoma is 3% per year. Poor prognostic features include advanced stage, age >60 years, elevated LDH, >4 nodal sites, and hemoglobin level <120 g/dL.[114,115]

In contrast to nodal FL, primary intestinal FL presents as multiple small polyps, often detected as an incidental finding on endoscopy performed for another indication. It is usually localized disease with an excellent prognosis, even without treatment. The histological features are similar to nodal lymphomas and therefore do not reveal the origin; hence, careful staging is imperative.[54]

FL is composed of germinal center B cells (both centrocytes and centroblasts/large transformed cells) in a predominantly follicular pattern with closely packed follicles effacing the nodal architecture. It is histologically graded according to the proportion of large cells (centroblasts) present per high-powered field. Grading is given from 1 to 3A or 3B, with the latter indicating a higher number of centroblasts present and has been shown to predict clinical outcome. Patients with more large cells follow a more aggressive clinical course, with a higher likelihood of transforming to a DLBCL. The majority of cases of intestinal FL fall into the grade 1 or 2 category. The t(14;18)(q32;q21) and BCL2 gene rearrangement cytogenetically characterize FL, present in more than 80% of cases.[54]

Treatment involves a combination of modalities including a "watch and wait" surveillance approach, localized radiotherapy, single-agent rituximab, high-dose chemotherapy with autologous stem-cell transplant and in select patients, and allogeneic transplantation, depending on the clinical course of disease. Many therapies have been incorporated into routine care based on improved response rates, or lengthened PFS in large randomized studies. However, it is uncertain as to whether these surrogate endpoints confer improvements in OS due to the indolent nature of the disease. There is considerable overlap for active regimens with other B-cell lymphomas: CHOP, CVP, FC, FCM, bendamustine and chlorambucil are all utilized, usually in combination with rituximab. Rituximab maintenance therapy, administered 3-monthly for 2 years after achieving a response with CHOP or R-CHOP, has improved survival in relapsed FL[116] and PFS after first-line rituximab plus chemotherapy and,[117] hence, is standard in those requiring systemic treatment.

Key Patient Consent Issues

- Prognosis of GI lymphomas varies considerably depending on histological subtype and stage and therefore should be carefully assessed before relaying this information to the patient.
- Aims of treatment can be either curative or palliative, with short or durable remissions obtained in the latter. The aim of treatment should be made clear to the patient as well as the expected outcomes.
- Chemotherapy regimens used in lymphoma can have significant toxicity and an associated risk of mortality of which patients must be made aware. Infertility as a potential complication must be discussed and provisions for this prior to commencement of treatment should be made, where possible, through referral to a fertility clinic.
- Hereditary forms of GI lymphoma are extremely rare and therefore no formal familial screening programs exist.

Acknowledgments

The authors would like to acknowledge Dr. Gary Cook and Dr. Bhupinder Sharma for providing PET images.

References

1. Freeman, C., Berg, J.W., Cutler, S.J. (1972) Occurrence and prognosis of extranodal lymphomas. *Cancer*, **29**, 252–260.
2. Otter, R., Bieger, R., Kluin, P.M. *et al.* (1989) Primary gastrointestinal non-Hodgkin's lymphoma in a population-based registry. *Br J Cancer*, **60**, 745–750.
3. Salem, P., el-Hashimi, L., Anaissie, E. *et al.* (1987) Primary small intestinal lymphoma in adults. A comparative study of IPSID versus non-IPSID in the Middle East. *Cancer*, **59**, 1670–1676.
4. Doglioni, C., Wotherspoon, A.C., Moschini, A. *et al.* (1992) High incidence of primary gastric lymphoma in northeastern Italy. *Lancet*, **339**, 834–845.
5. Isaacson, P., Wright, D.H. (1983) Malignant lymphoma of mucosa-associated lymphoid tissue. A distinctive type of B-cell lymphoma. *Cancer*, **52**, 1410–1416.
6. The Non-Hodgkin's Lymphoma Classification Project (1997) A clinical evaluation of the International Lymphoma Study Group classification of non-Hodgkin's lymphoma. *Blood*, **89**, 3909–3918.

7. Wotherspoon, A.C., Ortiz-Hidalgo, C., Falzon, M.R. *et al.* (1991) *Helicobacter pylori*-associated gastritis and primary B-cell gastric lymphoma. *Lancet*, **338**, 1175–1176.

8. Steinbach, G., Ford, R., Glober, G. *et al.* (1999) Antibiotic treatment of gastric lymphoma of mucosa-associated lymphoid tissue. An uncontrolled trial. *Ann Intern Med*, **131**, 88–95.

9. Algood, H.M., Cover, T.L. (2006) *Helicobacter pylori* persistence: an overview of interactions between *H. pylori* and host immune defenses. *Clin Microbiol Rev*, **19**, 597–613.

10. Hyjek, E., Smith, W.J., Isaacson, P.G. (1988) Primary B-cell lymphoma of salivary glands and its relationship to myoepithelial sialadenitis. *Hum Pathol*, **19**, 766–776.

11. Hyjek, E., Isaacson, P.G. (1988) Primary B cell lymphoma of the thyroid and its relationship to Hashimoto's thyroiditis. *Hum Pathol*, **19**, 1315–1326.

12. Koch, P., del Valle, F., Berdel, W.E. *et al.* (2001) Primary gastrointestinal non-Hodgkin's lymphoma: II. Combined surgical and conservative or conservative management only in localized gastric lymphoma—results of the prospective German Multicenter Study GIT NHL 01/92. *J Clin Oncol*, **19**, 3874–3883.

13. Thieblemont, C., Bastion, Y., Berger, F. *et al.* (1997) Mucosa-associated lymphoid tissue gastrointestinal and nongastrointestinal lymphoma behavior: analysis of 108 patients. *J Clin Oncol*, **15**, 1624–1630.

14. Zucca, E., Bertoni, F., Roggero, E. *et al.* (2000) The gastric marginal zone B-cell lymphoma of MALT type. *Blood*, **96**, 410–419.

15. Zucca, E., Conconi, A., Pedrinis, E. *et al.* (2003) Nongastric marginal zone B-cell lymphoma of mucosa-associated lymphoid tissue. *Blood*, **101**, 2489–2495.

16. Hitchcock, S., Ng, A.K, Fisher, D.C. *et al.* (2002) Treatment outcome of mucosa-associated lymphoid tissue/marginal zone non-Hodgkin's lymphoma. *Int J Radiat Oncol Biol Phys*, **52**, 1058–1066.

17. Taal, B.G., Boot, H., van Heerde, P. *et al.* (1996) Primary non-Hodgkin lymphoma of the stomach: endoscopic pattern and prognosis in low versus high grade malignancy in relation to the MALT concept. *Gut*, **39**, 556–561.

18. Wotherspoon, A.C., Doglioni, C., Diss, T.C. *et al.* (1993) Regression of primary low-grade B-cell gastric lymphoma of mucosa-associated lymphoid tissue type after eradication of *Helicobacter pylori*. *Lancet*, **342**, 575–577.

19. Rohatiner, A., d'Amore, F., Coiffier, B. *et al.* (1994) Report on a workshop convened to discuss the pathological and staging classifications of gastrointestinal tract lymphoma. *Ann Oncol*, **5**, 397–400.

20. Ruskone-Fourmestraux, A., Dragosics, B., Morgner, A. *et al.* (2003) Paris staging system for primary gastrointestinal lymphomas. *Gut*, **52**, 912–913.

21. Remstein, E.D., Kurtin, P.J., James, C.D. *et al.* (2002) Mucosa-associated lymphoid tissue lymphomas with t(11;18)(q21;q21) and mucosa-associated lymphoid tissue lymphomas with aneuploidy develop along different pathogenetic pathways. *Am J Pathol*, **161**, 63–71.

22. Liu, H., Ye, H., Ruskone-Fourmestraux, A. *et al.* (2002) T(11;18) is a marker for all stage gastric MALT lymphomas that will not respond to *H. pylori* eradication. *Gastroenterology*, **122**, 1286–1294.

23. Ott, G., Katzenberger, T., Greiner, A. *et al.* (1997) The t(11;18)(q21;q21) chromosome translocation is a frequent and specific aberration in low-grade but not high-grade malignant non-Hodgkin's lymphomas of

the mucosa-associated lymphoid tissue (MALT-) type. *Cancer Res*, **57**, 3944–3948.

24. Ye, H., Liu, H., Attygalle, A. *et al.* (2003) Variable frequencies of t(11;18) (q21;q21) in MALT lymphomas of different sites: significant association with CagA strains of *H. pylori* in gastric MALT lymphoma. *Blood*, **102**, 1012–1018.

25. Bayerdorffer, E., Oertel, H., Lehn, N. *et al.* (1989) Topographic association between active gastritis and *Campylobacter pylori* colonisation. *J Clin Pathol*, **42**, 834–839.

26. Lehours, P., Ruskone-Fourmestraux, A., Lavergne, A. *et al.* (2003) Which test to use to detect *Helicobacter pylori* infection in patients with low-grade gastric mucosa-associated lymphoid tissue lymphoma? *Am J Gastroenterol*, **98**, 291–295.

27. Eck, M., Greiner, A., Schmausser, B. *et al.* (1999) Evaluation of *Helicobacter pylori* in gastric MALT-type lymphoma: differences between histologic and serologic diagnosis. *Mod Pathol*, **12**, 1148–1151.

28. Carbone, P.P., Kaplan, H.S., Musshoff, K. *et al.* (1971) Report of the Committee on Hodgkin's Disease Staging Classification. *Cancer Res*, **31**, 1860–1861.

29. Musshoff, K. (1977) Clinical staging classification of non-Hodgkin's lymphomas (author's transl). *Strahlentherapie*, **153**, 218–221.

30. Aviles, A., Nambo, M.J., Neri, N. *et al.* (2005) Mucosa-associated lymphoid tissue (MALT) lymphoma of the stomach: results of a controlled clinical trial. *Med Oncol*, **22**, 57–62.

31. Fischbach, W., Goebeler, M.E., Ruskone-Fourmestraux, A. *et al.* (2007) Most patients with minimal histological residuals of gastric MALT lymphoma after successful eradication of *Helicobacter pylori* can be managed safely by a watch and wait strategy: experience from a large international series. *Gut*, **56**, 1685–1687.

32. de Boer, J.P., Hiddink, R.F., Raderer, M. *et al.* (2008) Dissemination patterns in non-gastric MALT lymphoma. *Haematologica*, **93**, 201–206.

33. Raderer, M., Streubel, B., Woehrer, S. *et al.* (2005) High relapse rate in patients with MALT lymphoma warrants lifelong follow-up. *Clin Cancer Res*, **11**, 3349–3352.

34. Cheson, B.D., Bennett, J.M., Kopecky, K.J. *et al.* (2003) Revised recommendations of the International Working Group for Diagnosis, Standardization of Response Criteria, Treatment Outcomes, and Reporting Standards for Therapeutic Trials in Acute Myeloid Leukemia. *J Clin Oncol*, **21**, 4642–4629.

35. Tomita, N., Kodaira, T., Tachibana, H. *et al.* (2009) Favorable outcomes of radiotherapy for early-stage mucosa-associated lymphoid tissue lymphoma. *Radiother Oncol*, **90**, 231–235.

36. Tsang, R.W., Gospodarowicz, M.K., Pintilie, M. *et al.* (2003) Localized mucosa-associated lymphoid tissue lymphoma treated with radiation therapy has excellent clinical outcome. *J Clin Oncol*, **21**, 4157–4164.

37. Schechter, N.R., Portlock, C.S., Yahalom, J. (1998) Treatment of mucosa-associated lymphoid tissue lymphoma of the stomach with radiation alone. *J Clin Oncol*, **16**, 1916–1921.

38. Conconi, A., Martinelli, G., Thieblemont, C. *et al.* (2003) Clinical activity of rituximab in extranodal marginal zone B-cell lymphoma of MALT type. *Blood*, **102**, 2741–2745.

39. Martinelli, G., Laszlo, D., Ferreri, A.J. *et al.* (2005) Clinical activity of rituximab in gastric marginal zone non-Hodgkin's lymphoma resistant to or not eligible for anti-*Helicobacter pylori* therapy. *J Clin Oncol*, **23**, 1979–1983.

40. Raderer, M., Jager, G., Brugger, S. *et al.* (2003) Rituximab for treatment of advanced extranodal marginal zone B cell lymphoma of the mucosa-associated lymphoid tissue lymphoma. *Oncology*, **65**, 306–310.

41. Wohrer, S., Troch, M., Zwerina, J. *et al.* (2007) Influence of rituximab, cyclophosphamide, doxorubicin, vincristine and prednisone on serologic parameters and clinical course in lymphoma patients with autoimmune diseases. *Ann Oncol*, **18**, 647–651.

42. Salar, A., Domingo-Domenech, E., Estany, C. *et al.* (2009) Combination therapy with rituximab and intravenous or oral fludarabine in the first-line, systemic treatment of patients with extranodal marginal zone B-cell lymphoma of the mucosa-associated lymphoid tissue type. *Cancer*, **115**, 5210–5217.

43. Levy, M., Copie-Bergman, C., Molinier-Frenkel, V. *et al.* (2010) Treatment of t(11;18)-positive gastric mucosa-associated lymphoid tissue lymphoma with rituximab and chlorambucil: clinical, histological, and molecular follow-up. *Leuk Lymphoma*, **51**, 284–290.

44. Hammel, P., Haioun, C., Chaumette, M.T. *et al.* (1995) Efficacy of single-agent chemotherapy in low-grade B-cell mucosa-associated lymphoid tissue lymphoma with prominent gastric expression. *J Clin Oncol*, **13**, 2524–2549.

45. Levy, M., Copie-Bergman, C., Gameiro, C. *et al.* (2005) Prognostic value of translocation t(11;18) in tumoral response of low-grade gastric lymphoma of mucosa-associated lymphoid tissue type to oral chemotherapy. *J Clin Oncol*, **23**, 5061–5066.

46. Zinzani, P.L., Stefoni, V., Musuraca, G. *et al.* (2004) Fludarabine-containing chemotherapy as frontline treatment of nongastrointestinal mucosa-associated lymphoid tissue lymphoma. *Cancer*, **100**, 2190–2194.

47. Jager, G., Neumeister, P., Quehenberger, F. *et al.* (2006) Prolonged clinical remission in patients with extranodal marginal zone B-cell lymphoma of the mucosa-associated lymphoid tissue type treated with cladribine: 6 year follow-up of a phase II trial. *Ann Oncol*, **17**, 1722–1723.

48. Zucca, E., Conconi, A., Martinelli, G. *et al.* (2010) Chlorambucil plus rituximab produces better event-free survival in comparison with chlorambucil alone in the treatment of malt lymphoma: 5-year analysis of the 2-arms part of the IELSG-19 Randomized Study. Proceedings of the 52nd ASH Annual Meeting, *Blood*, **118**, Abstr 432.

49. Al-Saleem, T., Zardawi, I.M. (1979) Primary lymphomas of the small intestine in Iraq: a pathological study of 145 cases. *Histopathology*, **3**, 89–106.

50. Parsonnet, J., Isaacson, P.G. (2004) Bacterial infection and MALT lymphoma. *N Engl J Med*, **350**, 213–215.

51. Al-Saleem, T., Al-Mondhiry, H. (2005) Immunoproliferative small intestinal disease (IPSID): a model for mature B-cell neoplasms. *Blood*, **105**, 2274–2280.

52. Rambaud, J.C. (1983) Small intestinal lymphomas and alpha-chain disease. *Clin Gastroenterol*, **12**, 743–766.

53. Al-Bahrani, Z.R., Al-Mondhiry, H., Bakir, F. *et al.* (1983) Clinical and pathologic subtypes of primary intestinal lymphoma. Experience with 132 patients over a 14-year period. *Cancer*, **52**, 1666–1672.

54. Swerdlow, S.H., Campo, E., Haris, N.L. *et al.* (2008) *WHO Classification of Tumours of Haematopoietic and Lymphoid Tissues*, 4th ed, IARC Press, Lyon.

55. Ben-Ayed, F., Halphen, M., Najjar, T. *et al.* (1989) Treatment of alpha chain disease. Results of a prospective study in 21 Tunisian patients by the Tunisian-French Intestinal Lymphoma Study Group. *Cancer*, **63**, 1251–1256.

56. Doe, W.F. (1975) Alpha chain disease clinicopathological features and relationship to so-called Mediterranean lymphoma. *Br J Cancer Suppl*, **2**, 350–355.

57. Salimi, M., Spinelli, J.J. (1996) Chemotherapy of Mediterranean abdominal lymphoma. Retrospective comparison of chemotherapy protocols in Iranian patients. *Am J Clin Oncol*, **19**, 18–22.

58. Rambaud, J.C., Halphen, M., Galian, A. *et al.* (1990) Immunoproliferative small intestinal disease (IPSID): relationships with alpha-chain disease and "Mediterranean" lymphomas. *Springer Semin Immunopathol*, **12**, 239–250.

59. Gough, K.R., Read, A.E., Naish, J.M. (1962) Intestinal reticulosis as a complication of idiopathic steatorrhoea. *Gut*, **3**, 232–239.

60. Fairley, N.H., Mackie, F.P. (1937) The clinical and biochemical syndrome in lymphadenoma and allied disease involving the mesenteric lymph glands. *Br Med J*, **1**, 3972–3980.

61. O'Farrelly, C., Feighery, C., O'Briain, D.S. *et al.* (1986) Humoral response to wheat protein in patients with coeliac disease and enteropathy associated T cell lymphoma. *Br Med J (Clin Res Ed)*, **293**, 908–910.

62. Dube, C., Rostom, A., Sy, R. *et al.* (2005) The prevalence of celiac disease in average-risk and at-risk Western European populations: a systematic review. *Gastroenterology*, **128**, S57–S67.

63. Catassi, C., Bearzi, I., Holmes, G.K. (2005) Association of celiac disease and intestinal lymphomas and other cancers. *Gastroenterology*, **128**, S79–S86.

64. Daum, S., Ullrich, R., Heise, W. *et al.* (2003) Intestinal non-Hodgkin's lymphoma: a multicenter prospective clinical study from the German Study Group on Intestinal non-Hodgkin's Lymphoma. *J Clin Oncol*, **21**, 2740–2746.

65. Smedby, K.E., Akerman, M., Hildebrand, H. *et al.* (2005) Malignant lymphomas in coeliac disease: evidence of increased risks for lymphoma types other than enteropathy-type T cell lymphoma. *Gut*, **54**, 54–59.

66. Silano, M., Volta, U., Mecchia, A.M. *et al.* (2007) Delayed diagnosis of coeliac disease increases cancer risk. *BMC Gastroenterol*, **7**, 8.

67. Viljamaa, M., Kaukinen, K., Pukkala, E. *et al.* (2006) Malignancies and mortality in patients with coeliac disease and dermatitis herpetiformis: 30-year population-based study. *Dig Liver Dis*, **38**, 374–380.

68. Gale, J., Simmonds, P.D., Mead, G.M. *et al.* (2000) Enteropathy-type intestinal T-cell lymphoma: clinical features and treatment of 31 patients in a single center. *J Clin Oncol*, **18**, 795–803.

69. Egan, L.J., Walsh, S.V., Stevens, F.M. *et al.* (1995) Celiac-associated lymphoma. A single institution experience of 30 cases in the combination chemotherapy era. *J Clin Gastroenterol*, **21**, 123–129.

70. Domizio, P., Owen, R.A., Shepherd, N.A. *et al.* (1993) Primary lymphoma of the small intestine. A clinicopathological study of 119 cases. *Am J Surg Pathol*, **17**, 429–442.

71. Chott, A., Dragosics, B., Radaszkiewicz, T. (1992) Peripheral T-cell lymphomas of the intestine. *Am J Pathol*, **141**, 1361–1371.

72. d'Amore, F., Brincker, H., Gronbaek, K. *et al.* (1994) Non-Hodgkin's lymphoma of the gastrointestinal tract: a population-based analysis of incidence, geographic distribution, clinicopathologic presentation features, and prognosis. Danish Lymphoma Study Group. *J Clin Oncol*, **12**, 1673–1684.
73. Hadithi, M., Mallant, M., Oudejans, J. *et al.* (2006) 18F-FDG PET versus CT for the detection of enteropathy-associated T-cell lymphoma in refractory celiac disease. *J Nucl Med*, **47**, 1622–1627.
74. Sieniawski, M., Angamuthu, N., Boyd, K. *et al.* (2010) Evaluation of enteropathy-associated T-cell lymphoma comparing standard therapies with a novel regimen including autologous stem cell transplantation. *Blood*, **115**, 3664–3670.
75. Bishton, M.J., Haynes, A.P. (2007) Combination chemotherapy followed by autologous stem cell transplant for enteropathy-associated T cell lymphoma. *Br J Haematol*, **136**, 111–113.
76. Al-Toma, A., Verbeek, W.H., Visser, O.J. *et al.* (2007) Disappointing outcome of autologous stem cell transplantation for enteropathy-associated T-cell lymphoma. *Dig Liver Dis*, **39**, 634–641.
77. Doocey, R.T., Toze, C.L., Connors, J.M. *et al.* (2005) Allogeneic haematopoietic stem-cell transplantation for relapsed and refractory aggressive histology non-Hodgkin lymphoma. *Br J Haematol*, **131**, 223–230.
78. Dearden, C.E., Matutes, E. (2006) Alemtuzumab in T-cell lymphoproliferative disorders. *Best Pract Res Clin Haematol*, **19**, 795–810.
79. Gallamini, A., Zaja, F., Patti, C. *et al.* (2007) Alemtuzumab (Campath-1H) and CHOP chemotherapy as first-line treatment of peripheral T-cell lymphoma: results of a GITIL (Gruppo Italiano Terapie Innovative nei Linfomi) prospective multicenter trial. *Blood*, **110**, 2316–2323.
80. Jiang, L., Yuan, C.M., Hubacheck, J. *et al.* (2009) Variable CD52 expression in mature T cell and NK cell malignancies: implications for alemtuzumab therapy. *Br J Haematol*, **145**, 173–179.
81. Armitage, J.O., Weisenburger, D.D. (1998) New approach to classifying non-Hodgkin's lymphomas: clinical features of the major histologic subtypes. Non-Hodgkin's Lymphoma Classification Project. *J Clin Oncol*, **16**, 2780–2795.
82. Papaxoinis, G., Papageorgiou, S., Rontogianni, D. *et al.* (2006) Primary gastrointestinal non-Hodgkin's lymphoma: a clinicopathologic study of 128 cases in Greece. A Hellenic Cooperative Oncology Group study (HeCOG). *Leuk Lymphoma*, **47**, 2140–2146.
83. Copie-Bergman, C., Gaulard, P., Lavergne-Slove, A. *et al.* (2003) Proposal for a new histological grading system for post-treatment evaluation of gastric MALT lymphoma. *Gut*, **52**, 1656.
84. Ferreri, A.J., Freschi, M., Dell'Oro, S. *et al.* (2001) Prognostic significance of the histopathologic recognition of low- and high-grade components in stage I-II B-cell gastric lymphomas. *Am J Surg Pathol*, **25**, 95–102.
85. The International Non-Hodgkin's Lymphoma Prognostic Factors Project (1993) A predictive model for aggressive non-Hodgkin's lymphoma. *N Engl J Med*, **329**, 987–994.
86. Feugier, P., Van Hoof, A., Sebban, C. *et al.* (2005) Long-term results of the R-CHOP study in the treatment of elderly patients with diffuse large B-cell lymphoma: a study by the Groupe d'Etude des Lymphomes de l'Adulte. *J Clin Oncol*, **23**, 4117–4126.
87. Pfreundschuh, M., Schubert, J., Ziepert, M. *et al.* (2008) Six versus eight cycles of bi-weekly CHOP-14 with or without rituximab in elderly patients

with aggressive CD20+ B-cell lymphomas: a randomised controlled trial (RICOVER-60). *Lancet Oncol*, **9**, 105–116.

88. Habermann, T.M., Weller, E.A., Morrison, V.A. *et al.* (2006) Rituximab-CHOP versus CHOP alone or with maintenance rituximab in older patients with diffuse large B-cell lymphoma. *J Clin Oncol*, **24**, 3121–3127.

89. Pfreundschuh, M., Trumper, L., Osterborg, A. *et al.* (2006) CHOP-like chemotherapy plus rituximab versus CHOP-like chemotherapy alone in young patients with good-prognosis diffuse large-B-cell lymphoma: a randomised controlled trial by the MabThera International Trial (MInT) Group. *Lancet Oncol*, **7**, 379–391.

90. Costa, L.J., Feldman, A.L., Micallef, I.N. *et al.* (2008) Germinal center B (GCB) and non-GCB cell-like diffuse large B cell lymphomas have similar outcomes following autologous haematopoietic stem cell transplantation. *Br J Haematol*, **142**, 404–412.

91. Tilly, H., Lepage, E., Coiffier, B. *et al.* (2003) Intensive conventional chemotherapy (ACVBP regimen) compared with standard CHOP for poor-prognosis aggressive non-Hodgkin lymphoma. *Blood*, **102**, 4284–4289.

92. Boehme, V., Schmitz, N., Zeynalova, S. *et al.* (2009) CNS events in elderly patients with aggressive lymphoma treated with modern chemotherapy (CHOP-14) with or without rituximab: an analysis of patients treated in the RICOVER-60 trial of the German High-Grade Non-Hodgkin Lymphoma Study Group (DSHNHL). *Blood*, **113**, 3896–3902.

93. Miller, T.P., Dahlberg, S., Cassady, J.R. *et al.* (1998) Chemotherapy alone compared with chemotherapy plus radiotherapy for localized intermediate- and high-grade non-Hodgkin's lymphoma. *N Engl J Med*, **339**, 21–26.

94. Persky, D.O., Unger, J.M., Spier, C.M. *et al.* (2008) Phase II study of rituximab plus three cycles of CHOP and involved-field radiotherapy for patients with limited-stage aggressive B-cell lymphoma: Southwest Oncology Group study 0014. *J Clin Oncol*, **26**, 2258–2263.

95. Aviles, A., Castaneda, C., Cleto, S. *et al.* (2009) Rituximab and chemotherapy in primary gastric lymphoma. *Cancer Biother Radiopharm*, **24**, 25–28.

96. Raderer, M., Chott, A., Drach, J. *et al.* (2002) Chemotherapy for management of localised high-grade gastric B-cell lymphoma: how much is necessary? *Ann Oncol*, **13**, 1094–1098.

97. Bellan, C., De Falco, G., Lazzi, S. *et al.* (2003) Pathologic aspects of AIDS malignancies. *Oncogene*, **22**, 6639–6645.

98. Berretta, M., Cinelli, R., Martellotta, F. *et al.* (2003) Therapeutic approaches to AIDS-related malignancies. *Oncogene*, **22**, 6646–6659.

99. Harris, N.L., Jaffe, E.S., Stein, H. *et al.* (1994) A revised European-American classification of lymphoid neoplasms: a proposal from the International Lymphoma Study Group. *Blood*, **84**, 1361–1392.

100. Murphy, S.B., Hustu, H.O. (1980) A randomized trial of combined modality therapy of childhood non-Hodgkin's lymphoma. *Cancer*, **45**, 630–637.

101. Magrath, I., Adde, M., Shad, A. *et al.* (1996) Adults and children with small non-cleaved-cell lymphoma have a similar excellent outcome when treated with the same chemotherapy regimen. *J Clin Oncol*, **14**, 925–934.

102. Patte, C., Auperin, A., Gerrard, M. *et al.* (2007) Results of the randomized international FAB/LMB96 trial for intermediate risk B-cell non-Hodgkin lymphoma in children and adolescents: it is possible to reduce treatment for the early responding patients. *Blood*, **109**, 2773–2780.

103. Blum, K.A., Lozanski, G., Byrd, J.C. (2004) Adult Burkitt leukemia and lymphoma. *Blood*, **104**, 3009–3020.

104. Romaguera, J.E., Medeiros, L.J., Hagemeister, F.B. *et al.* (2003) Frequency of gastrointestinal involvement and its clinical significance in mantle cell lymphoma. *Cancer*, **97**, 586–591.

105. Oinonen, R., Franssila, K., Teerenhovi, L. *et al.* (1998) Mantle cell lymphoma: clinical features, treatment and prognosis of 94 patients. *Eur J Cancer*, **34**, 329–336.

106. Hoster, E., Dreyling, M., Klapper, W. *et al.* (2008) A new prognostic index (MIPI) for patients with advanced-stage mantle cell lymphoma. *Blood*, **111**, 558–565.

107. Mozos, A., Royo, C., Hartmann, E. *et al.* (2009) SOX11 expression is highly specific for mantle cell lymphoma and identifies the cyclin D1-negative subtype. *Haematologica*, **94**, 1555–1562.

108. Fernandez, V., Salamero, O., Espinet, B. *et al.* (2010) Genomic and gene expression profiling defines indolent forms of mantle cell lymphoma. *Cancer Res*, **70**, 1408–1418.

109. Schulz, H., Bohlius, J.F., Trelle, S. *et al.* (2007) Immunochemotherapy with rituximab and overall survival in patients with indolent or mantle cell lymphoma: a systematic review and meta-analysis. *J Natl Cancer Inst*, **99**, 706–714.

110. Dreyling, M., Lenz, G., Hoster, E. *et al.* (2005) Early consolidation by myeloablative radiochemotherapy followed by autologous stem cell transplantation in first remission significantly prolongs progression-free survival in mantle-cell lymphoma: results of a prospective randomized trial of the European MCL Network. *Blood*, **105**, 2677–2684.

111. Kluin-Nelemans, J.C., Hoster, E., Vehling-Kaiser, U., *et al.* (2011) Rituximab maintenance significantly prolongs duration of remission in elderly patients with mantle cell lymphoma. First results of a randomised trial of the european MCL network. European Haematology Association 16th annual congress. London, UK.

112. Shia, J., Teruya-Feldstein, J., Pan, D. *et al.* (2002) Primary follicular lymphoma of the gastrointestinal tract: a clinical and pathologic study of 26 cases. *Am J Surg Pathol*, **26**, 216–224.

113. Yoshino, T., Miyake, K., Ichimura, K. *et al.* (2000) Increased incidence of follicular lymphoma in the duodenum. *Am J Surg Pathol*, **24**, 688–693.

114. Solal-Celigny, P., Roy, P., Colombat, P. *et al.* (2004) Follicular lymphoma international prognostic index. *Blood*, **104**, 1258–1265.

115. Ardeshna, K.M., Smith, P., Norton, A. *et al.* (2003) Long-term effect of a watch and wait policy versus immediate systemic treatment for asymptomatic advanced-stage non-Hodgkin lymphoma: a randomised controlled trial. *Lancet*, **362**, 516–522.

116. van Oers, M.H., Klasa, R., Marcus, R.E. *et al.* (2006) Rituximab maintenance improves clinical outcome of relapsed/resistant follicular non-Hodgkin lymphoma in patients both with and without rituximab during induction: results of a prospective randomized phase 3 intergroup trial. *Blood*, **108**, 3295–3301.

117. Salles, G.A., Seymour, J.F., Feugier, P. *et al.* (2010) Rituximab maintenance for 2 years in patients with untreated high tumor burden follicular lymphoma after response to immunochemotherapy. *J Clin Oncol*, **28**, 8004.

Index

Handbook of Gastrointestinal Cancer, First Edition. Edited by Janusz Jankowski and Ernest Hawk.
© 2013 John Wiley & Sons, Ltd. Published 2013 by John Wiley & Sons, Ltd.